D0868156

OXFORD MEDICAL PUBLICATIONS

Oxford Handbook of
Clinical Haematology

Oxford University Press makes no representation, express or implied, that the drug dosages in this book are correct. Readers must therefore always check the product information and clinical procedures with the most up-to-date published product information and data sheets provided by the manufacturers and the most recent codes of conduct and safety regulations. The authors and the publishers do not accept responsibility or legal liability for any errors in the text or for the misuse or misapplication of material in this work.

▶ Except where otherwise stated (eg Paediatric Haematology), drug doses and recommendations are for the non-pregnant adult who is not breast-feeding.

Oxford Handbook of
Clinical Haematology

D. Provan
Senior Lecturer in Haematology,
Southampton University Hospitals NHS Trust, Southampton, UK

M. Chisholm
Senior Lecturer in Haematology,
Southampton University Hospitals NHS Trust, Southampton, UK

A. S. Duncombe
Consultant Haematologist,
Southampton University Hospitals NHS Trust, Southampton, UK

C. R. J. Singer
Consultant Haematologist, Royal United Hospital, Bath, UK

A. G. Smith
Consultant and Honorary Senior Lecturer in Haematology,
Southampton University Hospitals NHS Trust, Southampton, UK

RC 636
.O94
1998

OXFORD
UNIVERSITY PRESS

INDIANA UNIVERSITY
LIBRARY
NORTHWEST

OXFORD
UNIVERSITY PRESS

Great Clarendon Street, Oxford OX2 6DP

Oxford University Press is a department of the University of Oxford.
It furthers the University's objective of excellence in research, scholarship,
and education by publishing worldwide in

Oxford   New York

Athens Auckland Bangkok Bogotá Buenos Aires Calcutta
Cape Town Chennai Dar es Salaam Delhi Florence Hong Kong Istanbul
Karachi Kuala Lumpur Madrid Melbourne Mexico City Mumbai
Nairobi Paris São Paolo Singapore Taipei Tokyo Toronto Warsaw

with associated companies in Berlin Ibadan

Oxford is a registered trade mark of Oxford University Press
in the UK and in certain other countries

Published in the United States
by Oxford University Press, Inc., New York

© D. Provan, M. Chisholm, A. S. Duncombe, C. R. J. Singer, and A. G. Smith,
1998

The moral rights of the author have been asserted
Database right Oxford University Press (maker)

First published 1998
Reprinted 1999

All rights reserved. No part of this publication may be reproduced,
stored in a retrieval system, or transmitted, in any form or by any means,
without the prior permission in writing of Oxford University Press,
or as expressly permitted by law, or under terms agreed with the appropriate
reprographics rights organization. Enquiries concerning reproduction
outside the scope of the above should be sent to the Rights Department
Oxford University Press, at the address above.

You must not circulate this book in any other binding or cover
and you must impose this same condition on any acquirer

A catalogue record for this book is available from the British Library
Library of Congress Cataloguing in Publication Data

1 3 5 7 9 10 8 6 4 2

ISBN 0 19 262903 4

Typeset by AMA DataSet Ltd, Preston, Lancs, UK
Printed in Great Britain on acid free paper by The Bath Press, Bath, UK

Foreword

The Concise Oxford Dictionary defines a handbook as 'a short manual or guide'. Modern haematology is a vast field which involves almost every other medical speciality and which, more than most, straddles the worlds of the basic biomedical sciences and clinical practice. Since the rapidly proliferating numbers of textbooks on this topic are becoming denser and heavier with each new edition, the medical student and young doctor in training are presented with a daunting problem, particularly as they try to put these fields into perspective. And those who try to teach them are not much better placed; on the one hand they are being told to decongest the curriculum, while on the other they are expected to introduce large slices of molecular biology, social science, ethics and communication skills, not to mention a liberal sprinkling of poetry, music and art.

In this over-heated educational scene the much maligned 'handbook' could well stage a come-back and gain new respectability, particularly in the role of a friendly guide. In the past this genre has often been viewed as having little intellectual standing, of no use to anybody except the panic-stricken student who wishes to try to make up for months of mis-spent time in a vain, one-night sitting before their final examination. But given the plethora of rapidly changing information that has to be assimilated, the carefully prepared précis is likely to play an increasingly important role in medical education. Perhaps even that ruination of the decent paragraph and linchpin of the pronouncements of medical bureaucrats, the 'bullet-point', may become acceptable, albeit in small doses, as attempts are made to highlight what is really important in a scientific or clinical field of enormous complexity and not a little uncertainty.

In this short account of blood diseases the editors have done an excellent service to medical students, as well as doctors who are not specialists in blood diseases, by summarising in simple terms the major features and approaches to diagnosis and management of most of the blood diseases that they will meet in routine clinical practice or in the tedious examinations that face them. And in condensing this rapidly expanding field they have, remarkably, managed to avoid one of the great difficulties and pitfalls of this type of teaching; in trying to reduce complex issues down to their bare bones, it is all too easy to introduce inaccuracies.

One word of warning from a battle-scarred clinician however. A précis of this type suffers from the same problem as a set of multiple-choice questions. Human beings are enormously complex organisms, and sick ones are even more complicated; during a clinical lifetime the self-critical doctor will probably never encounter a 'typical case' of anything. Thus the outlines of the diseases that are presented in this book must be used as approximate guides, and no more. But provided they bear this in mind, students will find that it is a very valuable summary of modern haematology; the addition of the Internet sources is a genuine and timely bonus.

D. J. WEATHERALL
April 1998

Preface

This small volume is intended to provide the essential core knowledge required to assess patients with possible disorders of the blood, organise relevant investigations and initiate therapy where necessary. By reducing extraneous information as much as possible, and presenting key information for each topic, a basic understanding of the pathophysiology is provided and this, we hope, will stimulate readers to follow this up by consulting the larger haematology textbooks.

We have provided both a patient-centred and disease-centred approach to haematological disease, in an attempt to provide a form of 'surgical sieve', hopefully enabling doctors in training to formulate a differential diagnosis before consulting the relevant disease-orientated section.

We have provided a full review of haematological investigations and their interpretation, handling emergency situations, and included the commonly used protocols in current use on Haematology Units, hopefully providing a unified approach to patient management.

There are additional sections relating to patient support organisations and Internet resources for further exploration by those wishing to delve deeper into the subject of blood and its diseases.

Obviously with a subject as large as clinical haematology we have been selective about the information we chose to include in the handbook. We would be interested to hear of diseases or situations not covered in this handbook. If there are inaccuracies within the text we accept full responsibility and welcome comments relating to this.

DP
MC
ASD
CRJS
AGS

1998

Acknowledgements

We are indebted to many of our colleagues for providing helpful suggestions and for proofreading the text. In particular we wish to thank Dr Helen McCarthy, Specialist Registrar in Haematology; Dr Jo Piercy, Specialist Registrar in Haematology; Dr Tanay Sheth, SHO in Haematology, Southampton; Sisters Clare Heather and Ann Jackson, Haematology Day Unit, Southampton General Hospital; Dr Mike Williams, Specialist Registrar in Anaesthetics; Dr Frank Boulton, Wessex Blood Transfusion Service, Southampton; Dr Paul Spargo, Consultant Anaesthetist, Southampton University Hospitals; Dr Sheila Bevin, Staff Grade Paediatrician; Dr Mike Hall, Consultant Neonatologist; Dr Judith Marsh, Consultant Haematologist, St George's Hospital, London; Joan Newman, Haematology Transplant Coordinator, Southampton; Professor Sally Davies, Consultant Haematologist, Imperial College School of Medicine, Central Middlesex Hospital, London; Dr Denise O'Shaughnessy, Consultant Haematologist, St Peter's Hospital, Chertsey.

Warm thanks are also extended to Oxford University Press for taking this project on in the first place, and for providing constant encouragement and help throughout the entire project.

Typographical notes – the entire book was typeset using Quark Express™ 3.32. Body text is Adobe Garamond with headings/subheadings in Frutiger. Symbols comprise Universal Greek w. Math Pi, Zapf Dingbats, Universal News w. Commercial Pi.

Symbols and abbreviations

▶	important
▶▶	very important
↓	decreased
↑	increased
↔	normal
♂:♀	male: female ratio
1°	primary
2°	secondary
2,3 DPG	2,3 diphosphoglycerate
2-CDA	2-chlorodeoxyadenosine
Ab	antibody
ACD	acid-citrate-dextrose
ACL	anticardiolipin antibody
ADP	adenosine 5-diphosphate
Ag	antigen
AIDS	acquired immunodeficiency syndrome
AIHA	autoimmune haemolytic anaemia
ALL	acute lymphoblastic leukaemia
AML	acute myeloid leukaemia
ANA	antinuclear antibodies
APCR	activated protein C resistance
APL	antiphospholipid antibody
APML	acute promyelocytic leukaemia
APS	antiphospholipid syndrome
APTT	activated partial thromboplastin time
APTT ratio	activated partial thromboplastin time ratio
ARMS	amplification refractory mutation system
AT (ATIII)	antithrombin III
ATLL	adult T cell leukaemia/lymphoma
ATP	adenosine triphosphate
ATRA	all-trans retinoic acid
B-CLL	B-cell chronic lymphocytic leukaemia
bd	*bis die* (twice daily)
BEAM	BCNU, etoposide, cytarabine (ara-C), melphalan
BFU-E	burst-forming unit-erythroid
BM	bone marrow
BMJ	British Medical Journal
BMT	bone marrow transplant(ation)
BNF	British National Formulary
BP	blood pressure
BPL	BioProducts Laboratory
Ca	carcinoma
Ca^{2+}	calcium
cALL	common acute lymphoblastic leukaemia
CD	cluster designation
CDA	congenital dyserythropoietic anaemia
cDNA	complementary DNA
CGL	chronic granulocytic leukaemia

CHAD	cold haemagglutinin disease
CHOP	cyclophosphamide, adriamycin, vincristine, prednisolone
CJD	Creutzfeldt Jacob disease (nv = new variant)
Cl^-	chloride
CLL	chronic lymphocytic ('lymphatic') leukaemia
CML	chronic myeloid leukaemia
CMML	chronic myelomonocytic leukaemia
CMV	cytomegalovirus
CNS	central nervous system
COAD	chronic obstructive airways disease
COMP	cyclophosphamide, vincristine, methotrexate, prednisolone
CRP	C-reactive protein
CT	computed tomography
CVP	cyclophosphamide, vincristine, prednisolone
CVS	cardiovascular system
CXR	chest x-ray
CytaBOM	cytarabine, bleomycin, vincristine, methotrexate
d	day
DAT	direct antiglobulin test
dATP	deoxy ATP
DBA	Diamond-Blackfan anaemia
DCT	direct Coombs test
DDAVP	desamino D-arginyl vasopressin
DFS	disease-free survival
DIC	disseminated intravascular coagulation
dl	decilitre
DNA	deoxyribonucleic acid
DRVVT	dilute Russell's viper venom test
DTT	dilute thromboplastin time
DVT	deep vein thrombosis
DXT	radiotherapy
EACA	epsilon aminocaproic acid
EBV	Epstein-Barr virus
ECG	electrocardiograph
EDTA	ethylenediamine tetraacetic acid
EFS	event-free survival
ELISA	enzyme-linked immunosorbent assay
Epo	erythropoietin
ESR	erythrocyte sedimentation rate
ET	essential thrombocythaemia
FAB	French–American–British
FACS	fluorescence-activated cell sorter
FBC	full blood count (complete blood count, CBC)
FDP	fibrin degradation products
Fe	iron
$FeSO_4$	ferrous sulphate
FFP	fresh frozen plasma
FISH	fluorescence *in situ* hybridisation
FIX	factor IX
fl	femtolitres
FL	follicular lymphoma
FOB	faecal occult blood

Symbols and abbreviations

FVIII	factor VIII
FVL	factor V Leiden
g	gram
G6PD	glucose-6-phosphate dehydrogenase
G-CSF	granulocyte colony stimulating factor
GIT	gastrointestinal tract
GM-CSF	granulocyte macrophage colony stimulating factor
GPI	glycosylphosphatidylinositol
GvHD	graft versus host disease
h	hour
HAV	hepatitis A virus
Hb	haemoglobin
HbA	haemoglobin A
HbA$_2$	haemoglobin A$_2$
HbF	haemoglobin F (fetal Hb)
HbH	haemoglobin H
HBsAg	hepatitis B surface antigen
HBV	hepatitis B virus
HCL	hairy cell leukaemia
HCO$_3^-$	bicarbonate
Hct	haematocrit
HCV	hepatitis C virus
HDN	haemolytic disease of the newborn
HE	hereditary elliptocytosis
HELLP	haemolysis, elevated liver enzymes and low platelets
HHT	hereditary haemorrhagic telangiectasia
HIV	human immunodeficiency virus
HLA	human leucocyte antigen
H/LMW	high/low molecular weight
HMP	hexose monophosphate shunt
HPA	human platelet antigen
HPFH	hereditary persistence of fetal haemoglobin
HPP	hereditary pyropoikilocytosis
HTLV-1	human T-lymphotropic virus type 1
HUS	haemolytic uraemic syndrome
IAGT	indirect antiglobulin test
ICH	intracranial haemorrhage
IDA	iron deficiency anaemia
IFN-α	interferon alpha
Ig	immunoglobulin
IgA	immunoglobulin A
IgD	immunoglobulin D
IgE	immunoglobulin E
IgG	immunoglobulin G
IgM	immunoglobulin M
IL-1	interleukin-1
IM	intramuscular
INR	International normalized ratio

inv	chromosomal inversion
ITP	idiopathic thrombocytopenic purpura
ITU	Intensive Therapy Unit
iu/IU	International units
IV	intravenous
IVI	intravenous infusion
IVIg	intravenous immunoglobulin
kg	kilogram
l	litre
LA	lupus anticoagulant
LAP	leucocyte alkaline phosphatase (score)
LDH	lactate dehydrogenase
LFTs	liver function tests
LGL	large granular lymphocyte
LP	lumbar puncture
MACOP-B	methotrexate, doxorubicin, cyclophosphamide, vincristine, bleomycin, prednisolone
MAHA	microangiopathic haemolytic anaemia
m-BACOD	methotrexate, bleomycin, adriamycin (doxorubicin), cyclophosphamide, vincristine, dexamethasone
MCH	mean cell haemoglobin
MCHC	mean corpuscular haemoglobin concentration
MCP	mitoxantrone, chlorambucil, prednisolone
M-CSF	macrophage colony-stimulating factor
MCV	mean cell volume
MDS	myelodysplastic syndrome
MetHb	methaemoglobin
mg	milligram
MGUS	monoclonal gammopathy of undetermined significance
MHC	major histocompatibility complex
MI	myocardial infarction
min(s)	minute(s)
MM	multiple myeloma
MoAb	monoclonal antibody
MPD	myeloproliferative disease
MPO	myeloperoxidase
MPV	mean platelet volume
MRI	magnetic resonance imaging
mRNA	messenger ribonucleic acid
Mst II	a restriction enzyme
MUD	matched unrelated donor (transplant)
Na^+	sodium
NADP	nicotinamide adenine diphosphate
NADPH	nicotinamide adenine diphosphate (reduced)
NAIT	neonatal alloimmune thrombocytopenia
NEJM	New England Journal of Medicine
NHL	non-Hodgkin's lymphoma
NRBC	nucleated red blood cells
NSAIDs	non-steroidal antiinflammatory drugs
OCP	oral contraceptive pill
od	*omni die* (once daily)
PaO_2	partial pressure of O_2 in arterial blood

Symbols and abbreviations

PAS	periodic acid–Schiff
PB	peripheral blood
PC	protein C
PCC	prothrombin complex concentrate
PCL	plasma cell leukaemia
PCP	*Pneumocystis carinii* pneumonia
PCR	polymerase chain reaction
PCV	packed cell volume
PE	pulmonary embolism
PET	pre-eclamptic toxaemia
Ph	Philadelphia chromosome
PIVKA	protein induced by vitamin K absence
PK	pyruvate kinase
PLL	prolymphocytic leukaemia
PML	promyelocytic leukaemia
PNH	paroxysmal nocturnal haemoglobinuria
PO	*per os* (by mouth)
PPP	primary proliferative polycythaemia
ProMACE	prednisolone, doxorubicin, cyclophosphamide, etoposide
PRV	polycythaemia rubra vera
PS	protein S
PT	prothrombin time
PTP	post-transfusion purpura
qds	*quater die sumendus* (to be taken 4 times a day)
℞	recipe (treat with)
RA	refractory anaemia
RAEB	refractory anaemia with excess blasts
RAEB-t	refractory anaemia with excess blasts in transformation
RAR	retinoic acid receptor
RARα	retinoic acid receptor α
RARS	refractory anaemia with ring sideroblasts
RBCs	red blood cells
RCC	red blood cell count
RCM	red cell mass
RDW	red cell distribution width
RES	reticuloendothelial system
RFLP	restriction fragment length polymorphism
Rh	Rhesus
rhG-CSF	recombinant human granulocyte colony stimulating factor
rHuEPO	recombinant human erythropoietin
RiCoF	ristocetin cofactor
RIPA	ristocetin-induced platelet aggregation
RT-PCR	reverse transcriptase polymerase chain reaction
s	seconds
SC	subcutaneous
SCA	sickle cell anaemia
SCD	sickle cell disease
SCID	severe combined immunodeficiency

SCT	stem cell transplant
SLE	systemic lupus erythematosus
SLVL	splenic lymphoma with villous lymphocytes
SmIg	surface membrane immunoglobulin
SOB	short of breath
stat	*statim* (immediate; as initial dose)
SVC	superior vena cava
SVCO	superior vena caval obstruction
T°	temperature
t½	half-life
T4	thyroxine
TB	tuberculosis
TCR	T-cell receptor
tds	*ter die sumendum* (to be taken 3 times a day)
TdT	terminal deoxynucleotidyl transferase
TENS	transcutaneous nerve stimulation
TFT	thyroid function test(s)
TIAs	transient ischaemic attacks
TIBC	total iron binding capacity
TNF	tumour necrosis factor
topo II	topoisomerase II
TPA	tissue plasminogen activator
TRAP	tartrate-resistant acid phosphatase
TSH	thyroid-stimulating hormone
TT	thrombin time
TTP	thrombotic thrombocytopenic purpura
TXA	tranexamic acid
U & E	urea and electrolytes
u/U	units
UC	ulcerative colitis
URTI	upper respiratory tract infection
USS	ultrasound scan
VAD	vincristine adriamycin dexamethasone regimen
VIII:C	Factor VIII clotting activity
Vit K	vitamin K
VTE	venous thromboembolism
vWD	von Willebrand's disease
vWF	von Willebrand factor
vWFAg	von Willebrand factor antigen
WBC	white blood count
WM	Waldenström's macroglobulinaemia
XDPs	cross-linked fibrin degradation products
μg	microgram

Contents

Clinical approach 1

History taking in patients with haematological disease

Approach to patient with suspected haematological disease

An accurate history combined with a careful physical examination are fundamental parts of clinical assessment. Although the likely haematological diagnosis may be apparent from tests carried out before the patient has been referred, it is nevertheless essential to assess the clinical background fully – this may influence the eventual plan of management, especially in older patients.

It is important to find out early on in the consultation what the patient may already have been told prior to referral, or what he/she thinks the diagnosis may be. Often fear and anxiety about diagnoses such as leukaemia, haemophilia or HIV infection.

Presenting symptoms and their duration

A full medical history needs to be taken to which is added direct questioning on relevant features associated with presenting symptoms:

- Non-specific symptoms such as fatigue, fevers, weight loss.
- Symptoms relating to anaemia eg reduced exercise capacity, recent onset of breathlessness and nature of its onset, or worsening of angina, presence of ankle oedema.
- Symptoms relating to neutropenia eg recurrent oral ulceration, skin infections, oral sepsis.
- Evidence of compromised immunity eg recurrent oropharyngeal infection.
- Details of potential haemostatic problems eg easy bruising, bleeding episodes, rashes.
- Anatomical symptoms, eg abdominal discomfort (splenic enlargement or pressure from enlarged lymph nodes), CNS symptoms (from spinal compression).
- Past medical history, ie detail on past illnesses, information on previous surgical procedures which may suggest previous haematological problems (eg may suggest an underlying bleeding diathesis) or be associated with haematological or other sequelae, eg splenectomy.
- Drug history: ask about prescribed and non-prescribed medications.
- Allergies. Since some haematological disorders may relate to chemicals or other environmental hazards specific questions should be asked about occupational factors and hobbies.
- Transfusion history: ask about whether the patient has been a blood donor and how much he/she has donated. May occasionally be a factor in iron deficiency anaemia. History of previous transfusion(s) and their timing is also critical in some cases, eg post-transfusion purpura.
- Tobacco and alcohol consumption is essential; both may produce significant haematological morbidity.
- Travel: clearly important in the case of suspected malaria but also relevant in considering other causes of haematological abnormality, including HIV infection.
- Family history also important, especially in the context of inherited haematological disorders.

A complete history for a patient with a haematological disorder should provide all the relevant medical information to aid diagnosis and clinical assessment, as well as helping the haematologist to have a working assessment of the patient's social situation. A well taken history also provides a basis for good communication which will often prove very important once it comes to discussion of the diagnosis.

Physical examination

Forms part of the clinical assessment of the haematology patient. Specific attention paid to:

General examination – eg evidence of weight loss, pyrexia, pallor (not a reliable clinical measure of anaemia), jaundice, cyanosis or abnormal pigmentation or skin rashes.

The mouth – ulceration, purpura, gum bleeding or infiltration, and the state of the patient's teeth. Hands and nails may show features associated with haematological abnormalities, eg koilonychia in chronic iron deficiency (rare).

Record – weight, height, T°, pulse and blood pressure; height and weight give important baseline data against which sequential measurements can subsequently be compared. In myelofibrosis, for example, evidence of significant weight loss in the absence of symptoms may be an indication of clinical progression.

Examination – of chest and abdomen should focus on detecting the presence of lymphadenopathy, hepatic and/or splenic enlargement. Node sizes and the extent of organ enlargement should be carefully recorded.

Lymph node enlargement – often recorded in centimetres, eg 3cm × 3cm × 4cm; sometimes more helpful to compare the degree of enlargement with familiar objects eg pea. Record extent of liver or spleen enlargement as maximum distance palpable from the lower costal margin.

Erythematous margins of infected skin lesions – mark these to monitor treatment effects.

Bones and joints – recording of joint swelling and ranges of movement are standard aspects of haemophilia care. In myeloma areas of bony tenderness & deformity are commonly present.

Optic fundi – examination is a key clinical assessment in the haematology patient. May yield the only objective evidence of hyperviscosity in paraproteinaemias (see Emergencies p420) or hyperleucocytosis (see Emergencies p420) such as in eg CML. Regular examination for haemorrhages should form part of routine observations in the severely myelosuppressed patient; rarely changes of opportunistic infection such as candidiasis can be seen in the optic fundi.

Neurological examination – fluctuations of conscious level and confusion are clinical presentations of hyperviscosity. Isolated nerve palsies in a patient with acute leukaemia are highly suspicious of neurological involvement or disease relapse. Peripheral neuropathy and long tract signs are well recognised complications of B_{12} deficiency.

Splenomegaly

Many causes. Clinical approach depends on whether splenic enlargement is present as an isolated finding or with other clinical abnormalities eg jaundice or lymphadenopathy. Mild to moderate splenomegaly have a much greater number of causes than massive splenomegaly.

Causes of splenomegaly

Infection	Viral	EBV, CMV, hepatitis
	Bacterial	SBE, miliary tuberculosis, *Salmonella, Brucella*
	Protozoal	Malaria, Toxoplasma, Leishmaniasis
Haemolytic	Congenital	Hereditary spherocytosis, hereditary elliptocytosis
		Sickle cell disease (infants), thalassaemia
		Pyruvate kinase deficiency, G6PD deficiency
	Acquired	AIHA (idiopathic or 2°)
Myeloproliferative & leukaemic		Myelofibrosis, CML, Polycythaemia rubra vera
		Essential thrombocythaemia, acute leukaemias
Lymphoproliferative		CLL, hairy cell leukaemia, Waldenström's,
		SLVL, other NHL, Hodgkin's disease,
		ALL & lymphoblastic NHL
Autoimmune disorders		Rheumatoid arthritis, SLE, hepatic cirrhosis
Storage disorders		Gaucher's disease, histiocytosis X
		Niemann Pick disease
Miscellaneous		Metastatic cancer, cysts, amyloid,
		portal hypertension, portal vein thrombosis,
		tropical splenomegaly

Clinical approach essentially involves a working knowledge of the possible causes of splenic enlargement and determining the more likely causes in the given clinical circumstances by appropriate further investigation. There are fewer causes of massive splenic enlargement, ie the spleen tip palpable below the level of the umbilicus.

Massive splenomegaly

- Myelofibrosis.
- Chronic myeloid leukaemia.
- Lymphoproliferative disease – CLL and variants including SLVL & marginal zone lymphoma.
- Tropical splenomegaly.
- Leishmaniasis.
- Gaucher's disease.
- Thalassaemia major.

Lymphadenopathy

Occurs in a range of infective or neoplastic conditions; less frequently enlargement occurs in active collagen disorders. May be isolated, affecting a single node, localised, involving several nodes in an anatomical lymph node grouping or generalised, where nodes are enlarged at different sites. As well as enlargement in the easily palpable areas (cervical, axillary & iliac) node enlargement may be hilar or retroperitoneal and identifiable only by imaging. Isolated/localised lymphadenopathy usually results from local infection or neoplasm. Generalised lymphadenopathy may result from systemic causes, especially when symmetrical, as well as infection or neoplasm. Rarely drug associated (eg phenytoin).

Causes

- **Infective**
  - *bacterial* — Tonsillitis, cellulitis, tuberculous infections & primary syphilis usually produce isolated or localised node enlargement
  - *viral* — EBV, CMV, Rubella, HIV
  - *other* — *Toxoplasma*, histoplasmosis and *Chlamydia*
- **Neoplastic** — Hodgkin's disease (typically isolated or localised lymphadenopathy), NHL isolated, generalised or localised, CLL, metastatic carcinoma, acute leukaemia (ALL especially, but occasionally AML)
- **Collagen** — and other systemic disorders, eg rheumatoid arthritis, SLE, sarcoidosis

History and examination – points to elicit

- Age.
- Onset of symptoms, whether progressing or not.
- Systemic symptoms, weight loss (>10% body weight loss in <6 months).
- Night sweats.
- Risk factors for HIV infection.
- Local or systemic evidence of infection.
- Evidence of systemic disorder such as rheumatoid arthritis.
- Evidence of malignancy; if splenic enlargement present then lymphoreticular neoplasm is more likely.
- Specific disease related features eg pruritus and alcohol induced lymph node pain associated with Hodgkin's disease.
- Determine the duration of enlargement ± associated symptoms, whether nodes are continuing to enlarge and whether tender or not. Distribution of node enlargement should be recorded as well as size of node.

Investigations

1. FBC and peripheral blood film examination.
2. ESR or plasma viscosity.
3. Screening test for infectious mononucleosis and serological testing for other viruses.
4. Imaging – eg chest radiography and abdominal ± pelvic USS to define hilar, retroperitoneal & para-aortic nodes. CT scanning may also be helpful.
5. Microbiology eg blood cultures, indirect testing for TB and culture of biopsied or aspirated lymph node material.

6. Lymph node biopsy for definitive diagnosis especially if a neoplastic cause is suspected. Aspiration of enlarged lymph nodes is generally unsatisfactory in providing effective diagnostic material.
7. Bone marrow examination should be reserved for staging in confirmed lymphoma or leukaemia cases – it is not commonly a useful primary investigation of lymphadenopathy.

Unexplained anaemia

Evaluate with the combined information from clinical history, physical examination and results of investigations.

History – focus on

- Duration of symptoms of anaemia – short duration of dyspnoea and fatigue etc. suggests recent bleeding or haemolysis.
- Specific questioning on blood loss – include system related questions eg GIT & gynaecological sources, ask about blood donation.
- Family history – eg in relation to hereditary problems such as HS or ethnic Hb disorders such as thalassaemia or HbSS.
- Past history – eg association of gastrectomy with later occurrence of Fe and/or B_{12} deficiency.
- Drug history – including prescribed and non-prescribed medication.
- Dietary factors – mainly relates to folate and Fe deficiency, rarely B_{12} in vegans. Fe deficiency always occurs because Fe losses exceed intake (it is extremely rare in developed countries for diet to be the sole cause of Fe deficiency).

Examination

- May identify indirectly helpful signs eg koilonychia in chronic Fe deficiency (rare), jaundice in haemolytic disorders.
- Lymphadenopathy suggesting lymphoreticular disease or viral infection.
- Hepatosplenomegaly in lymphoproliferative or myeloproliferative disorders.

Full blood count

Laboratory investigation of anaemia is discussed fully in section 2. Anaemia in adult ♂ if Hb <13.0g/dl and in adult ♀ if Hb <11.5g/dl

MCV useful for initial anaemia evaluation

↓ MCV (<76fl)	Fe deficiency
	α & β thalassaemia
	Anaemia of chronic disorders
Normal MCV (78–98 fl)	Recent bleeding
	Anaemia of chronic disorders
	Most non-haematinic deficiency causes
	Combined Fe + B_{12}/folate deficiency
↑ MCV (>100fl)	Folate or B_{12} deficiency
	Liver disease
	Marrow dysplasia & failure syndromes including aplastic anaemia
	2° to antimetabolite drug therapy eg hydroxyurea

The need for film examination, reticulocyte counting, additional tests on the FBC sample such as checking for Heinz bodies is based on the initial clinical and FBC findings. The findings from the initial FBC examination have a major influence in determining the nature and urgency of further clinical investigation. Serum ferritin level will identify iron deficiency and focus on the need for detailed investigation for blood loss which, for adult males and postmenopausal females, will frequently require large bowel examination with colonoscopy or barium enema, and gastroscopy. BM examination may occasionally be required.

Anaemia is not a diagnosis – it is an abnormal clinical finding requiring an explanation for its cause. There is no place for empirical use of Fe therapy for management and treatment of 'anaemia' in modern medical practice.

Patient with elevated haemoglobin

Finding a raised Hb concentration requires a systematic clinical approach for differential diagnosis and further investigation. Initially it is essential to check whether the result ties in with the known clinical findings – if unexpected the FBC should be re-checked to exclude a mix-up over samples or a sampling artefact. Dehydration and diuretic therapy may increase the Hct and these should be excluded in the initial phase of assessment.

Having ascertained that the raised Hb concentration is genuine the issue is whether there is a genuine increase in red cell mass or not, and the explanation for the elevated Hb.

Anoxia is a major stimulus to RBC production and will result in an increase in erythropoietin with consequent erythrocytosis.

History and examination should assess

- Recent travel and residence at high altitude (>3000m).
- COAD, other hypoxic respiratory conditions, cyanotic congenital heart disease, other cardiac problems causing hypoxia.
- Smoking – heavy cigarette smoking causes ↑ carboxyHb levels leading to ↑ RBC mass to compensate for loss of O_2 carrying capacity.
- Ventilatory impairment 2° to gross obesity, alveolar hypoventilation (Pickwickian syndrome).
- Possibility of high affinity Hb abnormalities arises if there is a FH of polycythaemia, otherwise requires assessment through Hb analysis.
- If obvious secondary causes excluded possibilities include:

Spurious polycythaemia – pseudopolycythaemia or Gaisbock's syndrome, associated features can include cigarette smoking, obesity, hypertension & excess alcohol consumption; sometimes described as 'stress polycythaemia'.

Primary proliferative polycythaemia (polycythaemia rubra vera) – plethoric facies, history of pruritus after bathing or on change of environmental temperature and presence of splenomegaly are helpful clinical findings to suggest this diagnosis.

Inappropriate erythropoietin excess – occurs in a variety of benign and malignant renal disorders. Recorded as a rare complication of some tumours including hepatoma, uterine fibroids and cerebellar haemangioblastoma.

Part of clinical assessment must also include an evaluation of thrombotic risk; previous thrombosis or a family history of such problems increase the urgency of investigation and appropriate treatment

See p188–192.

Elevated WBC

Leucocytosis is defined as elevation of the white cell count >2 SD above the mean. The detection of leucocytosis should prompt immediate scrutiny of the automated WBC differential (generally accurate except in leukaemia) and the other FBC parameters. Blood film should be examined and a manual differential count performed. Important to evaluate leucocytosis in terms of the age-related absolute normal ranges for neutrophils, lymphocytes, monocytes, eosinophils and basophils (see p592, 598) and the presence of abnormal elements: immature granulocytes, blasts, nucleated red cells and 'atypical cells'.

Leukaemoid reaction – leucocytosis >50 × 10^9/l defines a neutrophilia with marked 'left shift' (band forms, metamyelocytes, myelocytes and occasionally promyelocytes and myeloblasts in the blood film). Differential diagnosis is chronic granulocytic leukaemia (CGL) and in children, juvenile CML. Primitive granulocyte precursors are also frequently seen in the blood film of the infected or stressed neonate, and any seriously ill patient eg on ITU.

Leucoerythroblastic blood film – contains myelocytes, other primitive granulocytes, nucleated red cells and often tear drop red cells is due to bone marrow invasion by tumour, fibrosis or granuloma formation and is an indication for a bone marrow biopsy. Other causes include anorexia and haemolysis.

Leucocytosis due to blasts – suggests diagnosis of acute leukaemia and is an indication for cell typing studies and bone marrow examination.

FBC, blood film, white cell differential count and the clinical context in which the leucocytosis is detected will usually indicate whether this is due to a 1° haematological abnormality or reflects a 2° response.

▶ It is clearly important to seek a history of symptoms of infection and examine the patient for signs of infection or an underlying haematological disorder.

Neutrophilia
- 2° to acute infection is most common cause of leucocytosis.
- Usually modest (uncommonly >30 × 10^9/l), associated with a left shift and occasionally toxic granulation or vacuolation of neutrophils.
- Chronic inflammation causes less marked neutrophilia often associated with monocytosis.
- Moderate neutrophilia may occur following steroid therapy, heatstroke and in patients with solid tumours.
- Mild neutrophilia may be induced by stress (eg immediate postoperative period) and exercise.
- May be seen in the immediate aftermath of a myocardial infarction or major seizure.
- Frequently found in states of chronic bone marrow stimulation (eg chronic haemolysis, ITP) and asplenia.
- Primary haematological causes of neutrophilia are less common. CML is often the cause of extremely high leucocyte counts (>200 × 10^9/l), predominantly neutrophils with marked left shift, basophilia and occasional myeloblasts. A low LAP score and the presence of the Ph chromosome on karyotype analysis are usually helpful to differentiate CGL from a leukaemoid reaction.

- Less common are juvenile CML, transient leukaemoid reaction in Down's syndrome, hereditary neutrophilia and chronic idiopathic neutrophilia.

Bone marrow examination is rarely necessary in the investigation of a patient with isolated neutrophilia. Investigation of a leukaemoid reaction, leuco-erythroblastic blood film and possible CGL or juvenile CML are firm indications for a bone marrow aspirate and trephine biopsy. Bone marrow culture, including culture for atypical mycobacteria and fungi, may be useful in patients with persistent pyrexia or leucocytosis.

Lymphocytosis

- Lymphocytosis $>4.0 \times 10^9/l$.
- Normal infants and young children <5 have a higher proportion and concentration of lymphocytes than adults.
- Rare in acute bacterial infection except in pertussis (may $>50 \times 10^9/l$).
- Acute infectious lymphocytosis also seen in children, usually associated with transient lymphocytosis and a mild constitutional reaction.
- Characteristic of infectious mononucleosis but these lymphocytes are often large and atypical and the diagnosis may be confirmed with a heterophil agglutination test.
- Similar atypical cells may be seen in patients with CMV and hepatitis A infection.
- Chronic infection with brucellosis, tuberculosis, secondary syphilis and congenital syphilis may cause lymphocytosis.
- Lymphocytosis is characteristic of CLL, ALL and occasionally NHL.

Where primary haematological cause suspected, immunophenotypic analysis of the peripheral blood lymphocytes will often confirm or exclude a neoplastic diagnosis. BM examination is indicated if neoplasia is strongly suspected and in any patient with concomitant neutropenia, anaemia or thrombocytopenia.

Reduced WBC

Although not entirely synonymous, it is uncommon for absolute leucopenia (WBC $<4.0 \times 10^9$/l) to be due to isolated deficiency of any cell other than the neutrophil though in marked leucopenia several cell lines are often affected.

▶ Neutropenia

Defined as a neutrophil count $<2.0 \times 10^9$/l. The propensity to infective complications is closely related to the absolute neutrophil count. More severe when neutropenia due to impaired production from chemotherapy or marrow failure rather than to peripheral destruction or maturation arrest where there is often a cellular marrow with early neutrophil precursors and normal monocyte counts. Type of infection determined by the degree and duration of neutropenia. Ongoing chemotherapy further increases the risk of serious bacterial and fungal opportunistic infection and the presence of an indwelling intravenous catheter increases the incidence of infection with coagulase negative *Staphylococci* and other skin commensals. Patients with chronic immune neutropenia may develop recurrent stomatitis, gingivitis, oral ulceration, sinusitis and peri-anal infection.

Neutrophil count	Risk of infection
1.0–1.5×10^9/l	No significant increased risk of infection.
0.5–1.0	Some increase in risk; some fevers can be treated as an outpatient.
<0.5	Major increase in risk; treat all fevers with broad spectrum IV antibiotics as an inpatient.

The history and physical examination provide a guide to the subsequent management of a patient with neutropenia. Simple observation is appropriate initially for an asymptomatic patient with isolated mild neutropenia who has an unremarkable history and examination. If there has been a recent viral illness or the patient can discontinue a drug which may be the cause, follow-up over a few weeks may see resolution of the abnormality.

Investigations

BM examination – if there is concomitant anaemia or thrombocytopenia, if there is a history of significant infection or if lymphadenopathy or organomegaly are detected on examination. Usually unhelpful in patients with an isolated neutropenia $>0.5 \times 10^9$/l. However, if neutropenia persists, bone marrow aspiration, biopsy, cytogenetics and serology for collagen diseases, anti-neutrophil antibodies, HIV and immunoglobulins should be performed.

Differential diagnoses

Isolated neutropenia may be the presenting feature of myelodysplasia, aplastic anaemia, Fanconi's anaemia or acute leukaemia but these conditions will usually be associated with other haematological abnormalities.

Post-infectious (most usually post-viral) neutropenia may last several weeks and may be followed by prolonged immune neutropenia.

Severe sepsis particularly at the extremes of life.

Drugs – cytotoxic agents, and many others, notably phenothiazines, many antibiotics, NSAIDs, antithyroid agents and psychotropic agents. Recovery of neutrophils usually starts within a few days of stopping the offending drug.

Autoimmune neutropenia due to anti-neutrophil antibodies may occur in isolation or in association with haemolytic anaemia, immune thrombocytopenia or SLE.

Felty's syndrome neutropenia is accompanied by seropositive rheumatoid arthritis, and splenomegaly.

Chronic benign neutropenia of infancy and childhood is associated with fever and infection but resolves by age 4, probably also has an immune basis.

Benign familial neutropenia is a feature of rare families and of certain racial groups, notably negroes, is associated with mild neutropenia but no propensity to infection.

Chronic idiopathic neutropenia is a diagnosis of exclusion, associated with severe neutropenia but often a benign course.

Cyclical neutropenia is a condition of childhood onset and dominant inheritance characterised by severe neutropenia, fever, stomatitis and other infections occurring with a periodicity of ~4 weeks.

Hereditary causes (less common) include Kostmann syndrome (see p380), Shwachman-Diamond-Oski syndrome (see p380), Chediak-Higashi syndrome (see p379), reticular dysgenesis and dyskeratosis congenita.

Management

Febrile episodes should be managed according to the severity of the neutropenia (see table) and the underlying cause (bone marrow failure is associated with more life threatening infections). Broad spectrum IV antibiotics may be required and empirical systemic antifungal therapy may be required in those who fail to respond to antibiotics. Prophylactic antibiotic and antifungal therapy may be helpful in some patients with chronic neutropenia as may rhG-CSF. Antiseptic mouthwash is of value and regular dental care is important.

▶ Lymphocytopenia

Lymphocytopenia ($<1.5 \times 10^9/l$) may be seen in acute infections, cardiac failure, pancreatitis, tuberculosis, uraemia, lymphoma, carcinoma, SLE and other collagen disease, corticosteroid therapy, radiation, chemotherapy and anti-lymphocyte globulin. Most common cause of chronic severe lymphocytopenia in recent years has been HIV infection (see p328).

Chronic severe lymphocytopenia ($<0.5 \times 10^9/l$) is associated both with opportunistic infections notably *Candida* species, *Pneumocystis carinii*, CMV, Herpes zoster, *Mycoplasma* spp., *Cryptosporidium* and Toxoplasmosis and with an increased incidence of neoplasia particularly NHL, Kaposi's sarcoma and skin and gastric carcinoma.

Elevated platelet count

Thrombocytosis is defined as a platelet count >450 × 10^9/l. May be due to a *primary* myeloproliferative disorder (MPD) or a *secondary* reactive feature. If the platelet count is markedly elevated a patient with a myeloproliferative disorder has a risk of haemorrhage (due to the production of dysfunctional platelets), or thrombosis, or both. The patient's history may reveal features of the condition to which the elevated platelet count is secondary. Clinical examination may provide similar clues or reveal the presence of palpable splenomegaly which suggests a myeloproliferative disorder. FBC may provide useful information: marked leucocytosis with left shift (in the absence of a history of infection), basophilia or an elevated haematocrit and red cell count are highly suggestive of a myeloproliferative disorder when associated with thrombocytosis. Unusual for reactive thrombocytosis to cause a platelet count >1000 × 10^9/l. *Note:* platelet counts below this may occur in myeloproliferative disorders.

Differential diagnosis

Myeloproliferative disorders	*Conditions associated with thrombocytosis*
Primary thrombocythaemia	Haemorrhage
Polycythaemia rubra vera	Trauma
Chronic granulocytic leukaemia	Surgery
Idiopathic myelofibrosis	Iron deficiency anaemia
	Malignancy (ca lung, ca breast, Hodgkin's disease)
	Acute & chronic infection
	Inflammatory disease eg, rheumatoid arthritis, UC
	Post-splenectomy

Investigation
- BM aspirate may show megakaryocyte abnormalities in MPD.
- BM trephine biopsy may show clusters of abnormal megakaryocytes and increased reticulin or fibrosis in MPD.

Management
- In reactive thrombocytosis treat the underlying condition.
- Unusual for treatment to ↓ the platelet count to be necessary in a patient with reactive thrombocytosis.
- Consider low dose aspirin (or if contraindicated, dipyridamole).
- Reactive thrombocytosis is generally transient.
- If secondary to iron deficiency – review FBC after iron therapy: the platelet count normalises if thrombocytosis was due to iron deficiency.
- Iron deficiency may have masked PRV – this will be revealed by iron therapy.
- If impossible to define the cause of thrombocytosis then a watch and wait policy should be followed in an asymptomatic patient.
- If MPD is suspected – see *Essential thrombocythaemia*.

Reduced platelet count

Thrombocytopenia is defined as platelet count $<150 \times 10^9$/l. Although there is no precise platelet count at which a patient will or will not bleed, most patients with a count $>50 \times 10^9$/l are asymptomatic. The risk of spontaneous haemorrhage increases significantly $<20 \times 10^9$/l. Purpura is most common presenting symptom and is usually found on the lower limbs and areas subject to pressure. May be followed by bleeding gums, epistaxis or more serious life-threatening haemorrhage. A patient with newly diagnosed severe thrombocytopenia with or without purpura is a medical emergency and should be admitted for further investigation and treatment.

Confirm low platelet count by examination of the blood sample for clots and the blood film for platelet aggregates (causing pseudothrombocytopenia). History and examination will determine the clinical severity of the thrombocytopenia and should also reveal the duration of symptoms, presence of any prodromal illness, causative medication or underlying disease.

Determine whether the cause of thrombocytopenia is failure of production or increased consumption. FBC may be helpful as the mean platelet volume (MPV) is often elevated in the latter group (large platelets may also be seen on the blood film). May also reveal additional haematological abnormalities (normocytic anaemia or neutropenia) suggestive of a bone marrow disorder. A coagulation screen should also be performed. Examination of the bone marrow is the definitive investigation in all patients with moderate or severe thrombocytopenia – may reveal normal megakaryocytes or compensatory hyperplasia in peripheral destruction syndromes or marrow hypoplasia or infiltration. Tests for platelet antibodies are unreliable but an autoimmune screen may be helpful to exclude lupus.

Failure of production	*Increased consumption*
Drugs & chemicals (see p316)	ITP (see p312)
Viral infection	Drugs (see p316)
Radiation	DIC (see p422)
Aplastic anaemia (see p118)	Infection
Leukaemia	Massive haemorrhage & transfusion (see p432)
	SLE
Marrow infiltration (see p403)	CLL & lymphoma (see p152, 164)
Megaloblastic anaemia (see p56–60)	Heparin (see p502)
HIV (see p328)	TTP (see p438)
	Hypersplenism (see p316)
	Post-transfusion purpura (see p416)
	HIV (see p328)

Management

Treat underlying condition. Most patients with a platelet count $>40 \times 10^9$/l require no specific therapy. Avoid aspirin. In the event of life-threatening haemorrhage platelet transfusion should be administered to thrombocytopenic patients *with the exception of those with heparin-induced thrombocytopenia and TTP*.

Clinical approach

Easy bruising

Evaluation of a patient who complains of easy bruising involves a detailed history, physical examination with particular attention to any current haemorrhagic lesions and the performance of basic haemostatic investigations. More common in ♀ and often difficult to evaluate. Also a frequent complaint in the elderly.

History

Careful attention to the history is essential to the diagnosis of all the haemorrhagic disorders and one must attempt to define the nature of the bruising in a patient with this complaint. Note: many normal healthy people believe that they have excessive bleeding or bruising. Conversely some people with haemorrhagic disorders and abnormal bleeding histories will not volunteer the information unless asked directly or indeed may consider their bleeding to be normal. Remember that excessive bruising may be a manifestation of a blood vessel disorder rather than a coagulopathy or platelet disorder.

Ask about

Presenting complaint How long and how frequently has easy bruising occurred? Is it ecchymoses or purpura? How extensive are bruises? Are they located in areas subject to trauma (eg limbs) or pressure (eg waist band)? Do petechiae occur? Are bruises painful? Is there a palpable knot or cord? How long to resolution? How many currently?

Associated symptoms

Has there been gum bleeding? Has the patient experienced prolonged bleeding after skin trauma, dental extraction, childbirth or surgery? Has there been any other form of haemorrhage, eg epistaxis, menorrhagia, joint or soft tissue haematoma, haematemesis, melaena, haemoptysis or haematuria? Is there a history of poor wound healing?

Family history

Has any other family member a history of excessive bleeding or bruising?

Drug history

Is the patient on any medication (remember self medication of vitamins and food supplements), most notably aspirin, anticoagulant therapy?

Systematic enquiry

Is there evidence of a disorder associated with a haemorrhagic tendency eg hepatic or renal failure, malabsorption, leukaemia, connective tissue disorder or amyloid?

Physical examination

Haemorrhagic skin lesions are likely to be present in a patient with a serious problem and their distribution will often indicate the extent to which they are likely to be related to trauma. Senile purpura is almost invariably on the hands and forearms. True purpura is easily differentiated from erythema and telangiectasis by pressure. Petechiae are highly suggestive of a platelet or vascular disorder whilst palpable purpura is associated with anaphylactoid purpura. In addition there may be other physical findings which may indicate an underlying disorder, eg splenomegaly or lymphadenopathy in leukaemia, signs of hepatic failure, telangiectasia in Osler-Rendu-Weber syndrome or hyperextensible joints and paper thin scars in Ehlers-Danlos syndrome.

Basic haemostatic investigations

All patients should be investigated except those in whom history and examination has given strong grounds for believing that they are normal and in whom there is a history of a normal response to a haemostatic challenge eg surgery or dental extraction.

Screening tests

- FBC and blood film.
- APTT.
- PT.
- Thrombin clotting time and/or fibrinogen.
- Bleeding time.

If these investigations are normal there is no indication for further haemostatic investigations unless the history provides strong grounds for believing that there is indeed a haemostatic disorder. The appropriate further investigation of the haemostatic mechanism is discussed in Section 9.

Differential diagnoses

- Common diagnoses
  - Simple easy bruising (Purpura simplex)
  - Trauma (including non-accidental injury in children)
  - Senile purpura
- Haemostatic defects
  - Thrombocytopenia
  - Platelet function defects
  - Coagulation abnormalities (rarely)
- Vascular defects
  - Corticosteroid excess
  - Collagen diseases
  - Uraemia
  - Dysproteinaemias
  - Anaphylactoid purpura
  - Ehlers-Danlos disease

Recurrent thromboembolism

A hypercoagulable state should be suspected in all patients with recurrent thromboembolic disease, family history of thrombosis, thrombosis at a young age or at an unusual site (in addition to recurrent thromboembolism) associated with inherited thrombophilia. Further important aspects of the history are precipitating factors at the time of thrombosis and lifestyle considerations eg smoking, exercise and obesity. Clinical examination may reveal signs suggestive of an associated underlying condition.

Hypercoagulable states

Inherited
Activated Protein C Resistance (Factor V Leiden).
Protein C deficiency.
Protein S deficiency.
Antithrombin III deficiency and some very rare abnormalities of fibrinogen, plasminogen and plasminogen activator.

Acquired
Immobilisation.
Oral contraceptive or oestrogen therapy.
Postpartum.
Old age.
Postoperative.
Malignancy (notably Ca pancreas).
Nephrotic syndrome.
Myeloproliferative disorders.
Antiphospholipid syndrome (lupus anticoagulant).
Hyperviscosity.
Paroxysmal nocturnal haemoglobinuria.
Thrombotic thrombocytopenic purpura.
Heparin-induced thrombocytopenia.

Laboratory Investigation
See Thrombophilia p278.

Pathological fracture

Fracture in a bone compromised by the presence of a pathological process resulting in fracture occurring following relatively minor trauma. Most commonly due to local neoplastic involvement or osteoporosis.

Haematological causes
- Local bony damage.
- Myelomatous deposits.
- Lymphoma.
- Metastatic carcinoma (± marrow infiltration); breast, prostate and lung are commoner primary sites.
- Gaucher's disease.
- Sickle cell anaemia.
- Homozygous thalassaemia.
- Osteoporosis from prolonged corticosteroid therapy eg for autoimmune disease.

Clinically
Presentation as local pain, discomfort and restriction of mobility.

Diagnosis
Confirmed by X-ray or other imaging.

Management
- Awareness of risk/possibility and early diagnosis.
- Analgesia.
- Orthopaedic – immobilisation & support as appropriate for nature & site of injury, surgical intervention including pinning or other fixation.
- Radiotherapy – local management of fracture 2° to local malignancy.
- Mobilisation – physiotherapy.
- Treatment of underlying condition predisposing to fracture.

Raised ESR

The ESR remains an established, empirical test clinically useful as a method for identifying and monitoring the acute phase response. It is influenced by changes in fibrinogen, α-macroglobulins and immunoglobulins which enhance red cell aggregation *in vitro*.

Plasma viscosity is also an effective measure of acute phase reactants and can be used as an alternative to the ESR in clinical practice; increases in ESR and plasma viscosity generally parallel each other.

Normal ranges
- 0–10mm/h for ♂ 18–65 years.
- 1–20mm/h for ♀ 18–65 years.
- Upper limits of normal increase by 5–10mm/h for patients >65 years.
- Other factors eg Hct influence the ESR.
- Should be regarded as semiquantitative.
- Marked elevations are clinically significant.
- Modest elevations can be more problematic to interpret.

The main advantages to the ESR are its low cost and technical simplicity allied to the absence of a more accurate, inexpensive and technically simple alternative.

Causes of raised ESR

Pregnancy	Increases in pregnancy; maximal in 3rd trimester
Infections	Acute and chronic infections, including TB *Note:* ↑ ESR also occurs in HIV infection
Collagen disorders	Rheumatoid, SLE, polymyalgia rheumatica, vasculitides etc (including temporal arteritis); ESR useful as nonspecific monitor of disease activity
Other inflammatory processes	Inflammatory bowel disease, sarcoidosis, post-MI
Neoplastic conditions	Carcinomatosis, NHL, Hodgkin's disease and paraproteinaemias (benign & malignant)

Investigations

Given the wide range of situations in which a raised ESR can arise, further investigation depends on a carefully conducted history and examination. In the absence of likely causes from these, simple initial laboratory and radiology assessments to include urinalysis, full blood count and film examination, urea, electrolytes, plasma protein electrophoresis, an autoimmune profile and CXR should represent a practical and pragmatic primary diagnostic screen.

See p530.

Serum or urine paraprotein

Differential diagnosis

Common
- Monoclonal gammopathy of undetermined significance (MGUS).
- Myeloma.
- Solitary plasmacytoma.
- Lymphoproliferative disorders eg CLL, NHL, Waldenström's.

Less common
- Autoimmune disorders eg RA, SLE.
- Polymyalgia rheumatica.

Rare
- AL amyloid (primary amyloid).
- Plasma cell leukaemia.
- Heavy chain disease.

Discriminating clinical features

MGUS – no symptoms or signs, normal FBC and biochemical profile, paraprotein level < 30g/l and stable, no immuneparesis (rarely present), BM plasma cells <10%, no lytic lesions.

Plasmacytoma – localised bone pain, low paraprotein level, isolated bony lesion.

Myeloma – symptoms and signs of anaemia or hyperviscosity (see p420); bone pain or tenderness, raised Ca^{2+}, creatinine, urate; high β-2microglobulin and low albumin; immuneparesis; *paraprotein >30g/l of IgG or >20g/l of IgA or heavy Bence-Jones proteinuria; BM >10% plasma cells; lytic bone lesions on x-ray.* Minimum diagnostic criteria are at least 2 of emboldened items.

Plasma cell leukaemia – as Myeloma but fulminant history. Plasma cells seen on blood film.

Heavy chain disease – rare, characterised by a single heavy chain only in serum or urine electrophoresis. Presence of any light chain excludes.

Amyloid – myriad clinical features. Diagnosis on biopsy of affected site or, if inaccessible, by BM or rectal biopsy – characteristic fibrils stain with Congo Red and show green birefringence in polarised light.

CLL and NHL – systemic symptoms eg fever, night sweats, weight loss. Lymphadenopathy or hepatosplenomegaly likely. Confirm on BM or node biopsy.

Waldenström's – as for CLL but with symptoms or signs of hyperviscosity (see p212).

Autoimmune disorders – suggested by joint pain, skin rashes, multisystem disease. Confirm on autoimmune profile including Rheumatoid Factor, ANA, ANCA.

See p206.

Anaemia in pregnancy

Physiological changes red cell & plasma volume occur during pregnancy.

- Red cell mass ↑ by ≤30%.
- Plasma volume ↑ ≤60%.
- Net effect to ↑ blood volume by ≤50% with lowering of the normal Hb concentration to 10.0–11.0g/dl during pregnancy. MCV increases during pregnancy.
- Iron deficiency is a common problem and cause of anaemia in pregnancy.

Cause of increased requirements	Amount of additional Fe
↑ red cell mass	~500mg
fetal requirements	~300mg
placental requirements	~5mg
basal losses over pregnancy (1.0–1.5mg/day)	~250mg

These result in a total requirement of ≤1000mg Fe requiring an average daily intake of 3.5–4.0mg/d. Average Western diet provides <4.0mg Fe/d so that balance is marginal during pregnancy. Diets with Fe mainly in non-haem form provide less Fe available for absorption. Thus a high risk of developing Fe deficiency anaemia which is exacerbated if preconception Fe stores are reduced.

Folate requirements are increased during pregnancy because of increased cellular demands; folate levels tend to drop during pregnancy.

Prophylaxis recommendation to give 40–60mg elemental Fe/d which will increase availability of dietary absorbable Fe and protect against chronic Fe deficiency; debated whether supplements required by all pregnant women or only for those in at-risk socio-economic and nutritionally deficient groups. Folate supplementation is recommended for all and also appears to reduce incidence of neural tube defects.

- Dilutional anaemia – Hb seldom <10.0g/dl (requires no therapy).
- Fe deficiency – may occur with normal MCV because of ↑ MCV associated with pregnancy; check serum ferritin and give Fe replacement; assess and treat the underlying cause.
- Blood loss – sudden ↓ in Hb may signify fetomaternal bleeding or other forms of concealed obstetric bleeding.
- Folate deficiency – macrocytic anaemia in pregnancy almost invariably will be due to folate deficiency (B_{12} deficiency is extremely rare during pregnancy).
- Microangiopathic haemolysis/DIC may be seen in eclampsia or following placental abruption or intrauterine death. HELLP syndrome (p34) is rare but serious cause of anaemia.
- Anaemia may also arise during pregnancy from other unrelated causes and should be investigated appropriately.

Thrombocytopenia in pregnancy

A normal uncomplicated pregnancy is associated with a platelet count in the normal range though up to 10% of normal deliveries may be associated with mild thrombocytopenia (>100 × 10^9/l). Detection of thrombocytopenia in a pregnant patient requires consideration not only of the diagnoses listed in the previous section but also the conditions associated with pregnancy which cause thrombocytopenia. An additional important consideration is the possible effect on the fetus and its delivery.

If thrombocytopenia is detected late in pregnancy, most women will have a platelet count result from booking visit (at 10–12 weeks) for comparison. Mild thrombocytopenia (100–150 × 10^9/l) detected for the first time during an uncomplicated pregnancy is not associated with any risk to the fetus nor does it require special obstetric intervention other than hospital delivery.

Non-immune thrombocytopenia

- Thrombocytopenia may develop in association with pregnancy-induced hypertension, pre-eclampsia or eclampsia. Successful treatment of hypertension may be associated with improvement in thrombocytopenia which is believed to be due to consumption. Treatment of hypertension, pre-eclampsia or eclampsia may necessitate delivery of the fetus who is not at risk of thrombocytopenia.
- HELLP syndrome (haemolysis, elevated liver enzymes and low platelets) may occur in pregnancy.
- A number of obstetric complications, notably retention of a dead fetus, abruptio placentae and amniotic fluid embolism, are associated with DIC (see p422).

Immune thrombocytopenia may occur in pregnancy and women with chronic ITP may become pregnant. Therapeutic considerations must include an assessment of the risk to the fetus of transplacental passage of antiplatelet antibody causing fetal thrombocytopenia and a risk of haemorrhage before or during delivery. There is no reliable parameter for the assessment of fetal risk which, although relatively low, is most significant in women with pre-existing chronic ITP.

Women with a platelet count <50 × 10^9/l due to ITP should receive standard prednisolone therapy (see p314). If prednisolone fails or is contraindicated, IVIg should be administered and may need to be repeated at 3 week intervals. Splenectomy should be avoided (high rate of fetal loss). Enthusiasm has waned for assessing the fetal platelet count during pregnancy by cordocentesis followed by platelet transfusion. Fetal scalp sampling in early labour is unreliable and hazardous. Some experts recommend the administration of dexamethasone to the mother for 3 weeks before delivery to have a beneficial effect on the fetal platelet count. Delivery should occur in an Obstetric Unit with Paediatric support and the neonate's platelet count should be monitored for several days as delayed falls in the platelet count occur.

Prolonged bleeding after surgery

Prolonged bleeding following surgery often requires urgent haematological opinion and investigation. Usually the cause of the bleeding is surgical, ie due to local factors, and not a reflection of any underlying systemic bleeding disorder.

History and clinical assessment

- Past history in relation to previous haemostatic challenges, eg previous surgery, dental extractions. Ask specific questions about whether blood transfusion was required.
- Presence of specific clinical problems eg impaired liver or renal function.
- Recent drug history – especially aspirin or NSAIDs which can affect platelet function. Also enquire about cytotoxic drugs and anticoagulants.
- Family history of bleeding problems especially after surgery.
- Nature of the surgery and intrinsic haemorrhagic risks of procedure.
- Whether surgery was elective or emergency (in emergency surgery known risk factors are less likely to have been corrected).
- Check case record or ask surgeon/anaesthetist for information on intra-operative bleeding, technical problems etc.
- Whether surgery involves a high risk of triggering DIC, eg pancreatic or major hepatobiliary surgery.
- Detailed physical examination is not usually practical but bruising, ecchymoses or purpura should be assessed especially if remote from the site of surgery.
- What blood products have been used and over how long? Transfusion of several units of RBCs over a short period of time will dilute available clotting factors.
- Review preoperative investigation results and other information available in the record on past procedures and/or investigations.

Investigation

- Ensure samples not taken from heparinised line.
- FBC with platelet count and blood film examination.
- PT, APTT and fibrinogen.
  With normal platelets and coagulation screen bleeding is usually surgical and the patient should be supported with blood and urgent surgical re-exploration undertaken. Platelet function abnormalities may occur with aspirin/NSAIDs, uraemia, or extracorporeal circuits. Prolongation of both PT and APTT suggests massive bleeding and inadequate replacement, DIC, underlying liver disease or oral anticoagulants. Disproportionate, isolated increases in either PT or APTR are more likely to indicate previously undiagnosed clotting factor deficiencies. A low platelet count may reflect dilution and consumption from bleeding or DIC if platelets were known to be normal preoperatively.

Treatment

- Low platelets or platelet function abnormalities:
  Give 1–2 adult doses of platelets stat.
- DIC–give 2 adult doses of platelets are 4 units FFP (10–20 units of cryoprecipitate if fibrinogen low) and recheck PT, APTT and FBC.
- Anticoagulant effect:
  Heparin–reverse with protamine sulphate.
  Warfarin– reverse with FFP or PCC.

- Empirical tranexamic acid or aprotinin may be tried if bleeding continues despite the above.

Positive sickle test (HbS solubility test)

The decreased solubility of deoxyHbS forms the basis of this test. Blood is added to a buffered solution of a reducing agent eg sodium dithionate. HbS is precipitated by the solution and produces a turbid appearance. *Note*: does not discriminate between sickle cell *trait* and *homozygous disease.*

Use

This is a quick screening test (takes ~20 mins), often used preoperatively to detect HbS.

Action if sickle test +ve

- Delay elective operation until established whether *disease* or *trait*.
- Ask about family history of sickle cell anaemia or symptoms of SCA.
- FBC and film

Sickle cell trait	FBC–normal or reduced MCV & MCH, no anaemia
	Film–normal (may be microcytosis or target cells)
Sickle cell disease	FBC–Hb~7-8g/dl (range ~4–11g/dl)
	Film–sickled RBCs, target cells, polychromasia,
	basophilic stippling, NRBC (hyposplenic features in adults)

- Hb electrophoresis.
- Group and antibody screen serum.

False +ve results

- Low Hb.
- Severe leucocytosis.
- Hyperproteinaemia.
- Unstable Hb.

False –ve results

- Infants <6 months.
- HbS <20% (eg following exchange blood transfusion).

Sickle test not recommended as a screening test in pregnancy as it will not detect other Hb variants that interact with HbS eg β thalassaemia trait. Standard Hb electrophoresis of at-risk groups should be performed (and of all pregnant women if a high local ethnic population).

The peripheral film in anaemias

Morphological abnormalities and variants

Microcytic RBCs	Fe deficiency, thalassaemia trait & syndromes, congenital sideroblastic anaemia, anaemia of chronic disorders.
Macrocytic RBCs	Alcohol/liver disease (round macrocytes), MDS, pregnancy and newborn, compensated haemolysis, B_{12} or folate deficiency, hydroxyurea and antimetabolites (oval macrocytes), acquired sideroblastic anaemia, hypothyroidism, chronic respiratory failure, aplastic anaemia.
Dimorphic RBCs	Fe deficiency responding to iron, mixed Fe and B_{12}/folate deficiency, sideroblastic anaemia, post-transfusion.
Polychromatic RBCs	Response to blood loss or haematinic treatment, haemolysis, marrow infiltration.
Spherocytes	HS, haemolytic disorders eg warm AIHA, delayed transfusion reaction, ABO HDN, DIC and MAHA, post-splenectomy.
Pencil/rod cells	Fe deficiency anaemia, thalassaemia trait & syndromes, PK deficiency.
Elliptocytes	Hereditary elliptocytosis, MPD and MDS.
Fragmented red cells	MAHA, DIC, renal failure, HUS, TTP.
Teardrop RBCs	Myelofibrosis, metastatic marrow infiltration, MDS.
Sickle cells	Sickle cell anaemia, other sickle syndromes (not sickle trait).
Target cells	Liver disease, Fe deficiency, thalassaemia, HbC syndromes.
Crenated red cells	Usually storage or EDTA artifact. Genuine RBC crenation may be seen post-splenectomy and in renal failure.
Burr cells	Renal failure.
Acanthocytes	Hereditary acanthocytosis, a-β-lipoproteinaemia, McLeod red cell phenotype, PK deficiency, chronic liver disease (esp. Zieve's syndrome).
Bite cells	G6PD deficiency, oxidative haemolysis.
Basophilic stippling	Megaloblastic anaemia, lead poisoning, MDS, haemoglobinopathies.
Rouleaux	Chronic inflammation, paraproteinaemia, myeloma.
Increased reticulocytes	Bleeding, haemolysis, marrow infiltration, severe hypoxia, response to haematinic therapy.
Heinz bodies	Not seen in normals (removed by spleen), small numbers seen post-splenectomy, oxidant drugs, G6PD deficiency, sulphonamides, unstable Hb (Hb Zurich, Köln).
Howell-Jolly bodies	Composed of DNA, generally removed by the spleen, dyserythropoietic states eg B_{12} deficiency, MDS, post-splenectomy, hyposplenism.
H bodies	HbH inclusions, denatured HbH (β_4 tetramer), stain with methylene blue, seen in HbH disease ($--/-\alpha$), less prominent in α thalassaemia trait, not present in normal subjects.
Hyposplenic blood film	Howell-Jolly bodies, target cells, occasional nucleated RBCs, lymphocytosis, macrocytosis, acanthocytes.

Red cell disorders

Anaemia in renal disease

Anaemia is consistently found in the presence of chronic renal failure. Severity generally relates to the degree of renal impairment. The dominant mechanism is inadequate production of erythropoietin. Other contributory factors include suppressive effects of uraemia and reduction in RBC survival. Uraemia impairs platelet function leading to blood loss and Fe deficiency. Small amounts of blood are inevitably left in the tubing following dialysis so that blood loss and Fe deficiency are further contributory factors in dialysis patients. Folate is lost in dialysis and supplementation is required to avoid deficiency. Aluminium toxicity (from trace amounts in dialysis fluids) and osteitis fibrosa from hyperparathyroidism are rare contributory factors.

Laboratory features
- Hb typically 5.0–10.0g/dl.
- MCV normal.
- Blood film – mostly normochromic RBCs; schistocytes and acanthocytes present. No specific abnormalities in WBC or platelets.
- Microangiopathic haemolytic changes present in vasculitic collagen disorders with renal failure and classically in HUS & TTP.

Management
- Short term treatment with RBC transfusion, based on *symptoms* (not Hb).
- Correction of Fe and folic acid deficiencies.
- Erythropoietin (Epo) will correct anaemia in almost all patients.
  Start at 50–100units/kg SC ×3/week. Response apparent <10 weeks; reduced doses required as maintenance. Renal Association Guidelines have been produced for application and monitoring of Epo therapy. Although expensive it improves quality of life and avoids transfusion dependency and iron overload.

Side effects of Epo
- Raised BP.
- Thrombotic tendency.

Anaemia in endocrine disease

Anaemia and other haematological effects occur as associated features in disordered endocrine states. The abnormalities will typically correct as the endocrine abnormality is corrected.

Pituitary disorders

Deficiency/hypopituitarism is associated with normochromic, normocytic anaemia; associated leucopenia may also occur. Findings correct as normal function is restored, usually by appropriate replacement therapy.

Thyroid disorders

Hypothyroidism may produce a mild degree of anaemia; MCV is usually raised but may be normal. Corrects on restoration of normal thyroid function. Menorrhagia occurs in hypothyroidism and can result in associated Fe deficiency. B_{12} levels should be checked because of the association with other autoimmune disorders (including pernicious anaemia).

Thyrotoxicosis may be associated with mild degrees of normochromic anaemia in 20% cases which corrects as function is normalised. Erythroid activity is increased but a disproportionate increase in plasma volume means either no change in Hb concentration or mild anaemia. Haematinic deficiencies occur and need to be excluded.

Adrenal disorders

Hypoadrenalism results in normochromic, normocytic anaemia; the plasma volume is also reduced which masks the true degree of associated anaemia. The abnormalities are corrected by replacement mineralocorticoids.

Hyperadrenalism (Cushing's) results in erythrocytosis with a typical net increase in Hb (by 1–2g/dl). Occurs whether Cushing's is primary or iatrogenic. Mechanism is unclear.

Parathyroid disorders – hyperparathyroidism may be associated with anaemia from impairment of erythropoietin production, or in some cases from secondary marrow sclerosis.

Sex hormones – androgens stimulate erythropoiesis and are occasionally used to stimulate red cell production in aplastic anaemia. The influence of androgens explains the higher levels on Hb in adult males than females.

Diabetes mellitus when poorly controlled may be associated with anaemia; however the majority of haematological abnormalities in diabetes mellitus result from secondary disease related complications, eg renal failure.

Anaemia in joint disease

Rheumatoid arthritis, psoriatic arthropathy and osteoarthritis may be complicated by anaemia which requires systematic evaluation. Various factors may contribute to anaemia, commonly more than one is present, especially in rheumatoid arthritis. Some of the mechanisms that give rise to anaemia in rheumatoid also apply in other connective tissue disease, eg SLE, polyarteritis nodosa, etc.

Anaemia of chronic disorders (ACD)

The clinical problem is to being able to recognise the presence of other contributory factors in pathogenesis of the anaemia. There is impaired marrow utilisation of iron and a lower than expected rise in erythropoietin suggesting some inhibition in its pathway. Marrow also appears less responsive to erythropoietin. Elevated levels of IL-1 have been identified. Detailed studies suggest a synergistic effect of IL-1 with T-cells to produce γ-interferon which can suppress erythroid activity. May also be elevated levels of TNF which has an inhibitory effect on erythropoiesis mediated by the release of β-interferon from marrow stromal cells.

Typical features of ACD

- Hb range 7.0–11.0 g/dl.
- MCV is usually ↔ or moderately ↓ (occasionally indices may be identical to those found in iron deficiency).
- Ferritin usually ↔ but may be ↑.
- Serum iron ↔ or ↓; TIBC ↔ or ↓.
- Serum transferrin receptor levels normal.
- Bone marrow Fe stores plentiful.

Management

Supportive transfusion in symptomatic patients; coexistent Fe deficiency should be excluded and treated. Minority may be suitable for/responsive to erythropoietin therapy.

Bleeding/Fe deficiency

Usually secondary to use of NSAIDs – consider/exclude other causes of blood loss which may occur in this patient group.

Additional mechanisms in rheumatoid disease include

Autoimmune phenomena	Warm antibody AIHA in association with rheumatoid and other collagen disorders; film will show reticulocytosis and +ve DAT
	Red cell aplasia
Drug related problems	Chronic blood loss (caused by medication) – *see above*
	Drug side effects eg macrocytosis from antimetabolite immunosuppressives, eg azathioprine and methotrexate, oxidative haemolysis secondary to dapsone or sulphasalazine (occurs in normal individuals as well as those with G6PD deficiency)
	Anaemia secondary to gold therapy for rheumatoid arthritis
	Idiosyncratic reactions – unexplained/unforeseeable reactions such as marrow aplasia
	Rare autoimmune haemolysis due to mefenamic acid, diclofenac or ibuprofen
2° to other organ problems	Hypersplenism, Felty's syndrome in rheumatoid, renal failure in SLE or polyarteritis

Anaemia in gastrointestinal disease

Anaemia occurs in GIT disorders through mechanisms of blood loss, chronic disorder anaemia, specific disease related complications or drug side effects/idiosyncrasy occurring singly or in various combinations.

Blood loss

Acute	Immediately following acute haemorrhage – RBC indices usually normal Normochromic anaemia
Acute on chronic	RBC indices show low normal or marginally ↓, especially MCV Drop in Hb is > expected for fall in Hb Film shows mixture of normochromic & hypochromic RBCs ('dimorphic')
Chronic	RBC indices show established chronic Fe deficiency features ↓ MCV, MCH, platelets often↑

Anaemia in GIT disorders can be simply considered against some of the commoner problems arising through the GIT:

Oesophageal – bleeding from peptic oesophagitis, association of oesophageal web and chronic Fe deficiency.

Gastric – pernicious anaemia and B_{12} deficiency, late effects of partial/total gastrectomy producing B_{12} and/or Fe deficiency. Microangiopathic haemolytic anaemia from metastatic adenocarcinoma.

Small bowel malabsorption states, eg Fe and/or folate deficiency 2° to coeliac disease, malabsorption from other problems including inflammatory bowel disease; hyposplenism secondary to coeliac with or without ↑ platelets.

Large bowel – blood loss anaemia from inflammatory bowel disorders, *note*: these may also be associated with chronic disorder anaemia. Rare occurrence of autoimmune haemolysis associated with ulcerative colitis.

Pancreas – chronic disorder anaemia associated with carcinoma or chronic pancreatitis, DIC associated with acute pancreatitis.

Liver – see p52.

Drug related anaemia arises through

- Upper GIT irritation causing blood loss – aspirin, NSAIDs, corticosteroids.
- Bleeding due to specific drugs eg warfarin and heparin.
- Drug induced haemolysis, eg oxidative (Heinz body) haemolysis due to sulphasalazine or dapsone.
- Production impairment, eg aplasia secondary to mesalazine.

Anaemia in liver disease

Anaemia is common in chronic liver disorders. May be more than one cause for anaemia but mechanisms include:

- Chronic disorder/secondary anaemia – part of marrow response to chronic inflammatory processes.
- Macrocytosis ± anaemia: specific effects on membrane lipids cause ↑ in MCV.
- Alcohol – direct toxic effect on erythropoiesis with ↑ MCV.
- Folate deficiency: seen in alcoholic liver disease → nutritional deficiency and/or direct effect of alcohol on folate metabolism.
- Blood loss from oesophageal varices → acute or chronic anaemia.
- Hypersplenism – portal hypertension can produce marked splenic enlargement leading to hypersplenism.
- Haemolytic anaemias eg
  - autoimmune in association with chronic active hepatitis
  - Zieve's syndrome (hypertriglyceridaemia + self-limiting haemolysis due to acute alcohol excess)
  - viral hepatitis may provoke oxidative haemolysis in those with G6PD deficiency
  - acute liver failure – DIC and MAHA may occur
  - acanthocytosis: acute haemolytic anaemia with acanthocytosis (spur cell anaemia). rare. Usually late stage liver disease, with poor prognosis.

Iron deficiency anaemia

Microcytic anaemia is common and commonest cause is chronic iron deficiency.

Iron physiology & metabolism

Normal (western) diet provides $\cong 15$mg of iron/d, of which 5–10% is absorbed in duodenum and upper jejunum. Ferrous (Fe^{2+}) iron is better absorbed than ferric (Fe^{3+}) iron. Total body iron store $\cong$ 4g. Around 1mg of iron/d lost in urine, faeces, sweat and cells shed from the skin and GIT. Iron deficiency is commoner in $\female$ of reproductive age since menstrual losses account for ~20mg Fe/month and in pregnancy an additional 500–1000mg Fe may be lost.

Causes of iron deficiency

Reproductive system	Menorrhagia.
GI tract	Oesophagitis, oesophageal varices, hiatus hernia (ulcerated), peptic ulcer, inflammatory bowel disease, haemorrhoids, carcinoma: stomach, colorectal, (rarely angiodysplasia, hereditary haemorrhagic telangiectasia).
Malabsorption	Coeliac disease, atrophic gastritis (*note:* may also result *from* Fe deficiency), gastrectomy.
Physiological	Growth spurts, pregnancy.
Dietary	Vegans, elderly.
Genito-urinary system	Haematuria (uncommon cause).
Others	PNH, frequent venesection.
Worldwide	Commonest cause is Hookworm infestation.

Assessment

Clinical history review possible sources of blood loss, especially GIT loss.

Menstrual loss quantitation may be difficult; ask about number of tampons used per day, how often these require changing, and duration.

Other sources of blood loss eg haematuria and haemoptysis should be apparent on initial assessment but should be reassessed. Ask patient if he/she has been a blood donor – regular blood donation over many years may cause chronic iron store depletion.

Drug therapy eg NSAIDs and corticosteroids may cause GI irritation and blood loss.

Past medical history eg previous gastric surgery ($\rightarrow$ malabsorption). Ask about previous episodes of anaemia and treatments with iron.

In patients with iron deficiency assume underlying cause is blood loss until proved otherwise. In developed countries pure dietary iron lack causing iron deficiency is almost unknown.

Examination

- General examination including assessment of mucous membranes (eg hereditary haemorrhagic telangiectasia).
- Seek possible sources of blood loss.
- Abdominal examination, rectal examination and sigmoidoscopy mandatory.
- Gynaecological examination also required.

Laboratory tests

- Hb $\downarrow$.
- $\downarrow$ MCV (<76fl) and $\downarrow$ MCHC (*note:* $\downarrow$ MCV in thalassaemia and ACD).

- Red cell distribution width (RDW): ↑ in iron deficiency states with a greater frequency than in ACD or thalassaemia trait.
- Ferritin ± measurement of iron/TIBC.
  Ferritin assay preferred – a low serum ferritin identifies the presence of iron deficiency but as an acute phase protein it can be ↑, masking iron deficiency. ↓ iron and ↑ TIBC indicates iron deficiency.
- Examination of BM aspirate (iron stain) is occasionally useful.
- Theoretically FOB testing may be of value in iron deficiency but results can be misleading. False +ve results seen in high dietary meat intake.

Treatment of iron deficiency

Simplest, safest and cheapest treatment is oral ferrous salts, eg $FeSO_4$ (Fe gluconate and fumarate equally acceptable). Provide an oral dose of elemental iron of 150–200mg/d. Side effects in 10–20% patients (eg abdominal distension, constipation and/or diarrhoea) – try ↓ the daily dose to bd or od. Liquid iron occasionally necessary, eg children or adults with swallowing difficulties. Increasing dietary iron intake has no routine place in the management of iron deficiency except where intake is grossly deficient.

Response to replacement

A rise of Hb of 2.0g/dl over 3 weeks is expected. MCV will ↑ concomitantly with Hb. Reticulocytes may ↑ in response to iron therapy but is not a reliable indicator of response.

Duration of treatment

Generally ~6 months. After Hb and MCV are normal continue iron for at least 3 months to replenish iron stores.

Failure of response

- Is the diagnosis of iron deficiency correct?
  – *consider chronic disorder anaemia or thalassaemia trait*
- Is there an additional complicating illness?
  – *chronic infection, collagen disorder or neoplasm*
- Is the patient complying with prescribed medication?
- Is the preparation of iron adequate in dosage and/or formulation?
- Is the patient continuing to bleed excessively?
- Is there possible malabsorption?
- Are other concomitant haematinic deficiencies (eg B_{12} or folate) present?
- Reassess patient: ?evidence of continued blood loss or malabsorption.

Parenteral iron

Occasionally of value in genuine iron intolerance, if compliance is a problem, or if need to replenish stores rapidly eg in pregnancy or prior to major surgery. *Note:* Hb will rise no faster than with oral iron.

Intravenous iron Iron may be administered IV as iron hydroxide sucrose complex.

Intramuscular iron eg iron sorbitol citrate. Usually ~10–20 IM injections over several week period *(note:* injections painful and lead to long-term skin discoloration at the injection site).

Vitamin B$_{12}$ deficiency

B$_{12}$ deficiency presents with macrocytic, megaloblastic anaemia ranging from mild to severe (Hb <6.0g/dl). Symptoms are those of chronic anaemia, ie fatigue, dyspnoea on effort, etc. Neurological symptoms may also be present – classically peripheral paraesthesiae and disturbances of position and vibration sense. Occasionally neurological symptoms occur with no/minimal haematological upset. If uncorrected, the patient may develop subacute combined degeneration of the spinal cord → permanently ataxic.

Pathophysiology

B$_{12}$ (along with folic acid) is required for DNA synthesis; B$_{12}$ is also required for neurological functioning. B$_{12}$ is absorbed in terminal ileum after binding to Intrinsic Factor produced by gastric parietal cells. Body stores of B$_{12}$ are 2–3mg (sufficient for 3 years). B$_{12}$ is found in meats, fish, eggs and dairy produce. Strictly vegetarian (vegan) diets are low in B$_{12}$ although not all vegans develop clinical evidence of deficiency.

Presenting haematological abnormalities

- Macrocytic anaemia (MCV usually >110fl). In extreme cases RBC anisopoikilocytosis can result in MCV values lying just within normal range.
- RBC changes include oval macrocytosis, poikilocytosis, basophilic stippling, Howell-Jolly bodies, circulating megaloblasts.
- Hypersegmentation of neutrophils.
- Leucopenia and thrombocytopenia common.
- Bone marrow shows megaloblastic change; marked erythroid hyperplasia with predominance of early erythroid precursors, open atypical nuclear chromatin patterns, mitotic figures and 'giant' metamyelocytes.
- Iron stores usually increased.
- Serum B$_{12}$ ↓.
- Serum/red cell folate usually ↔ or ↑.
- LDH levels markedly ↑ reflecting ineffective erythropoiesis.
- Autoantibody screen in pernicious anaemia: 80–90% show circulating gastric parietal cell antibodies, 55% have circulating intrinsic factor antibodies.

Causes of B$_{12}$ deficiency

Pernicious anaemia	Commonest, due to autoimmune gastric atrophy resulting in loss of intrinsic factor production required for absorption of B$_{12}$. Incidence increases >40 years and often associated with other autoimmune problems, eg hypothyroidism.
Following total gastrectomy	May develop after major partial gastrectomy.
Ileal disease	Resection of ileum, Crohn's disease.
Blind loop syndromes	Eg diverticulae or localised inflammatory bowel changes allowing bacterial overgrowth which then competes for available B$_{12}$.
Fish tapeworm	Diphyllobothrium latum.
Other malabsorptive problems	Tropical sprue, coeliac disease.
Dietary deficiency	Eg vegans.

Management of B_{12} deficiency

1. Identification and correction of cause if possible.
2. Above investigations are undertaken and a test of B_{12} absorption is carried out (eg Schilling Test). Urinary excretion of a test dose of B_{12} labelled with trace amounts of radioactive cobalt is compared with excretion of B_{12} bound to Intrinsic Factor; the test is done in two parts. B_{12} malabsorption corrected by Intrinsic Factor is diagnostic of pernicious anaemia (in absence of previous gastric surgery).
3. Management – hydroxycobalamin 1mg IM and folic acid PO should be given immediately.
4. Supportive measures – bed rest, O_2 and diuretics may be needed while awaiting response. Transfusion is best avoided but 2 units of concentrated RBCs may be used for patients *severely* compromised by anaemia (risk of precipitating cardiac failure); *hypokalaemia* is occasionally observed during the immediate response to B_{12} and serum [K^+] should be monitored.
5. Response apparent in 3–5d with reticulocyte response of >10%; normoblastic conversion of marrow erythropoiesis in 12–24 hours. Patients frequently describe a subjective improvement within 24 hours.
6. B_{12} replacement therapy – initially hydroxocobalamin 5 × 1mg IM should be given during the first 2 weeks, thereafter maintenance injections are needed 3-monthly.
7. Long term follow-up depends on the primary cause. Pernicious anaemia patients require lifelong treatment and should be checked annually with a full blood count and thyroid function; the incidence of gastric cancer is twice as high in these patients compared to the normal population.
8. Broad spectrum antibiotics should be given to suppress bacterial overgrowth in blind loop syndrome ± local surgery if appropriate. Long term IM B_{12} may be the pragmatic solution if blind loop cannot be corrected.

Toh B-T, Van Driel IR, Gleeson PA 1997 NEJM **337** 1441

Folate deficiency

Folate deficiency represents the other main deficiency cause of megaloblastic anaemia; haematological features indistinguishable from those of B_{12} deficiency. Distinction is on basis of demonstration of reduced red cell and serum folate.

▶▶ Megaloblastic anaemia patients should *never* receive empirical treatment with folic acid alone. **If they lack B_{12}, folic acid is capable of precipitating subacute combined degeneration of the cord**.

Pathophysiology

Adult body folate stores comprise 10–15mg; normal daily requirements are 0.1–0.2mg, ie sufficient for 3–4 months. Folate absorption from dietary sources is rapid; proximal jejunum is main site of absorption. Main dietary sources of folate are liver, green vegetables, nuts and yeast. Western diets contain ~0.5–0.7mg folate/d but availability may be lessened as folate is readily destroyed by cooking, especially in large volumes of water. Folate coenzymes are an essential part of DNA synthesis, hence the occurrence of megaloblastic change in deficiency.

Diagnosis

Haematology identical to B_{12} deficiency – macrocytic, megaloblastic anaemia. Other findings also similar to B_{12} except parietal cell and intrinsic factor auto-antibodies usually –ve. Reduced folate levels – *serum* folate levels reflect recent intake, *red cell folate* levels give a more reliable indication of folate status.

Causes of folate deficiency

Decreased intake	Poor nutrition, eg in poverty or old age, 'skid row' alcoholics.
↑ requirements/losses	Pregnancy, ↑ cell turnover, eg haemolysis, exfoliative dermatitis, renal dialysis.
Malabsorption	Coeliac disease, tropical sprue, Crohn's and other malabsorptive states.
Drugs	Phenytoin, barbiturates, valproate, oral contraceptives, nitrofurantoin. May induce folate malabsorption.
Antifolate drugs	Methotrexate, trimethoprim, pentamidine. *Antagonise* folate *cf.* induce deficiency.
Alcohol	Poor nutrition *plus* a direct depressant effect on folate levels which can precipitate clinical folate deficiency.

Management

1. Treatment & support of severe anaemia as for B_{12} deficiency.
2. Folic acid 5mg/d PO (never on its own – see above), unless patient known to have fully normal B_{12} level.
3. Treatment/correction of underlying cause, eg in coeliac disease folate levels and absorption normalize once patient established on gluten-free diet. Long term supplementation advised in chronic haemolysis eg HbSS or HS.

Prophylactic folate supplements recommended in pregnancy and other states of increased demand eg prematurity.

Other causes of megaloblastic anaemia

Megaloblastic anaemia not due to actual deficiency of either B_{12} or folate is uncommon, but may occur in the following situations.

Congenital

- Transcobalamin II deficiency – absence of the key B_{12} transport protein results in severe megaloblastic anaemia (will correct with parenteral B_{12}).
- Congenital intrinsic factor deficiency – autosomal recessive, results in failure to produce intrinsic factor. Presents as megaloblastic anaemia up to age of 2 years and responds clinically to parenteral B_{12}.
- Inborn errors of metabolism – errors in folate pathways, also occurs in orotic aciduria and Lesch-Nyan syndrome.
- Megaloblastosis commonly present in the congenital dyserythropoietic anaemias (see p366).

Acquired

- MDS – often present in sideroblastic anaemia (RARS).
- Acute leukaemia – megaloblastic-like erythroid dysplasia in AML M6.
- Drug induced – secondary to antimetabolite drugs including 6-mercaptopurine, cytosine arabinoside, zidovudine and hydroxyurea.
- Anaesthetic agents – transient megaloblastic change after nitrous oxide.
- Alcohol excess – may result in megaloblastic change in absence of measurable folate deficiency.
- Vitamin C deficiency – occasionally results in megaloblastic change.

Red cell disorders

Anaemia in other deficiency states

Iron, folate or vitamin B_{12} deficiencies account for the majority of clinically significant deficiency syndromes resulting in anaemia. Anaemia is recognised as a complication in other vitamin deficiencies and in malnutrition.

Vitamin A deficiency
Produces chronic disorder like iron deficiency anaemia with ↓ MCV & MCH.

Vitamin B_6 (pyridoxine) deficiency
Can produce hypochromic microcytic anaemia; sideroblastic change may occur. Pyridoxine is given to patients on antituberculous therapy with Isoniazid which is known to interfere with vitamin B_6 metabolism and cause sideroblastic anaemia.

Vitamin C deficiency
Occasionally associated with macrocytic anaemia (± megaloblastic change in 10%); since the main cause of vitamin C deficiency is inadequate diet or nutrition there may be evidence of other deficiencies.

Vitamin E deficiency
Occasionally seen in the neonatal period in low birth weight infants – results in haemolytic anaemia with abnormal RBC morphology.

Starvation
Normochromic anaemia ± leucopenia occurs in anorexia nervosa; features are not associated with any specific deficiency; bone marrow is typically hypocellular.

Haemolytic syndromes

Definition
Any situation in which there is a reduction in red cell life-span due to increased destruction. Failure of compensatory marrow response results in anaemia. Predominant site of RBC destruction is red pulp of the spleen.

Classification – 3 major types
1. Hereditary *vs.* Acquired
2. Immune *vs.* Non-immune
3. Extravascular *vs.* Intravascular

Hereditary cause suggested if history of anaemia refractory to treatment in infancy ± FH eg other affected members, anaemia, gallstones, jaundice, splenectomy. *Acquired* haemolytic anaemia is suggested by sudden onset of symptoms or signs in adulthood. *Intravascular* haemolysis – takes place in peripheral circulation *cf.* *extravascular* haemolysis which occurs in RES.

Hereditary
- Red cell membrane disorders eg HS and hereditary elliptocytosis.
- Red cell enzymopathies eg G6PD and PK deficiencies.
- Abnormal Hb eg thalassaemias and sickle cell disease, unstable Hbs.

Acquired – *immune*

Alloimmune
- HDN
- RBC transfusion incompatibility

Autoimmune
- Warm AIHA – 1° or 2° to SLE, CLL, drugs
- Cold – Mycoplasma or EBV infection,
- Cold haemagglutinin disease (CHAD)
- Lymphoproliferative disorders
- Paroxysmal cold haemoglobinuria (PCH)

Acquired – *non-immune*
- MAHA
- TTP/HUS
- Hypersplenism
- Prosthetic heart valves
- March haemoglobinuria
- Sepsis
- Malaria
- Paroxysmal nocturnal haemoglobinuria

Clinical features
Symptoms of anaemia eg breathlessness, fatigue. Urinary changes eg red or dark brown of haemoglobinuria. Symptoms of underlying disorder.

Confirm haemolysis is occurring
- Check FBC.
- Peripheral blood film – polychromasia, spherocytosis, fragmentation (schistocytes), helmet cells, echinocytes.
- ↑ reticulocytes.
- ↑ serum bilirubin (unconjugated).
- ↑ LDH.
- Low/absent serum haptoglobin (bind free Hb).
- Schumm's test (for intravascular haemolysis).
- Urinary haemosiderin (implies chronic intravascular haemolysis eg PNH).

Red cell disorders

Discriminant diagnostic features

Establish whether immune or non-immune – check DAT

?Immune if DAT +ve check IgG and C_3 specific reagents – suggest warm and cold antibody respectively. Screen serum for red cell alloantibodies.

?Cold antibody present – examine blood film for agglutination, check MCV on initial FBC sample and again after incubation at 37°C for 2h. High MCV at room temperature due to agglutinates falls to normal at 37°C. Check anti-I and anti-i titres for confirmation. Check *Mycoplasma* IgM and EBV serology, and for presence of Donath Landsteiner antibody (cold reacting IgG antibody with anti-P specificity).

?Warm antibody present – IgG +ve DAT only suggestive – examine film for spherocytes (usually prominent), lymphocytosis or abnormal lymphs to suggest LPD. Examine patient for nodes.

?Intravascular haemolysis – check for urinary haemosiderin, Schumm's test.

?Sepsis – check blood cultures.

?Malaria – examine thick and thin blood films for parasites.

?Renal/liver abnormality – examine for hepatomegaly, splenomegaly, LFTs and U & Es.

?Low platelets – consider TTP/HUS.

?Haemoglobinopathy – check Hb electrophoresis.

?Red cell membrane abnormality – check family history and perform red cell fragility test.

?Red cell enzyme disorder – check family history and do G6PD and PK assay.

?PNH – check Ham's test, immunophenotyping (CD55 + CD59).

Treatment

Treat underlying disorder. Give folic acid and iron supplements if low.

Genetic control of haemoglobin production

Hb comprises 4 protein subunits (eg adult Hb = $2 \times \alpha + 2 \times \beta$ chains, $\alpha_2\beta_2$) each linked to a haem group. Production of different globin chains varies from embryo → adult to meet the particular environment at each stage. Globin genes are located on chromosomes 11 and 16. All globins related to α globin are located on chromosome 16; all those related to β globin are on chromosome 11. The sequence in which they are produced during development reflects their physical order on chromosomes such that ζ is the first α-like globin to be produced in life. After ζ expression stops, α production occurs ($\zeta \to \alpha$ switch). On chromosome 11 the arrangement of β-like globin genes follows the order (from left to right) $\epsilon \to \gamma \to \delta \to \beta$ mirroring the β-like globin chains produced during development. As embryo develops into fetus, ζ production stops and α is produced. The α globin combines with γ chains and produces $\alpha_2\gamma_2$ (fetal Hb or HbF). After birth γ production ↓ and δ and β chains are produced. Adults have predominantly HbA ($\alpha_2\beta_2$) although small amounts of HbA$_2$ ($\alpha_2\delta_2$) and HbF are produced.

Hb switching is physiological but mechanism unclear. HbF ($\alpha_2\gamma_2$) binds oxygen more tightly than adult haemoglobin, ensuring adequate oxygen delivery to the fetus which must extract its oxygen from mother's circulation. After birth the lungs expand and the oxygen is derived from the air, with β production replacing that of γ, leading to an increase in adult haemoglobin ($\alpha_2\beta_2$).

Haemoglobin	Globin chains	Amount
Embryo		
Hb Gower 1	$\zeta_2\epsilon_2$	42%*
Hb Gower 2	$\alpha_2\epsilon_2$	24%*
Hb Portland	$\zeta_2\gamma_2$	
*by 5th week		
Fetus		
HbF	$\alpha_2\gamma_2$	85%
HbA	$\alpha_2\beta_2$	5–10%
Adult		
HbA	$\alpha_2\beta_2$	97%
HbA$_2$	$\alpha_2\delta_2$	2.5%
HbF	$\alpha_2\gamma_2$	0.5%

Haemoglobin abnormalities

Fall into 2 major groups: *structural abnormalities* of Hb due to alterations in DNA coding for the globin protein leading to an abnormal amino acid in the globin molecule, eg sickle haemoglobin (β^S). Second group of Hb disorders results from imbalanced globin chain production–globins produced are structurally normal but their relative amounts are incorrect and lead to *the thalassaemias*.

Haemoglobinopathies result in significant morbidity and mortality on a worldwide scale. Patients with these disorders are also seen in Northern Europe and the UK, especially in areas with significant Greek, Italian, Afro-Caribbean and Asian populations.

Sickling disorders

Sickle cell anaemia (homozygous SS, $\beta^S\beta^S$), HbSC ($\beta^S\beta^C$), HbS/β^+ or $\beta°$ thalassaemia, and HbSD ($\beta^S\beta^D$) all produce significant symptoms but homozygous sickle cell anaemia is generally the most severe. The gene has remained at high frequency due to conferred resistance to malaria in heterozygotes. Inheritance is autosomal recessive.

Sickle cell anaemia (SCA HbSS)

Pathogenesis

Widespread throughout Africa, Middle East, parts of India and Mediterranean. Single base change in β globin gene, amino acid 6 (glu→val). In UK Afro-Caribbean population gene is found in ~1:10. RBCs containing HbS deform (elongate) under conditions of reduced oxygenation, and form characteristic sickle cells – do not flow well through small vessels, and are more adherent than normal to vascular endothelium, leading to vascular occlusion and sickle cell crises. Patients with SCA are the offspring of parents both of whom are carriers of the β^s gene, ie, they both have sickle cell trait, and homozygotes for the abnormal β^s gene demonstrate features of chronic red cell haemolysis and tissue infarction.

Clinical features

Highly variable. Many have few symptoms whilst others have severe and frequent crises, marked haemolytic anaemia and chronic organ damage. HbF level plays role in ameliorating symptoms. History may reveal a positive family history or past history of crises.

- **Infancy** – newborns have higher HbF level than normal adult, protected during first 8–20 weeks of life. Symptoms start when HbF level falls. SCA often diagnosed <1 year.
- **Infection** – high morbidity and mortality due to bacterial and viral infection. Pneumococcal septicaemia (*Streptococcus pneumoniae*) well-recognised. Other infecting organisms: meningococcus (*Neisseria meningitidis*), *Escherichia coli* and *Haemophilus influenzae* (hyposplenic).
- **Anaemia** – children and adults often severely anaemic (Hb ~6.0–9.0 g/dl). Anaemia is chronic and patients generally well-adapted until episode of decompensation (eg severe infection) occurs.

Sickle crises

- **Vaso-occlusive** – dactylitis, chest syndrome & girdle syndrome. Patients complain of severe bone, joint and abdominal pain. Bone pain affects long bones and spine, and is due to occlusion of small vessels. *Triggers:* infection, dehydration, alcohol, menstruation, cold and temperature changes – often no cause found.
- **Dactylitis** – mainly children. Metacarpals, metatarsals, backs of hands and feet swollen and tender (small vessel occlusion and infarction). Recurrent, can result in permanent radiological abnormalities in bones of the hands and feet (rare).
- **Acute chest syndrome** – common cause of death. Chest wall pain, sometimes with pleurisy, fever and SOB. Resembles infection, infarction or embolism. Requires prompt and vigorous treatment. Transfer to ITU if pO2 cannot be kept >70 mmHg on air. 10% mortality. Treat infection vigorously, often due to *S. pneumoniae, H. influenzae, Mycoplasma, Legionella.*
- **Aplastic crises** – sudden ↓ in marrow production (esp. red cells). Parvovirus B19 infection is cause (invades developing RBCs). Mostly

self-limiting and after 1–2 weeks the marrow begins to function normally. Top-up transfusion may be needed.

- *Haemolytic crises* – uncommon; markedly reduced red cell lifespan. May be drug-induced, 2° to infection (eg malaria) or associated G6PD deficiency.

- *Sequestration crises* – mainly children (30%). Pooling of large volumes of blood in spleen and/or liver. Severe hypotension and profound anaemia may result in death.

- **Other problems**
  – *Growth retardation* common in children, but adult may have normal height (weight tends to be lower than normal). Sexual maturation delayed.
  – *Locomotor* Avascular necrosis of the head of the femur or humerus, arthritis and osteomyelitis (*Salmonella* infection). Chronic leg ulceration is complication of many haemoglobinopathies including sickle cell anaemia. Ischaemia is main cause.
  – *Genitourinary* Renal papillary necrosis → haematuria and renal tubular defects. Inability to concentrate urine. Priapism in ~60% males. Less common if HbF↑. Frequent UTIs in women, CRF in adults.
  – *Spleen* Severe pain (infarction of splenic vessels). Spleen may enlarge in early life but after repeated infarcts diminishes in size (→ hyposplenism by 9–12 months of age). Splenic function is impaired.
  – *Gastrointestinal* Gallstones common (2° to chronic haemolysis). Derangement of LFTs (multifactorial).
  – *CVS* Murmurs (anaemia), tachycardia.
  – *Eye* Proliferative retinopathy (in 30%), blindness (esp. HbSC), retinal artery occlusion, retinal detachment.
  – *CNS* Convulsions, TIAs or strokes, sensory hearing loss (usually temporary).
  – *Psychosocial* Depression, socially withdrawn.

Laboratory features
Anaemia usual (Hb~6.0–9.0 g/dl in HbSS although may be much lower; HbSC have higher Hb). Reticulocytes may be ↑ (to ~10–20%) reflecting intense bone marrow production of RBCs. Anaemic symptoms usually mild since HbS has reduced O_2 affinity. MCV and MCH are normal, unless also thalassaemia trait (25% cases). Blood film shows marked variation in red cell size with prominent sickle cells and target cells; basophilic stippling, Howell-Jolly bodies and Pappenheimer bodies (hyposplenic features after infancy). Sickle cell test (eg sodium dithionate) will be positive. Does *not* discriminate between sickle cell *trait* and *homozygous disease*. Serum bilirubin often ↑ (due to excess red cell breakdown).

Confirmatory tests
Haemoglobin electrophoresis shows 80–99% HbS with no normal HbA. HbF may be elevated to about 15%. Parents will have features of sickle cell trait.

Screening
In at-risk groups pregnant woman should be screened early in pregnancy. If both parents of fetus are carriers offer prenatal/neonatal diagnosis. Affected babies should be given penicillin daily and be immunised against *Strep pneumoniae, Haemophilus influenzae* type b, and *Neisseria meningitidis*.

Prenatal diagnosis

May be carried out from first trimester (chorionic villus sampling from 10 weeks gestation) or second trimester (fetal blood sampling from umbilical cord or trophoblast DNA from amniotic fluid). DNA may be analysed using restriction enzyme digestion with Mst II and Southern blotting, RFLP analysis assessing both parental and fetal DNA haplotypes, oligonucleotide probes specific for sickle globin point mutation, or PCR amplification followed by restriction enzyme digestion of amplified DNA. ARMS (amplification refractory mutation system) PCR is useful in ambiguous cases. In late pregnancy fetal blood sampling may be used to confirm diagnosis.

Management

General

Lifelong prophylactic penicillin 250 mg bd PO with folate replacement. Pneumovax II vaccination advisable.

Management during pregnancy & anaesthesia

Anaesthesia should be carried out by experienced anaesthetist who is aware of complications of SCA. If the patient is unwell consider transfusion to Hb of 10 g/dl, but generally transfusion not necessary.

Management of crises

▶▶ See *Haematological Emergencies: Sickle Crisis* p440.

Red cell disorders

HbS – new therapies

Agents that elevate HbF levels

Recognised for some time that ↑ HbF levels ameliorate β thalassaemia and sickle cell disease. HbF reduces HbS polymerisation and hence sickling. HbF level of >10% reduces episodes of aseptic necrosis; levels >20% HbF are associated with fewer painful crises.

Hydroxyurea – several studies have shown that baboons treated with cytosine arabinoside showed ↑ HbF. Similar results obtained with hydroxyurea which has advantages over other cytotoxics eg, low risk of secondary malignancy with prolonged use. Hydroxyurea evaluated in a large number of clinical trials. Effects are dose-dependent and the highest elevation of HbF is seen at myelosuppressive doses.

Erythropoietin – leads to ↑ HbF but not widely used in the management of haemoglobinopathies. Evidence suggests that rHuEPO provides an additive effect when alternated with hydroxyurea. Dose required is high (1000–3000 iu/kg × 3d/week) with co-administration of Fe supplements.

5-azacytidine – inhibitor of methyltransferase, enzyme responsible for methylation of newly incorporated cytosines in DNA. Preventing methylation of the γ globin gene leads to ↑ HbF. ▶▶ Risk of developing 2° malignancy.

Short chain fatty acids – butyrate analogues are potent inducers of haemopoietic differentiation. Elevated concentrations of butyrate and other fatty acids in diabetic mothers is responsible for the persistently elevated HbF in the neonates born to such mothers. Initial studies involving the use of butyrate to increase HbF levels in patients with sickle cell anaemia appeared promising but subsequent studies have been disappointing.

Bone marrow transplantation – sibling donor transplants for sickle cell disease have been carried out in a number of centres. Since the mortality from sickle cell disease has dropped over recent years from 15% →1%, and with the advent of hydroxyurea therapy, there is a less compelling argument for BMT in sickle cell disease.

Gene therapy – potentially curative but experimental. Globin gene transfer has been attempted with variable results. Expression of exogenous gene has been at levels too low to be of benefit.

Sickle cell trait (HbAS)

Asymptomatic carriers have one abnormal β^s gene and one normal β gene (with 30 million carriers worldwide).

Clinical features

- Carriers are not anaemic and have no abnormal clinical features.
- Sickling rare unless O_2 saturation falls <40%. Crises have been reported with severe hypoxia (anaesthesia, unpressurised aircraft).
- Occasional renal papillary necrosis, haematuria and inability to concentrate the urine in adults.

Laboratory features

- Hb, MCV, MCH & MCHC normal (unless also α thalassaemia trait).
- HbS level 40–55% (if <40% then also α thalassaemia trait).
- Film may be normal or show microcytes and target cells.
- Sickle cell test will be +ve (HbSS and HbAS).

Carrier detection

Neither FBC nor film can be used for diagnostic purposes. Detection of the carrier state relies on haemoglobin electrophoresis (HbA ~50%; HbS ~50%).

▶ Care needed during anaesthesia (*avoid hypoxia*).

Other sickling disorders

HbSC

Milder than sickle cell anaemia but resembles it. Patients have fewer and milder crises. Retinal damage (microvascular, proliferative retinopathy) and blindness are major complications (30–35%). Arrange regular ophthalmological review by specialist. Aseptic necrosis of femoral head and recurrent haematuria are common. Increased risk of splenic infarcts and abscesses.

▶ Beware thrombosis and PE especially in pregnancy.

Clinical

Mild anaemia (Hb 8–14 g/dl) and splenomegaly common. Less haemolysis, fewer painful crises, fewer infections and less vaso-occlusive disease than SCA. Growth and development normal. Lifespan normal.

▶ *Pregnancy may be hazardous.*

Film

Prominent target cells with fewer NRBC than seen in SCA. Howell-Jolly and Pappenheimer bodies (hyposplenism). Occasional C crystals may be seen.

Diagnosis

Hb electrophoresis and family studies. MCV and MCH are much lower than in HbSS.

HbSD, HbSO$_{Arab}$

Milder than HbSS. Both rare. Interactions of these globins with HbS results in reduced polymerisation. HbD$_{Punjab}$ $^{(\beta 121\ glu \rightarrow\ gln)}$ and HbO$_{Arab}$ $^{(\beta 121\ glu \rightarrow\ lys)}$ cause little disease on their own although there may be mild haemolysis in the homozygote. These haemoglobins cause sickle cell disease when present with HbS.

HbSα thalassaemia

Common in Blacks. Lessens severity of SCA by reducing the concentration of Hb in red cells.

HbSβ thalassaemia

Caused by inheritance of β^S from one parent and β thalassaemia from the other. Sickle/β° thalassaemia is severe since no normal β globin chains are produced. Sickle/β⁺ thalassaemia is much milder having β globin in 5–15% of their Hb. Microcytosis and splenomegaly are characteristic. Family screening will confirm microcytosis and ↑ HbA$_2$ in one of the parents.

Management

Essentially as for HbSS with prompt treatment of crises (*see above*).

Other haemoglobinopathies

HbC disease ($\beta^{6\ glu \rightarrow lys}$)

West Africa. Patients have benign compensated haemolysis. Development is normal, splenomegaly is common. Gallstones are recognised complication. The Hb may be mildly ↓. MCV and MCH are ↓ and reticulocytes are ↑. Blood film shows prominent target cells and occasional HbC crystals. Hb electrophoresis shows mainly HbC with some HbF. HbA is absent. Red cells said to be 'stiff'. Care with anaesthesia.

HbC trait ($\beta^{6\ glu \rightarrow lys}$)

Asymptomatic. Hb is ↔. Film may be normal or show presence of target cells. HbC 30–40%.

HbD disease (eg D$_{Punjab}$ $\beta^{121\ glu \rightarrow gln}$)

Found in N W India, Pakistan and Iran. Film shows target cells.

HbD trait (eg D$_{Punjab}$ $\beta^{121\ glu \rightarrow gln}$)

Of little consequence other than interaction with HbS. Hb and MCV are ↔. Film normal or shows target cells.

HbE disease ($\beta^{26\ glu \rightarrow lys}$)

South East Asia (commonest Hb variant), India, Burma and Thailand. This Hb is moderately unstable when exposed to oxidants. May produce thalassaemic syndrome when mRNA splice mutants. There is mild anaemia, MCV and MCH are ↓, reticulocytes are ↔. Film shows target cells, hypochromic and microcytic red cells. There are few symptoms; underlying compensated haemolysis, mild jaundice. Liver and spleen size are normal. Treatment is not usually required.

HbE trait ($\beta^{26\ glu \rightarrow lys}$)

Asymptomatic. Indices similar to β thalassaemia trait. Hb usually ↔.

Unstable haemoglobins

Congenital Heinz body haemolytic anaemia caused by point mutations in globin genes. Hb precipitates in red blood cells → Heinz bodies. In normal Hb there are non-covalent bonds maintaining the Hb structure; loss of bonds leads to Hb denaturation and precipitation. Production of Heinz bodies leads to less deformable red cells with reduced lifespan.

Predominantly autosomal dominant; most patients are heterozygotes. Mainly affects β globin chain. Eg Hb Hammersmith (mutation involves amino acid in contact with haem pocket); Hb Bristol (replacement of nonpolar by polar amino acid with distortion of protein).

Clinical features
- Well compensated haemolysis.
- [Hb] may be ↔ if unstable Hb has high O_2 affinity.
- Haemolysis exacerbated by infection and oxidant drugs.
- Jaundice and splenomegaly are common.
- Some Hbs are unstable *in vitro* but show little haemolysis *in vivo*.

Investigation
- Hb ↔ or ↓.
- MCV often ↓.
- Film shows hypochromic RBCs, polychromatic RBCs, basophilic stippling.
- Heinz bodies seen post-splenectomy.
- Reticulocytes are ↑.
- Demonstrate unstable Hb using eg heat or isopropanol stability tests.
- Brilliant cresyl blue will stain Heinz bodies.
- Estimation of P_{50} may be helpful.
- DNA analysis of value in some cases.

Management

Most cases run benign course. Treatment seldom required. Gallstones common. Recommend regular folic acid supplementation. Splenectomy of value in some patients. Avoidance of precipitants of haemolysis advised.

Thalassaemias

Arise as a result of diminished or absent production of one or more globin chains. Net result is imbalanced globin chain production. Globins chains in excess precipitate within RBCs leading to chronic haemolysis in bone marrow and peripheral blood. Occur at high frequency in parts of Africa, the Mediterranean, Middle East, India and Asia. Found in high frequency in areas where malaria is endemic and thalassaemia trait probably offers some protection.

Named after affected gene eg in α thalassaemia the α globin gene is altered in such a way that either α globin synthesis is *reduced* (α⁺) or *abolished* (α°) from RBCs. Severity varies depending on type of mutation or deletion of the α or β globin gene.

α thalassaemia

Two α globin genes on each chromosome 16, with total of 4 α globin genes per cell (normal person is designated αα/αα). Like sickle cell anaemia, patients can either have mild α thalassaemia (α *thalassaemia trait*) where one or two α globin genes are affected or may have severe α thalassaemia if three or four of the genes are affected. α thalassaemia is generally the result of large deletions within α globin complex.

Silent α thalassaemia (–α/αα)
One gene deleted. Asymptomatic. ↓ MCV and MCH in minority.

α thalassaemia trait (αα/–– or –α/–α)
Asymptomatic carrier – recognised once other causes of microcytic anaemia are excluded (eg iron deficiency). Hb may be ↔ or minimally ↓. MCV and MCH are ↓. Absence of splenomegaly or other clinical findings. Requires no therapy.

Haemoglobin H disease (––/– α)
Three α genes deleted; only one functioning copy of the α globin gene/cell. Clinical features variable. May be moderate anaemia with Hb 8.0–9.0 g/dl. MCV and MCH are ↓. Hepatosplenomegaly, chronic leg ulceration and jaundice (reflecting underlying haemolysis). Infection, drug treatment and pregnancy may worsen anaemia.

Blood film shows hypochromia, target cells, NRBC and increased reticulocytes. Brilliant cresyl blue stain will show HbH inclusions (tetramers of β globin, β_4, that have polymerised due to lack of α chains). Hb pattern consists of 2–40% HbH (β_4) with some HbA, A_2 and F.

Treatment
Not usually required but prompt treatment of infection advisable. Give regular folic acid especially when pregnant. Splenectomy of value in some patients with HbH disease. Needs monitoring and may require blood transfusion.

Haemoglobin Bart's hydrops fetalis (––/––)
Common cause of stillbirth in Southeast Asia. All 4 α globin genes affected. γ chains form tetramers (γ_4) which bind oxygen very tightly, with resultant poor tissue oxygenation. Fetus is either stillborn (at 34–40 weeks gestation) or dies soon after birth. They are pale, distended, jaundiced and have marked hepatosplenomegaly and ascites. Haemoglobin is ~6.0 g/dl and the film shows

hypochromic red cells, target cells, increased reticulocytes and nucleated red cells. Haemoglobin analysis shows mainly HbBart's (γ_4) with a small amount of HbH (β_4); HbA, A_2 and F are absent.

β thalassaemia

Only 2 copies of β globin gene per cell. Abnormality in one β globin gene results in β *thalassaemia trait;* if both β globin genes affected the patient has β *thalassaemia major* or β *thalassaemia intermedia.* Unlike α thalassaemia, most β thalassaemias are due to single point mutations. Results in reduced β globin synthesis (β^+) or absent β globin production (β°). In β thalassaemia major, patients have severe anaemia requiring lifelong support with blood transfusion (with resultant iron overload). There is ineffective erythropoiesis. Not obvious at birth due to presence of HbF ($\alpha_2\gamma_2$) but as γ chain production diminishes and β globin production increases effects of the mutation become obvious. Children fail to thrive, and development is affected. Hepatosplenomegaly (due to production and destruction of red cells by these organs) is typical. Children also develop facial abnormalities as the flat bones of the skull and other bones attempt to produce red cells to overcome the genetic defect. Skull radiographs show 'hair on end' appearances reflecting the intense marrow activity in the skull bones.

Investigation and management

β thalassaemia trait
- Carrier state.
- Hb may be ↓ but is not usually <10.0g/dl.
- MCV ↓ to ~63–77fl.
- Blood film: microcytic, hypochromic RBCs; target cells often present. Basophilic stippling especially in mediterraneans.
- RCC ↑.
- HbA_2 ($\alpha_2\delta_2$) ↑ – provides useful diagnostic test for β thalassaemia trait.
- Occasionally confused with iron deficiency anaemia, however, in thalassaemia trait the serum iron and ferritin are normal (or increased) whereas in IDA they are reduced.

Treatment
Not usually required. Usually detected antenatally or on routine FBC pre-op.

β thalassaemia intermedia
- Denotes thalassaemia major not requiring regular blood transfusion; more severe than β thalassaemia trait but milder than β thalassaemia major.
- May arise through several mechanisms eg
  - *inheritance of mild β thalassaemia mutations* (eg homozygous β^+ thalassaemia alleles, compound heterozygote for two mild β^+ thalassaemia alleles, compound heterozygotes for mild plus severe β^+ thalassaemia alleles)
  - *elevation of HbF*
  - *coinheritance of α thalassaemia*
  - *coinheritance of β thalassaemia trait with eg HbLepore*
  - *severe β thalassaemia trait*

Clinical
- Present with symptoms similar to β thalassaemia major but with only moderate degree of anaemia.
- Hepatosplenomegaly.
- Iron overload is a feature.
- Some patients are severely anaemic (Hb ~6 g/dl) although not requiring regular blood transfusion, have impaired growth and development, skeletal deformities and chronic leg ulceration.

- Others have higher Hb (eg 10–12 g/dl) with few symptoms.

Management

Depends on severity. May require intermittent blood transfusion, iron chelation, folic acid supplementation, prompt treatment of infection, as for β thalassaemia major.

β thalassaemia major (Cooley's anaemia)

Patients have abnormalities of both β globin genes. Presents in childhood with anaemia and recurrent bacterial infection. There is extramedullary haemopoiesis with hepatosplenomegaly and skeletal deformities.

Clinical

- Moderate/severe anaemia (Hb ~3.0–9.0 g/dl).
- MCV and MCHC ↓.
- Reticulocytes ↑.
- Blood film: marked anisopoikilocytosis, target cells and nucleated red cells.
- Methyl violet stain shows RBC inclusions containing precipitated α globin.
- Hb electrophoresis shows mainly HbF ($\alpha_2\gamma_2$). In some β thalassaemias there may be a little HbA ($\alpha_2\beta_2$) if some β globin is produced.
- HbA_2 may be ↔ or mildly elevated.

Management

- Regular lifelong blood transfusion (every 2–4 weeks) to *suppress* ineffective erythropoiesis and allow normal growth and development in childhood.
- Leucocyte depleted transfusion required to reduce incidence of febrile transfusion reactions.
- Iron overload (*transfusion haemosiderosis*) is major problem – damages heart, endocrine glands, pancreas and liver. Desferrioxamine reduces iron overload (by promoting iron excretion in the urine and stool), and is given for 8–12h per day SC for 5 days of the week. Compliance may be difficult, especially in younger patients. Complications of desferrioxamine include retinal damage, cataract and infection with *Yersinia* spp.
- Splenectomy may be of value (eg if massive splenomegaly or increasing transfusion requirements) but best avoided until after the age of 5 years due to ↑ risk of infection. Infective episodes should be treated promptly with intravenous antibiotics.
- Bone marrow transplantation has been carried out using sibling donor HLA-matched transplants with good results in young patients with β thalassaemia major. The procedure carries a significant procedure-related morbidity and mortality, along with GvHD (see BMT section).

Screening

Screen mothers at first antenatal visit. If mother is thalassaemic carrier, screen father. If both carriers for severe thalassaemia offer prenatal diagnostic testing. Fetal blood sampling can be carried out at 18 weeks gestation and globin chain synthesis analysed. CVS at 10+ weeks gestation provides a source of fetal DNA that can be analysed in a variety of methods: Southern blotting, oligonucleotide probes or RFLP analysis may determine genotype of fetus. Moving towards PCR based techniques; likely to improve carrier detection.

Other thalassaemias

Heterozygous δβ thalassaemia

Produces a picture similar to β thalassaemia trait with ↑ HbF (5–20%) and microcytic RBCs; HbA_2 is ↔ or reduced.

Homozygous δβ thalassaemia

Homozygous condition is uncommon. There is failure of production of both δ and β globins. Milder than β thalassaemia major, ie β thalassaemia intermedia. Represents a form of thalassaemia intermedia. Hb8–11g/dl. Absence of HbA and HbA_2; only HbF is present (100%).

Heterozygous β thalassaemia/δβ thalassaemia

Similar to β thalassaemia major (but less severe). Hb produced is mainly HbF with small amount of HbA_2.

γδβ thalassaemia

Homozygote is not viable. Heterozygous condition is associated with haemolysis in neonatal period and thalassaemia trait in adults with ↔ HbF and HbA_2.

HbLepore

This abnormal Hb is the result of unequal crossing over of chromosomes. Affects β and δ globin genes with generation of a chimeric globin with δ sequences at NH_2 terminal and β globin at COOH terminal. Production of δβ globin is inefficient; there is absence of normal δ and β globins. The phenotype of the heterozygote is thalassaemia trait; the homozygote picture is thalassaemia intermedia.

Hereditary persistence of fetal haemoglobin

Heterogeneous groups of disorders caused by deletions or cross-overs involving β and γ chain production, or non-deletional forms due to point mutations upstream of the γ globin gene, with high levels of HbF production in adult life. There is ↓ δ and β chain production with enhanced γ chain production. Globin chain imbalance is much less marked than in β thalassaemia, resulting in milder disorder. There are few clinical effects.

May be *pancellular* (very high levels of HbF haemoglobin synthesis with uniform distribution in RBCs) or *heterocellular* (increased numbers of F cells).

Mechanism
Like δβ-thalassaemia, HPFH frequently arises from deletions of DNA, which remove or inactivate the β-globin gene (note: heterocellular HPFH may be result of mutations outside the β-globin gene).

Heterozygous HPFH
Anaemia may be mild or absent. Haematological indices are normal. There is balanced α/non-α globin chain synthesis. HbF level ~25%.

Hb patterns in haemoglobin disorders

	A	F	A$_2$	S	Other
			% Haemoglobin		
Normal	97	<1	2–3		
β thalassaemia trait	80–95	1–5	3–7		
β thalassaemia intermedia	30–50	50–70	0–5		
β thalassaemia major	0–20	80–100	0–13		
HPFH (black heterozygote)	60–85	15–35	1–3		
HPFH (black homozygote)		100			
α thalassaemia trait	85–95				Bart's 0-10% at birth
HbH disease	60–95				H 5–30%; Bart's 20-30% at birth
HbBart's hydrops					Bart's 80–90%
HbE trait	60–65	1–2	2–3		E 30–35
HbE disease	0	5–10	5		E 95
HbE/β thalassaemia	0	30-40	–		E 60-70
HbE/α thalassaemia	13				E 80
HbD trait	50–65	1–5	1–3		D 45-50
HbD disease		1–5	1–3		D 90-95
HbD/β thalassaemia	0-7	1-7			D 80-90
HbC trait	60-70				C 30-40
HbC disease		slight increase			C 95
sickle trait	55–70	1	3	30–45	
sickle cell anaemia	0	7	3	90	
sickle/β+ thalassaemia	5–30	5–15	–	60–85	
sickle/β0 thalassaemia	0	5–30	4–8	70–90	
sickle/D	0	1–5		50	D 50%
sickle/C	0	1	*	50–65	C 50%
HbLepore trait	80–90	1-3	2-2.5		Lepore 9-11%
HbLepore disease	0	70-90	0		Lepore 8-30%
HbLepore/β thalassaemia		70-90	2.5		Lepore 5-15%

Non-immune haemolysis

4 major groups

- Infections.
- Vascular (mechanical damage).
- Chemical damage.
- Physical damage.

Infection

Malaria – especially falciparum. Causes anaemia through marrow suppression, hypersplenism and RBC sequestration. In addition there is haemolysis due to destruction of parasitised RBCs by RES and intravascular haemolysis when sporozoites released from infected RBCs. Blackwater fever refers to severe acute intravascular haemolysis with haemoglobinaemia, ↓ Hb, haemoglobinuria and ARF.

Babesiosis – *Babesia* (RBC protozoan). Rapid onset of vomiting, diarrhoea, rigors, jaundice, ↑T°. Haemoglobinaemia, haemoglobinuria, ARF and death.

Clostridium perfringens – septicaemia and acute intravascular haemolysis.

Viral – especially viral haemorrhagic fevers eg Dengue, Yellow fever.

Mechanical

Cardiac – turbulence and shear stress following mechanical valve replacement. General feature of haemolysis: ↑ reticulocytes, LDH, plasma Hb, with ↓ haptoglobins ± platelets. Urinary haemosiderin +ve.

MAHA – see p108.

HUS/TTP – see p374.

March haemoglobinuria – with severe strenuous exercise eg running. Destruction of RBCs in soles of feet. Worse with hard soles and uneven hard ground. Mild anaemia. No specific features on film. May be associated GIT bleeding and ↓ ferritin (lost in sweat).

Chemical & physical

Oxidative haemolysis – chronic Heinz body intravascular haemolysis with dapsone or salazopyrine in G6PD deficient people or unstable Hb (and normals if dose high enough). Film: bite cells (RBC). Heinz bodies not prominent if intact spleen. Haemolysis well compensated.

MetHb – see p106.

Lead poisoning – moderate ↓ RBC lifespan. Anaemia mainly due to block in haem synthesis although lead also inhibits 5' NT. Basophilic stippling on film. Ring sideroblasts in BM.

O_2 – haemolysis in patients treated with hyperbaric O_2.

Insect bites – eg spider, bee sting (not common with snake bites).

Heat – eg burns, → severe haemolysis due to direct RBC damage.

Liver disease – reduced RBC lifespan in acute hepatitis, cirrhosis, Zieve's syndrome is an uncommon form of haemolysis – intravascular associated with acute abdominal pain (see p52).

Wilson's disease – autosomally inherited disorder of copper metabolism, with hepatolenticular, hepatocerebral degeneration.

PNH – see p120.

Hereditary acanthocytosis – a-β-lipoproteinaemia. Rare, inherited. Associated with retinitis pigmentosa, steatorrhoea, ataxia and mental retardation.

93

Hereditary spherocytosis

Most common inherited RBC membrane defect characterised by variable degrees of haemolysis, spherocytic RBCs with ↑ osmotic fragility.

Pathophysiology

Abnormal RBC cytoskeleton: partial deficiency of spectrin, ankyrin, band 3 or protein 4.2 (leads to ↓ binding to band 4.1 protein & ankyrin). Loss of lipid from RBC membrane → spherical (cf. biconcave) RBCs with reduced surface area → get trapped in splenic cords and have reduced lifespan. RBCs use more energy than normal in attempt to maintain cell shape. RBC membrane has ↑ Na^+ permeability (loses intracellular Na^+) and energy required to restore Na^+ balance. Red cells are less deformable than normal.

Epidemiology

In Northern Europeans 1:5000 people are affected. In most cases inheritance is autosomal dominant although autosomal recessive inheritance has been reported.

Clinical features

Presents at any age. Highly variable from asymptomatic to severely anaemic, but usually there are few symptoms. Well-compensated haemolysis; other features of haemolytic anaemia may be present eg splenomegaly, gallstones, mild jaundice. Occasional aplastic crises occur, eg with parvovirus B19 infection.

Diagnosis

- Positive family history of HS in many cases.
- Blood film shows ↑↑ spherocytic RBCs.
- Anaemia, ↑ reticulocytes, ↑ LDH, unconjugated bilirubin, urinary urobilinogen with ↓ haptoglobins. DAT –ve.

Osmotic fragility test – RBCs incubated in saline at various concentrations. Results in cell expansion and eventually rupture. Normal RBCs can withstand greater volume increases than spherocytic RBCs. Positive result (ie confirms HS) when RBCs lyse in saline at near to isotonic concentration, ie 0.6–0.8 g/dl (whereas normal RBCs will simply show swelling with little lysis). Osmotic fragility more marked in patients who have not undergone splenectomy, and if the RBCs are incubated at 37°C for 24h before performing the test.

Autohaemolysis test – since spherocytic RBCs use more glucose than normal RBCs (to maintain normal shape) red cells incubated in buffer or serum for 48h show lysis and release of Hb into solution, which can be measured. In HS RBCs release greater amounts of Hb cf. normal RBCs (3% vs. 1% in normal).

Complications

- Aplastic crisis (eg parvovirus B19 infection, but may be any virus); see temporary ↓↓ reticulocytes, Hb and Hct.
- Megaloblastic changes in folate deficiency.
- ↑ haemolysis during intercurrent illness eg infections.
- Gallstones (in 50% patients; occur even in mild disease).
- Leg ulceration.
- Extramedullary haemopoiesis.
- Iron overload if multiply transfused.

Exclude
Other causes of haemolytic anaemia eg immune-mediated, unstable Hbs and MAHA, which can give rise to spherocytic RBCs.

Treatment
Supportive treatment is usually all that is required, eg folic acid (5mg/d). In parvovirus crisis Hb drops significantly and blood transfusion may be required. Splenectomy is 'curative' but is reserved for patients who are severely anaemic or who have symptomatic moderate anaemia. Best avoided in patients <10 years old due to risk of ↑ fatal infection post-splenectomy.

▶ Remember pre-splenectomy vaccines and post-splenectomy antibiotics (see p494).

Hereditary elliptocytosis

Heterogeneous group of disorders with elliptical RBCs.

3 major groups
- Hereditary elliptocytosis.
- Spherocytic HE.
- Southeast Asian ovalocytosis.

Pathophysiology
Mutations in α or β spectrin. There may be partial, complete deficiency, or structural abnormality of protein 4.1, or absence of glycophorin C.

Epidemiology
In Northern Europeans 1:2500 are affected. Inheritance is autosomal dominant. More common in areas where malaria is endemic.

Clinical features
Most are asymptomatic. Well-compensated haemolysis. A few patients have chronic symptomatic anaemia. Homozygote more severely affected.

Diagnosis
- May have positive family history.
- Blood film shows ↑↑ elliptical or oval RBCs.
- Anaemia, ↑ reticulocytes, ↑ LDH, unconjugated bilirubin, urinary urobilinogen with ↓ haptoglobins. DAT is –ve.
- Osmotic fragility usually normal (unless spherocytic HE).
- Transient increase in haemolysis if intercurrent infection.

Complications
Usual complications of haemolytic anaemia eg gallstones, folate deficiency, etc.

Treatment
Supportive care: folic acid (5mg/d). Most patients require no treatment. In more severe cases consider splenectomy. Remember pre-splenectomy vaccines and post-splenectomy antibiotics (see p494).

Spherocytic HE
Elliptical and spherical 'sphero-ovalocytes' in peripheral blood. Haemolysis and ↑ osmotic fragility distinguish it from common hereditary elliptocytosis. Molecular basis is unknown.

Southeast Asian ovalocytosis
Caused by abnormal band 3 protein. RBCs are oval with 1–2 transverse ridges. Cells have ↑ rigidity and ↓ osmotic fragility. RBCs are more resistant to malaria than normal RBCs.

Glucose-6-phosphate dehydrogenase deficiency

G6PD is involved in pentose phosphate shunt → generates NADP and NADPH as well as glutathione (required for maintenance of Hb and RBC membrane integrity, and to reverse oxidant damage to red cell membrane and RBC components). G6PD deficiency is X–linked and clinically important cause of oxidant haemolysis. Affects ♂ predominantly; ♀ carriers have 50% normal G6PD activity. Occurs in West Africa, Southern Europe, Middle East and South East Asia.

Features:
- Haemolysis after exposure to oxidants or infection.
- Chronic non-spherocytic haemolytic anaemia.
- Acute episodes of haemolysis with fava beans (termed favism).
- Methaemoglobinaemia.
- Neonatal jaundice.

Mechanism Oxidants → denatured Hb → methaemoglobin → Heinz bodies → RBC less deformable → destroyed by spleen.

2 main forms of the enzyme: normal enzyme is termed G6PD-B, the most prevalent form worldwide; 20% Africans are type A. A and B differ by one amino acid. Mutant enzyme with normal activity = G6PD A(+), find only in blacks. G6PD A(–) is main defect in African origin; ↓ stability of enzyme *in vivo*; 5–15% normal activity. There are 400 or more variants but only 2 are relevant clinically: type A(–) = Africans (with 10% enzyme activity) and Mediterranean (with 1–3% activity).

Drug-induced haemolysis in G6PD deficiency
- Begins 1–3d after ingestion of drug.
- Anaemia most severe 7–10d after ingestion.
- Associated with low back and abdominal pain.
- Urine becomes dark (black sometimes).
- Red cells develop Heinz body inclusions (cleared later by spleen).
- Haemolysis is typically self-limiting.
- Implicated drugs:

Definite risk of haemolysis in G6PD deficient subjects	Possible risk of haemolysis in *some* G6PD deficient subjects
Antimalarial drugs	Aspirin (1g/d acceptable in most
Primaquine	G6PD def. subjects)
Pamaquine (not available in UK)	Chloroquine
	Probenecid
Analgesic drugs	Quinine & quinidine (acceptable in
Aspirin	acute malaria)
Phenacetin	
Others	
Dapsone	
Methylene blue	
Nitrofurantoin	
4-quinolones (eg Ciprofloxacin, nalidixic acid)	
Sulphonamides (eg Cotrimoxazole)	

- But heterogeneous; variable sensitivity to drugs.
- Risk and severity are DOSE-RELATED.

Haemolysis due to infection & fever
- 1–2d after onset of fever.
- Mild anaemia develops.
- Commonly seen in pneumonic illnesses.

Favism
- Hours/days after ingestion of fava beans (broad beans).
- Beans contain oxidants vicine and convicine → free radicals → oxidise glutathione.
- Urine becomes red or very dark.
- Shock may develop – *may be fatal.*

Neonatal jaundice
- May develop kernicterus (*possible permanent brain damage*).
- Rare in A(–) variants.
- More common in Mediterranean and Chinese variants.

Laboratory investigation
- In steady state (ie no haemolysis) the RBCs appear normal.
- Heinz bodies in drug-induced haemolysis (methyl violet stain).
- Spherocytes and RBC fragments on blood film if severe haemolysis.
- ↑ reticulocytes.
- ↑ LDH.
- ↑ unconjugated bilirubin.
- ↑ urinary urobilinogen.
- ↓ haptoglobins.
- DAT is –ve.

Diagnosis
Demonstrate enzyme deficiency. In suspected red cell enzymopathy, assay G6PD and PK first, then look for presence of unstable Hb (isopropanol stability test). Diagnosis is difficult during haemolytic episode since reticulocytes have ↑↑ levels of enzyme and may get erroneously normal result; wait until steady state (~6 weeks after episode of haemolysis). Family studies are helpful.

Management
- Avoid oxidant drugs – *see BNF.*
- Transfuse in severe haemolysis or symptomatic anaemia.
- IV fluids to maintain good urine output.
- ± exchange transfusion in infants.
- Splenectomy may be of value in severe recurrent haemolysis.
- Folic acid supplements (?proven value).
- Avoid iron unless definite iron deficiency.

Pyruvate kinase deficiency

Congenital non-spherocytic haemolytic anaemia, caused by deficiency of PK enzyme (involved in glycolytic pathway), leading to unstable enzyme with reduction in ATP generation in RBCs. O_2 curve is shifted to the right due to ↑ 2,3 DPG production.

Epidemiology

Autosomal recessive. Affected persons are homozygous or double heterozygotes.

Clinical features

Variable, with chronic haemolytic syndrome. May be apparent in neonate (if severe) or may present in later life.

Diagnosis

- Variable anaemia.
- Reticulocytes ↑↑.
- DAT –ve.
- LDH ↑.
- Serum haptoglobin ↓.
- Definitive diagnosis requires assay of PK level.

Complications

Aplastic crisis may be seen in viral infection (eg parvovirus B19).

Treatment

Dependent on severity. General supportive measures include daily folic acid (5mg/d). Transfusion may be required. Splenectomy may be of value if high transfusion requirements. In aplastic crisis (eg viral infection) support measures should be used.

Other red cell enzymopathies

Glycolytic pathway
- Hexokinase deficiency.
- Glucose phosphate isomerase deficiency.
- Phosphofructokinase deficiency.
- Aldolase deficiency.
- Triosephosphate isomerase deficiency.
- Phosphoglycerate kinase deficiency.

Epidemiology
Incidence <1 in 10^6. Inheritance is autosomal recessive (most double heterozygote) except for phosphoglycerate kinase deficiency (X-linked recessive).

Clinical features
Similar to PK deficiency although most are more severely affected for the degree of anaemia (glycolytic block results in ↓ 2,3 DPG and left shift of O_2 dissociation curve). PFK deficiency is associated with myopathy. TPI and PGK deficiencies are associated with progressive neurological deterioration.

Diagnosis
- *See pyruvate kinase deficiency.*
- Non-specific morphology with anisocytosis, macrocytosis and polychromasia.
- Definitive diagnosis requires assay of deficient enzyme (→ reference lab).

Complications
- *See pyruvate kinase deficiency.*

Treatment
Folic acid (5 mg/d). Transfusion may be required (beware Fe overload if high transfusion requirement). Role of splenectomy controversial.

Natural history
Similar to pyruvate kinase except TPI and PGK-TPI present in childhood and cause progressive paraparesis, most die <5 years old due to cardiac arrhythmias. PGK can cause exertional rhabdomyolysis and consequential renal failure. Those affected progressive neurological deterioration.

Nucleotide metabolism – pyrimidine 5' nucleotidase deficiency

Epidemiology
Autosomal recessive. *Note:* lead poisoning causes *acquired* pyrimidine 5' nucleotidase deficiency.

Clinical features
- Moderate anaemia (Hb ~10g/dl).
- ↑ Reticulocytes.
- ↑ bilirubin.
- Splenomegaly.

Diagnosis
- RBCs show prominent basophilic stippling.
- P5'N assay.

Treatment
Symptomatic, splenectomy is of limited value.

Drug-induced haemolytic anaemia

Large number of drugs shown to cause haemolysis of RBCs. Mechanisms variable. May be immune or non-immune.

- Some drugs interfere with lipid component of RBC membrane.
- Oxidation and denaturation of Hb: seen with eg sulphonamides, especially in G6PD deficient subjects, but may occur in normal subjects if drugs given in large doses eg
  - *dapsone*
  - *sulphasalazine*
- **Hapten mechanism** describes the interaction between certain drugs and the RBC membrane components generating antigens that stimulate antibody production. DAT +ve.
  - *penicillins*
  - *cephalosporins*
  - *tetracyclines*
  - *tolbutamide*
- **Autoantibody mediated haemolysis** is associated with warm antibody mediated AIHA. DAT +ve.
  - *cephalosporins*
  - *mefenamic acid*
  - *methyldopa*
  - *procainamide*
  - *ibuprofen*
  - *diclofenac*
  - *IFN-α*
- **Innocent bystander mechanism** occurs when drugs form immune complexes with antibody (IgM commonest) which then attach to RBC membrane. Complement fixation and RBC destruction occurs.
  - *quinine*
  - *quinidine*
  - *rifampicin*
  - *antihistamines*
  - *chlorpromazine*
  - *melphalan*
  - *tetracycline*
  - *probenecid*
  - *cefotaxime*

Laboratory features
As for autoimmune haemolytic anaemia, Hb ↓, reticulocytes ↑, etc.

Differential diagnosis
- Warm/cold autoimmune haemolytic anaemia.
- Congenital haemolytic disorders, eg HS, G6PD deficiency, etc.

Treatment
- Discontinue offending drug.
- Chose alternative if necessary.
- If DAT +ve with methyldopa no need to stop unless haemolysis.
- Corticosteroids generally unnecessary and of doubtful value.
- Transfuse in severe or symptomatic cases only.
- Outlook good with complete recovery usual.

Methaemoglobinaemia

The normal O_2 dissociation curve requires iron to be in the ferrous form (ie reduced, Fe^{2+}). Hb containing the ferric (oxidised, Fe^{3+}) form is termed methaemoglobin (MetHb). MetHb binds O_2 tightly leading to poor tissue oxygenation. May be congenital or acquired.

Congenital MetHb

HbM
α or β globin mutation in vicinity of Fe.
Fe becomes stabilised in Fe^{3+} form.
Heterozygote has 25% HbM.

MetHb reductase deficiency
Due to deficiency of NADH-cytochrome b_5 reductase. Autosomal recessive inheritance; symptoms mainly in homozygote.

Clinical features
Cyanosis from infancy. PaO_2 is normal. General health is good.

Acquired MetHb
Occurs when RBCs are exposed to oxidising agents, producing HbM. Implicated agents include: phenacetin, local anaesthetics (eg lignocaine), inorganic nitrates (NO_2). Patients may experience severe tissue ↑ hypoxia. HbM binds O_2 tightly and fails to release to tissues.

▶▶ HbM level ≥60% requires urgent medical attention.

Diagnosis
May be history of exposure to oxidant drugs or chemicals. Spectrophotometry or haemoglobin electrophoresis will demonstrate HbM. Assays for MetHb reductase are available.

Treatment
In patients with congenital symptomatic HbM give ascorbate or methylene blue. In acquired disorder remove oxidant, if present, and administer methylene blue.

▶ If severely affected consider exchange blood transfusion.

Microangiopathic haemolytic anaemia (MAHA)

Definition
Increased RBC destruction caused by mechanical red cell deformation. Caused by trauma or vascular endothelial abnormalities.

Causes
- TTP/HUS see p374, 438.
- PET/HELLP (haemolysis, elevated liver enzymes and low platelets).
- Malignant tumour circulations.
- Renal abnormalities eg acute glomerulonephritis, transplant rejection, cyclosporin.
- Vasculitidies eg Wegener's, PAN, SLE.
- DIC.
- Prosthetic heart valves.
- March haemoglobinuria.
- A-V malformations.
- Burns.

Clinical
- Varying degree of anaemia – most severe in DIC, TTP/HUS and HELLP.
- Often associated with ↓ platelets.
- Blood film shows marked RBC fragmentation, stomatocytes and spherocytes.
- Reticulocytosis often very marked.
- Signs of underlying disease should be sought.

Treatment
- Diagnose and treat underlying disease.
- Give folic acid and iron supplements if deficient.

Acanthocytosis

Abnormal RBC shape (thorn-like surface protrusions) seen in a number of conditions, inherited or acquired, affecting RBC membrane lipid structure. RBCs develop normally in marrow but once in plasma adopt characteristic shape. RBCs lose membrane and become progressively less elastic.

Inherited conditions resulting in significant acanthocytosis
- A-β-lipoproteinaemia.
- McLeod phenotype (lacking Kell antigen).
- In(Lu) phenotype.
- In association with abnormalities of band 3 protein.
- Hereditary hypobetalipoproteinaemia.

Acquired conditions resulting in significant acanthocytosis
- Severe liver disease.
- Myelodysplastic syndromes.
- Neonatal vitamin E deficiency.

Inherited conditions resulting in mild acanthocytosis
- McLeod phenotype heterozygote.
- Pyruvate kinase deficiency.

Acquired conditions resulting in mild acanthocytosis
- Post-splenectomy and hyposplenic states.
- Starvation including anorexia nervosa.
- Hypothyroidism.
- Panhypopituitarism.

A-β-lipoproteinaemia
Autosomal recessive. Congenital absence of β apolipoprotein. Cholesterol: phospholipid ratio ↑. RBC precursors normal. Usually obvious in early life with associated malabsorption of fat (including vitamins A, D, E and K). Sphingomyelin accumulates.

Haematological abnormalities
- Mild haemolytic anaemia.
- 50–90% circulating RBCs are acanthocytic.
- Reticulocytes mildly ↑.

McLeod phenotype
- ↓ expression of Kell antigen on RBC.
- Mild (compensated) haemolytic anaemia.
- 10–85% acanthocytic RBCs in peripheral blood.

Autoimmune haemolytic anaemia

RBCs react with autoantibody ± complement → premature destruction of RBCs by reticuloendothelial system.

Mechanism

RBCs coated in IgG, react with Fc receptors on RES macrophages → phagocytosis. If phagocytosis incomplete remaining portion of RBC continues to circulate as *spherocyte* (*note:* phagocytosis usually complete if complement involved).

Seen in

- Haemolytic blood transfusion reactions.
- Autoimmune haemolytic anaemia.
- Drug-induced haemolysis (some).

'Warm' antibody induced haemolysis	Idiopathic 2° to lymphoproliferative disease eg CLL, NHL
'Cold' antibody induced haemolysis	Idiopathic Cold haemagglutinin disease (CHAD) 2° to *Mycoplasma* infection Infectious mononucleosis Lymphoma
Paroxysmal cold haemoglobinuria	Idiopathic 2° to viral infection Congenital or tertiary syphilis

Warm antibody induced haemolysis

Extravascular RBC destruction by RES mediated by warm-reacting antibody. Most cases are idiopathic with no underlying pathology, but may be 2° to lymphoid malignancies eg CLL, or autoimmune disease such as SLE.

Epidemiology

Affects people >50 years of age mainly.

Clinical features

- Highly variable symptoms, asymptomatic or severely anaemic.
- Chronic compensated haemolysis.
- Mild jaundice common.
- Splenomegaly usual.

Diagnosis

- Anaemia.
- Spherocytes on peripheral blood film.
- Reticulocytes are ↑↑.
- Neutrophilia common.
- RBC coated with IgG, complement or both (detect using DAT).
- Autoantibody – often no specificity; occasionally reacts with Rhesus antigen.
- LDH ↑.
- Serum haptoglobin ↓.
- Exclude underlying lymphoma (BM, blood and marrow cell markers).
- Autoimmune profile – to exclude SLE or other connective tissue disorder.

Treatment

Prednisolone 1mg/kg/d PO tailing off after response noted (usually 1–2 weeks). If no response consider immunosuppression eg azathioprine (suitable for elderly but not younger patients – risk of 2° leukaemia) or cyclophosphamide. Splenectomy should be considered in selected cases. IVIg (0.4g/kg/d for 5d) useful in refractory cases, or where rapid response required.

Cold haemagglutinin disease (CHAD)

Describes syndrome associated with acrocyanosis in cold weather due to RBC agglutinates in blood vessels of skin. Caused by RBC antibody that reacts most strongly at temperatures <32°C. Complement is activated→RBC lysis →haemoglobinaemia & haemoglobinuria. May be idiopathic (1°) or 2° to infection with *Mycoplasma* or EBV (infectious mononucleosis).

Clinical features
- Elderly.
- Acrocyanosis (blue discoloration of extremities eg fingers, toes) in cold conditions.
- Chronic compensated haemolysis.
- Splenomegaly usual.

Diagnosis
- Anaemia.
- Reticulocytes are ↑↑.
- Neutrophilia common.
- Positive DAT – C$_3$ only.
- ± Autoantibodies – IgG or IgM
  - monoclonal in NHL
  - polyclonal in infection-related CHAD.
- IgM antibodies react best at 4°C (thermal amplitude 4–32°C).
- Specificity
  - anti-I (*Mycoplasma*)
  - anti-i (infectious mononucleosis) – causes little haemolysis in adults since RBCs have little anti-i (*cf.* newborn i >> I).
- LDH ↑.
- Serum haptoglobin ↓.
- ***Exclude underlying lymphoma*** (BM, blood and marrow cell markers).
- Autoimmune profile to exclude SLE or other connective tissue disorder.

Treatment
- Keep warm.
- Corticosteroids generally of little value.
- Chlorambucil or cyclophosphamide (greatest value when there is underlying B cell lymphoma, occasionally helpful in 1° CHAD).
- Plasma exchange may help in some cases.
- If blood transfusion required use in-line blood warmer.
- Splenectomy occasionally useful (*note:* liver is main site of RBC sequestration of C3b coated RBCs).
- Infectious CHAD generally self-limiting.

Natural history
Prolonged survival, spontaneous remissions not unusual, with periodic relapses.

Red cell disorders

Leucoerythroblastic anaemia

Definition
A form of anaemia characterised by the presence of immature white and red blood cells in the peripheral blood. Mature white cells and platelets are also often reduced.

Causes
Marrow infiltration by
- 2° malignancy: commonly breast, lung, prostate, thyroid, kidney and colon.
- Myelofibrosis (a primary myeloproliferative disorder see p198).
- Other haematological malignancy eg myeloma and Hodgkin's disease.
- Rarely, severe haemolytic or megaloblastic anaemia.

Marrow stimulation by
- Infection, inflammation, hypoxia, trauma (common in ITU patients).
- Massive blood loss.

Marrow infiltrative causes often have associated neutropenia ± thrombocytopenia. Marrow stimulative causes often have neutrophilia and thrombocytosis.

Investigations
- FBC and blood film. Typical film appearances are of increased polychromasia due to reticulocytosis, nucleated RBCs, poikilocytosis (tear drop forms common in infiltrative causes), myelocytes and band forms, occasionally even promyelocytes and blast cells.
- Clotting screen – where cause is 2° malignancy or infective, DIC may occur.

Bone marrow is usually diagnostic
- Hypercellular BM with normal cell maturation, typical of marrow stimulation causes.
- Infiltration with neoplastic cells of a 2° malignancy may be identified as abnormal clumps with characteristic morphology – immunohistochemistry may identify the primary source eg PSA for prostate.
- Increase in reticulin fibres running in parallel bundles identifies fibrotic infiltrative cause – usually myelofibrosis, but may occur with other haematological malignancy.

Treatment
- Diagnose and treat underlying cause if possible.
- Supportive transfusions as required, management of bone marrow failure (See p472).

Aplastic anaemia

Definition

A gross reduction or absence of haemopoietic precursors in all 3 cell lineages in bone marrow resulting in pancytopenia in peripheral blood. Although this encompasses all situations in which there is myelosuppression, the term is generally used to describe those in which spontaneous marrow recovery is unusual.

Incidence

Rare ~5 cases per million population annually. Wide age range, slight increase around age 25 years and >65 years. 10 × more common in Orientals.

Causes

Divided into categories where aplasia is regarded as:

- **Inevitable**

    TBI dose of >1.5 Gy (*note:* >8 Gy always fatal in absence of graft rescue).
    Chemotherapy eg high dose busulphan.

- **Hereditary**

    Fanconi syndrome – stem cell repair defect resulting in abnormalities of skin, facies, musculo-skeletal system and urogenital systems. BM failure often delayed until adulthood.

- **Idiosyncratic**

    Chronic benzene exposure.
    Drug-induced – but not dose related – mainly gold, chloramphenicol, phenylbutazone, NSAIDs, carbamazepine, phenytoin, mesalazine. Genetic predisposition demonstrated for chloramphenicol.

- **Post-viral**

    Parvoviral infections – classically red cell aplasia but may be all elements. Devastating in conjunction with chronic haemolytic anaemia eg aplastic sickle crisis.
    Hepatitis viruses A, B and C, CMV and EBV.

- **Idiopathic**

    Constitute the majority of cases.

Classification

- According to severity most clinically useful.
- Defines highest risk groups

Severe	2 of the following:	neutrophils <0.5 × 10^9/l
		platelets <20 × 10^9/l
		reticulocytes <1%
Very severe	neutrophils <0.2 × 10^9/l, and infection present	

Clinical features

Reflects the pancytopenia. Bleeding from mucosal sites common, with purpura, ecchymoses. Infections, particularly upper and lower respiratory tracts, skin, mouth, peri-anal. Bacterial and fungal infections common. Anaemic symptoms usually less severe due to chronic onset.

Diagnosis and investigation

- FBC and blood film show pancytopenia, MCV may be ↑, film morphology unremarkable.
- Reticulocytes usually absent.
- BM aspirate and trephine show gross reduction in all haemopoietic tissue replaced by fat spaces – important to exclude hypocellular MDS or leukaemia – the main differential diagnoses.

Red cell disorders

- Ham's test (acidified serum lysis test, see p538) or immunophenotyping with CD55 and CD59 is important to exclude PNH see p120.
- Specialised cytogenetics on blood to exclude Fanconi syndrome see p370.

Complications
- Progression to more severe disease.
- Evolution to PNH – occurs in 7%.
- Transformation to acute leukaemia occurs in 5–10%.

Treatment:
- Mild cases need careful observation only. More severe will need supportive treatment with red cell and platelet transfusions and antibiotics as needed. Blood products should be CMV –ve, and preferably leucodepleted to reduce risk of sensitisation.
- Specific treatment options are between allogeneic transplant and immuno-suppression.
- Sibling allogeneic transplant treatment of choice for those <50 with sibling donor. Should go straight to transplant avoiding immunosuppression and blood products if possible.
- Matched unrelated donor transplant should be considered in <25 age group.
- Immunosuppressive options include Anti-lymphocyte globulin (ALG) ± cyclosporin. Response to ALG may take 3 months. Refractory or relapsing patients may respond to a second course of ALG from another animal.
- Cyclosporin post-ALG looks promising.
- Androgens or Danazol may be useful in some cases.

Paroxysmal nocturnal haemoglobinuria

Definition
Acquired clonal abnormality of cell membranes rendering them more sensitive to complement-mediated lysis, most noticeable in RBCs. Cells lack phosphatidylinositol glycoproteins (PIG) transmembrane anchors.

Incidence
Rare. Aplastic anaemia is closely related.

Clinical features
- Chronic intravascular haemolytic anaemia particularly overnight (?due to lower blood pH). Infections trigger acceleration of haemolysis.
- WBC and platelet production also often ↓.
- Chronic haemolysis may induce nephropathy.
- Haemoglobinuria usually results in iron deficiency.
- ↑↑ tendency to venous thrombosis particularly at atypical sites eg hepatic vein (Budd Chiari syndrome), sagittal sinus thrombosis.
- Fatigue, dysphagia and impotence occasionally seen.

Diagnosis and treatment
- FBC, blood film – polychromasia and reticulocytosis (cf. AA).
- BM aspirate and trephine biopsy – usually hypoplastic with increased fat space but with erythropoietic nests or islands distinct from AA.
- Ham's test (acidified serum lysis) is invariably +ve.
- Urinary haemosiderin +ve.
- Cellular immunophenotype shows altered PIG proteins, CD55 and CD59.

Complications
- May progress to more severe aplasia.
- Transforms to acute leukaemia in 5%.
- Serious thromboses in up to 20%.

Treatment:
- Chronic disease – supportive care may be satisfactory in mild cases.
- Iron replacement usually required.
- Trial of steroid/androgens/Danazol may ↓ symptoms and transfusion need.
- ALG/cyclosporin may be indicated for more severe cases as for aplastic anaemia.
- Acute major thromboses should be treated aggressively with urgent thrombolysis and 10 days heparin. Long-term warfarin mandatory. Consider warfarin prophylaxis after any one clotting episode.
- Severe cases <50 years should be considered for sibling allogeneic transplant if they have a donor – consider MUD in <25 age group if no sibling donor.

Prognosis:
Median survival from diagnosis is 9 years. Major cause of mortality is thrombosis and marrow failure. Molecular genetic basis now established – could be a candidate disease for gene transplantation.

Pure red cell aplasia

Definition
A severe anaemia characterised by reticulocytes <1% in PB, <0.5% mature erythroblasts in BM but with normal WBC and platelets.

Incidence
Rare.

Classification

Congenital   Diamond Blackfan anaemia (DBA), see p368

Acquired   Childhood: Transient erythroblastopenia of childhood (TEC)

                Adults: *Primary:* Autoimmune or idiopathic
                        Secondary chronic: Thymoma, haematological malignancies especially CLL, pernicious anaemia, some solid tumours, SLE, RA, malnutrition with riboflavin deficiency
                        Secondary transient: Infections especially Parvovirus B19, CMV, HIV, many drugs

Clinical features
- Lethargy usually only symptom of the anaemia since slow onset.
- No abnormal physical signs except of any underlying disease.

Diagnosis and investigations
- FBC shows severe normochromic, normocytic anaemia with retics <1%. WBC and platelets normal.
- BM shows absence of erythroblasts but is normocellular (distinguishes from aplastic anaemia).

Treatment
- Treat underlying cause first if identified.
- Remove thymoma.
- If due to Parvovirus B19, try IVIg.
- Assume immune origin if no other cause found and give prednisolone 60mg od PO as starter dose ~40% response. Failure of response, try cyclosporin or ALG or azathioprine.

Prognosis
- 15% have spontaneous remission. 65% will respond to immunosuppression.
- 50% will relapse but 80% of relapsers will respond again.
- A few progress to AA or AML.

Iron overload

Iron is an essential metal but overload occurs when intake of iron exceeds requirements and occurs due to the absence in man of a physiological mechanism to excrete excess iron. Sustained ↑ Fe intake (dietary or parenteral) may result in iron accumulation, overload and potentially fatal tissue damage.

Timing and pattern of tissue damage is determined by rate of accumulation, the quantity of total body iron and distribution of iron between reticuloendothelial (RE) storage sites and vulnerable parenchymal tissue. Iron accumulation in parenchymal cells of the liver, heart, pancreas and other organs is major determinants of clinical sequelae.

Haemochromatosis
- Inherited (autosomal recessive) occurring in up to 0.5% population.
- Haemochromatosis locus is tightly linked to the HLA locus on chromosome 6p and up to 10% population are heterozygous.
- Single missense mutation found in the homozygous state in 80% of patients.
- The gene designated HFE is an MHC class Ib gene.
- Homozygotes develop symptomatic iron overload.

Caused by failure to regulate iron absorption from bowel causing progressive increase in total body iron. Parenchymal accumulation occurs initially in liver then pancreas, heart, skin and other organs rather than RE sites. Symptoms do not usually develop until middle age when body iron stores of ≥15–20g have accumulated. Environmental factors (eg alcohol use in males and menstruation in females) affect rate of accumulation and age at presentation. Clinical expression of haemochromatosis is seen 10 × more commonly in ♂. Only 25% of heterozygotes show evidence of minor increases in iron stores and clinical problems do not occur.

Clinical manifestations of iron overload only occur in homozygotes and presentation as 'bronze diabetes' is characteristic.

Clinical features of Fe overload (homozygous haemochromatosis)
• Skin pigmentation	Slate grey or bronze discolouration
• Hepatic dysfunction	Hepatomegaly, chronic hepatitis, fibrosis, cirrhosis, hepatocellular carcinoma (20–30%)
• Diabetes mellitus	Retinopathy, nephropathy, neuropathy, vascular complications
• Gonadal dysfunction	Hypogonadism, impotence
• Other endocrine dysfunction	Hypothyroidism, hypoparathyroidism, adrenal insufficiency
• Abdominal pain	Unknown aetiology (25%)
• Cardiac dysfunction	Cardiomyopathy, heart failure, dysrhythmias (10–15%)
• Chondrocalcinosis	Arthropathy

Evaluation of iron status
Most useful indirect measure of iron stores is serum ferritin estimation. Rises to maximum concentration of 4000µg/l and may underestimate extent of iron overload in some patients. *Note:* may be spuriously increased by infection, inflammation or neoplasia. The % transferrin saturation provides confirmatory

evidence but no measure of the extent of iron overload. Liver biopsy provides a direct albeit invasive measure of iron stores (% iron concentration by weight) and visual assessment of iron distribution, and the extent of tissue damage.

Diagnosis

May be difficult to differentiate haemochromatosis from iron overload 2° to other causes, particularly that associated with chronic liver disease. Recent identification of HFE gene will provide a tool for more definitive diagnosis and screening of relatives (previously performed by serum ferritin estimation).

Management

- Aim to reduce iron stores to normal levels and prevent complications of overload.
- Achieved by regular venesection (500ml blood) on weekly basis until iron deficiency develops (may take many months).
- Hb should be measured prior to each venesection and response to therapy can be monitored by intermittent measurement of the serum ferritin.
- Once iron deficiency develops a maintenance regimen can be commenced with venesection every 3–4 months.

Natural history

Cirrhosis and hepatocellular carcinoma are most common causes of death in patients with haemochromatosis and are due to hepatic iron accumulation. Cirrhosis does not usually develop until the hepatic iron concentration reaches 4000–5000 µg/g of liver (normal 50–500µg/g). Hepatocellular carcinoma is the cause of death in 20–30% but does not occur in the absence of cirrhosis which increases the risk over 200×. If venesection can be commenced prior to the development of cirrhosis and other complications of haemosiderosis the life expectancy is that of a normal individual. Reduction of iron overload by venesection has only a small effect on symptomatology which has already developed: skin pigmentation diminishes, liver function may improve, cardiac abnormalities may resolve, diabetes and other endocrine abnormalities may improve slightly, arthropathy is unaffected.

Transfusion haemosiderosis

Iron overload occurs in patients with transfusion-dependent anaemia, notably thalassaemia major, Blackfan-Diamond syndrome, aplastic anaemia and acquired refractory anaemia. In many of these conditions iron overload is aggravated by physiological mechanisms which promote increased dietary absorption of iron in response to ineffective erythropoiesis. Each unit of blood contains 250mg iron and average transfusion dependent adult receives 6–10g of iron/year. Distribution of iron is similar to haemochromatosis with primarily liver parenchymal cell accumulation followed by pancreas, heart and other organs. Cardiac deposition occurs in patients who have received 100 units blood (20g iron) without chelation, and is followed by damage to the liver, pancreas and endocrine glands.

Clinical features of iron overload in children who require transfusion support for hereditary anaemia are listed. Similar problems excluding those related to growth and sexual maturation develop in patients who commence a transfusion programme for acquired refractory anaemia in later life.

Features of transfusion haemosiderosis in hereditary anaemia
- Growth retardation in second decade.
- Hypogonadism – delayed or absent sexual maturation.
- Skin pigmentation – slate grey or bronze discolouration.
- Hepatic dysfunction – hepatomegaly, chronic hepatitis, fibrosis, cirrhosis, hepatocellular carcinoma.
- Diabetes mellitus.
- Other endocrine dysfunction – rarely hypothyroidism, hypoparathyroidism, adrenal insufficiency.
- Cardiac dysfunction – cardiomyopathy, heart failure, dysrhythmias.
- Death from heart disease in adolescence.

Management
- Iron chelation therapy by parenteral desferrioxamine is the only treatment for patients with transfusion haemosiderosis, who remain anaemic. Haemosiderosis due to previous transfusions in conditions where Hb now normal eg treated AML, may be venesected to remove iron.
- Regular treatment is required in transfusion dependent children if they are to avoid the consequences of iron overload in the second decade of life.
- SC administration of desferrioxamine by portable syringe pump over 9–12h on 5–7 nights/week is a common regimen.
- Ascorbic acid supplementation may help mobilise iron and increase excretion with desferrioxamine but can cause hazardous redistribution of storage iron.
- Early and regular desferrioxamine infusion ↓ hepatic iron and improves hepatic function, promotes growth and sexual development and protects against heart disease and early death.
- Much work has been expended in the search for an effective non-toxic oral chelator and deferiprone is currently under evaluation in clinical trials.

Natural history
The prognosis of the underlying haematological condition in transfusion-dependent elderly patients may eliminate the need for iron chelation. In others with a longer life expectancy, IV infusion of desferrioxamine with each blood transfusion may adequately delay the rate of iron accumulation.

Other causes of haemosiderosis

Dietary iron overload may also occur as a result of chronic over-ingestion of iron-containing traditional home-brewed fermented maize beverages peculiar to sub-Saharan Africa, which overwhelms physiological controls on iron absorption. Iron stores may >50g and iron is initially deposited in both hepatocytes and Kupffer cells but when cirrhosis develops, accumulates in the pancreas, heart and other organs. Over-ingestion of medicinal iron may possibly have a similar though less dramatic effect but is certainly harmful to patients with iron-loading disorders. The excessive iron absorption seen in patients with chronic liver disease is associated with accumulation in Kupffer cells rather than hepatic parenchyma. Rare congenital defects associated with iron overload have been reported.

White blood cell abnormalities 3

Neutrophilia

Neutrophils derived from same precursor as monocyte. Cytoplasm contains granules; nucleus has 3–4 segments. Functions include chemotaxis – neutrophils migrate to sites of inflammation by chemotactic factors eg complement components (C5a & C3), arachidonic acid metabolites, and peptides. Cytotoxic activity is via phagocytosis and destruction of particles/invading microorganisms (latter often antibody coated = *opsonised*). Granules contain cationic proteins → lyse gram negative bacteria, 'defensins', myeloperoxidase – interacts with H_2O_2 and HCl → hypochlorous acid (HOCl); lysozyme (hydrolyses bacterial cell walls); superoxide (O_2^-) and hydroxyl (OH^-) radicals. Neutrophil lifespan is ~1–2d in tissues.

Normal neutrophil count 2.0–7.5 $\times$ 10^9/l (neonate differs from adult; *see* Normal ranges).

Neutrophilia is defined as absolute neutrophil count >7.5 $\times$ 10^9/l.

Mechanisms
- Increased production.
- Accelerated/early release from marrow → blood.
- Demargination (marginal pool → circulating pool).

Causes
- Infection (bacterial, viral, fungal, spirochaetal, rickettsial).
- Inflammation (trauma, infarction, vasculitis, rheumatoid disease, burns).
- Chemicals eg drugs, hormones, toxins, haemopoietic growth factors eg G-CSF, GM-CSF, adrenaline, corticosteroids, venoms.
- Physical agents eg cold, heat, burns, labour, surgery, anaesthesia.
- Haematological eg myeloproliferative disease, CML, PRV, myelofibrosis.
- Other malignancies.
- Cigarette smoking.
- Post-splenectomy.
- Chronic bleeding.
- Idiopathic.

Investigation
Full history and examination. Ask about cigarette smoking, symptoms suggesting occult malignancy.

Other investigations
LAP/NAP score occasionally useful: ↑ in inflammatory disorders and most causes of neutrophilia but ↓ in CML & PNH.

Treatment
Usually treatment of underlying disorder is all that is required.

Leukaemoid reaction
May resemble leukaemia (hence name); see ↑ WBC (myeloblasts and promyelocytes prominent). Occurs in severe and/or chronic infection, metastatic malignancy.

Neutropenia

Defined as absolute peripheral blood neutrophil count of < 2.0×10^9/l.
Racial variation: blacks & Middle Eastern people may have neutrophil count of < 1.5×10^9/l.

Congenital neutropenia syndromes

Kostmann's syndrome: see Paediatric haematology, p380.

Chediak-Higashi: see Paediatric haematology, p378–379.

Shwachman-Diamond syndrome: see Paediatric haematology, p371, 380.

Miscellaneous: transcobalamin II deficiency, reticular dysgenesis.

Acquired neutropenia

Commonest causes:

Infection	Viral, eg influenza, HIV (inhibits progenitor cells), hepatitis, overwhelming bacterial sepsis
Drugs	Anticonvulsants (eg phenytoin) Antithyroid (eg carbimazole) Phenothiazines (eg chlorpromazine) Antiinflammatory agents (eg phenylbutazone) Antibacterial agents (eg cotrimoxazole) Others (gold, penicillamine, tolbutamide, mianserin, imipramine, cytotoxics)
Immune mediated	Autoimmune (antineutrophil antibodies) SLE Felty's syndrome (Rheumatoid arthritis + neutro-penia + splenomegaly; no correlation between spleen size and degree of neutropenia) Cyclical (3–4 week periodicity; often 21 day cycle, lasts 3–6 days)
As part of pancytopenia	
Bone marrow failure	Leukaemia, lymphoma, haematinic deficiency, anorexia
Splenomegaly (any cause)	

Clinical features – when severe neutropenia: throat/mouth infection, oral ulceration, septicaemia.

Diagnosis – examine peripheral blood film, check haematinics, autoimmune profile, anti-neutrophil antibodies, haematinics, bone marrow aspirate and trephine biopsy if indicated (eg severe or prolonged neutropenia, or features suggestive of infiltration of marrow failure syndrome).

Treatment consists of prompt antibiotic therapy if infection, IVIg and corticosteroids may be helpful but effects unpredictable. In seriously ill patients consider use of G-CSF (need to exclude underlying leukaemia before starting therapy with growth factors). Consider prophylaxis with low dose antibiotics (eg ciprofloxacin 250mg bd) and antifungal (eg fluconazole 100mg od) agents. Drug-induced neutropenia usually recovers on stopping suspected agent (may take 1–2 weeks).

Lymphocytosis and lymphocytopenia

Lymphocytes are small cells with high N:C ratio; some (eg natural killer cells) have prominent cytoplasmic granules. Two principal types: B and T lymphocyte. B cells express monoclonal surface (not cytoplasmic) IgM and often IgD. B cell stimulation through cross linkage of surface Ig molecules or via effector T cells causes their differentiation into plasma cells. Predominant role is humoral immunity via Ig secretion.

T cells are derived from stem cells that undergo maturation in thymus and express T cell receptor molecule (CD3) on cell surface. Responsible for cell-mediated immunity eg delayed hypersensitivity, graft rejection, contact allergy, and cytotoxic reactions against other cells.

Lymphocytosis (peripheral blood lymphocytes >4.5 × 10⁹/l)

- Leukaemias and lymphomas including: CLL, NHL, Hodgkin's disease, acute lymphoblastic leukaemia, hairy cell leukaemia, Waldenström's macroglobulinaemia, heavy chain disease, mycosis fungoides, Sézary syndrome, large granular lymphocyte leukaemia, adult T cell leukaemia lymphoma (ATLL).
- Infections eg EBV, CMV, *Toxoplasma gondii*, rickettsial infection, *Bordetella pertussis*, mumps, varicella, Coxsackie, rubella, hepatitis virus, adenovirus.
- 'Stress' eg myocardial infarction, sickle crisis.
- Trauma.
- Rheumatoid disease (occasionally).
- Adrenaline.
- Vigorous exercise.
- Post-splenectomy.
- β thalassaemia intermedia.

Lymphocytopenia (peripheral blood lymphocytes <1.5 × 10⁹/l)

- Malignant disease eg Hodgkin's disease, some NHL, non-haematopoietic cancers, angioimmunoblastic lymphadenopathy.
- MDS.
- Collagen vascular disease eg rheumatoid, SLE, GvHD.
- Infections eg HIV.
- Chemotherapy.
- Surgery.
- Burns.
- Liver failure.
- Renal failure (acute & chronic).
- Anorexia nervosa.
- Iron deficiency (uncommon).
- Aplastic anaemia.
- Cushing's.
- Sarcoidosis.
- Congenital disorders (rare) such as SCID, reticular dysgenesis, agammaglobulinaemia (Swiss type), thymic aplasia (di George's syndrome), ataxia telangiectasia.

Eosinophilia

Differential diagnosis

Common
- Drugs (huge list eg gold, sulphonamides, penicillin); erythema multiforme (Stevens-Johnson syndrome).
- Parasitic infections: hookworm, *Ascaris,* tapeworms, filariasis, amoebiasis, schistosomiasis.
- Allergic syndromes – asthma, eczema, urticaria.

Less common
- Pemphigus.
- Dermatitis herpetiformis (DH).
- Polyarteritis nodosa (PAN).
- Sarcoid.
- Tumours esp. Hodgkin's.
- Irradiation.

Rare
- Hypereosinophilic (Loeffler's) syndrome.
- Eosinophilic leukaemia.
- AML with eosinophilia esp. M4Eo (see p146).

Discriminating clinical features
- Drugs – history of exposure, time course of eosinophilia with resolution on cessation of drug.
- Allergic conditions – history of eczema, urticaria or typical rashes. Symptoms and signs of asthma.
- Parasites – history of exposure from foreign travel, symptoms and signs of iron deficiency anaemia (hookworm is commonest cause world-wide). Blood film may show filariasis. Stool microscopy and culture for ova, cysts and parasites for Amoebiasis, *Ascaris, Taenia,* schistosomiasis.
- Skin diseases – typical appearances confirmed by biopsy e.g. DH and Pemphigus.
- PAN – renal failure, neuropathy, angiography and ANCA positivity.
- Sarcoid – multi-system features with non-caseating granulomata in biopsy of affected tissue or on BM biopsy; high serum ACE.
- Hodgkin's – lymphadenopathy, hepatosplenomegaly – BM or node biopsy.
- Hypereosinophilic syndrome – history of allergy, cough, fever and pulmonary infiltrates on CXR, may be cardiac involvement. Eosinophils on blood film have normal morphology and granulation. Diagnosis on exclusion of similar causes.
- Eosinophilic leukaemia – eosinophils on blood film have abnormal morphology with hyperlobular and hypergranular forms. BM heavily infiltrated with same abnormal cells. Other signs of myeloproliferative disease may be present.
- AML M4 Eo – blasts with myelomonoblastic features on BM and blood film (see p146).

Basophilia and basopenia

Basophils are found in peripheral blood and marrow (= mast cells in tissues). Short lifespan (1–2d), cannot replicate. Degranulation results in hypersensitivity reactions (IgE F_c receptors trigger), flushing, etc.

Basophilia (peripheral blood basophils >0.1 × 10^9/l)

- Myeloproliferative disorders

  CGL
  Other chronic myeloid leukaemias
  PRV
  Myelofibrosis
  Essential thrombocythaemia
  Basophilic leukaemia.

- AML (rare).
- Hypothyroidism.
- IgE-mediated hypersensitivity reactions.
- Inflammatory disorders eg rheumatoid disease, ulcerative colitis.
- Drugs eg oestrogens.
- Infection eg viral.
- Irradiation.
- Hyperlipidaemia.

Basopenia (peripheral blood basophils <0.1 × 10^9/l)

- As part of generalised leucocytosis eg infection, inflammation.
- Thyrotoxicosis.
- Haemorrhage.
- Cushing's syndrome.
- Allergic reaction.
- Drugs eg progesterone.

Monocytosis and monocytopenia

Bone marrow monocytes give rise to blood monocytes and tissue macrophages. Part of reticuloendothelial system (RES). Other components of RES: lung alveolar macrophages; pleural and peritoneal macrophages; Kupffer cells in liver; histiocytes; renal mesangial cells; macrophages in lymph node, spleen and marrow.

Contain 2 sets of granules (i) lysosomal (acid phosphatase, arylsulphatase and peroxidase), and (ii) function of second set unknown.

Monocytosis (peripheral blood monocytes >0.8 × 10⁹/l)

Common
- Malaria, trypanosomiasis, typhoid (commonest world-wide causes).
- Post-chemotherapy or stem cell transplant esp. if GM-CSF used.
- Tuberculosis.
- Myelodysplasia (MDS).

Less common
- Infective endocarditis.
- Brucellosis.
- Hodgkin's lymphoma.
- AML (M4 or M5).

Discriminating clinical features
- Malaria: identification of parasites on thick and thin blood films.
- Trypanosomiasis: parasites seen on blood film, lymph node biopsy or blood cultures.
- Typhoid: blood culture, faecal and urine culture and BM culture.
- Infective endocarditis: cardiac signs and blood cultures.
- Tuberculosis: AFB seen and cultured in sputum, EMU, blood or BM, tuberculin positivity on intradermal challenge, caseating granulomata on biopsy of affected tissue or BM.
- Brucellosis: blood cultures and serology.
- Hodgkin's: lymphadenopathy, hepatosplenomegaly, eosinophilia, biopsy of node or BM.
- MDS: typical dysplastic features on blood film or BM (see p176).
- AML(M4 or M5): monoblasts on blood film and BM biopsy. Skin and gum infiltration common see p146.

Monocytopenia (peripheral blood monocytes <0.2 × 10⁹/l)
- Autoimmune disorders eg SLE.
- Hairy cell leukaemia.
- Drugs eg glucocorticoids, chemotherapy.

Mononucleosis syndromes

Definition
Constitutional illness associated with atypical lymphocytes in the blood.

Clinical features
Peak incidence in adolescence: may be subclinical or acute presentation consisting of fever, lethargy, sweats, anorexia, pharyngitis, lymphadenopathy (cervical > axillary > inguinal), tender splenomegaly ± hepatomegaly, palatal petechiae, maculopapular rash especially if given ampicillin. Rarely also pericarditis, myocarditis, encephalitis. Usually self-limiting illness but complications include lethargy persisting for months or years (chronic fatigue syndrome), depression, autoimmune haemolytic anaemia, thrombocytopenia, secondary infection and splenic rupture.

Causes
EBV, CMV, *Toxoplasma, Brucella*, Coxsackie and adenoviruses, HIV seroconversion illness.

Pathophysiology
In EBV related illness, EBV infection of B lymphocytes results in immortalisation and generates a T cell response (the *atypical lymphocytes*) which controls EBV proliferation. In severe immunodeficiency following prolonged use of cyclosporin, oligoclonal EBV-related lymphoma may develop which usually regresses with reduction of immunosuppressive therapy but may evolve to a monoclonal and aggressive lymphoma eg after MUD stem cell transplant. In malarial Africa, EBV infection is associated with an aggressive lymphoma – Burkitt's lymphoma see p166, 168, 392.

Diagnosis–haematological features
- Atypical lymphocytes on blood film (recognised by the dark blue cytoplasmic edge to cells and invagination (scalloping) around red blood cells).
- Usually lymphocytosis with mild neutropenia.
- Occasionally anaemia due to cold antibody mediated haemolysis (anti-i)–identify with cold haemagglutinin titre.
- Paul Bunnell/monospot test for presence of heterophile antibody +ve when cause is EBV but only in the first few weeks. False +ves can occur in lymphoma.
- ↑ bilirubin and abnormal LFTs.
- Serological testing should include EBV capsid Ag, CMV IgM, *Toxoplasma* titre, *Brucella* titre, HIV 1 and 2 Ag and Ab.
- Immunophenotype of peripheral blood B lymphocytes shows polyclonality (distinguishes from lymphoma and other lymphoproliferative disorders).

Treatment
Rest and symptom relief are mandatory. No other specific treatment has been shown to influence outcome.

Leukaemia and lymphoma 4

Acute myeloid leukaemia

Malignant tumour of haemopoietic precursor cells of non-lymphoid lineage, almost certainly arising in the bone marrow.

Incidence

~1 in 10,000 annually. Increasing frequency with age (median 60 years). Cause unclear – association with heavy radiation dose exposure eg post-Chernobyl disaster, chronic benzene exposure, alkylating agents and hereditary predisposition in Down's and Fanconi's syndromes, pre-existing myeloproliferative disorders.

Classification – morphological (French-American-British, FAB)

M0 – Undifferentiated

M1 – Early myeloblastic (minimal differentiation)

M2 – late myeloblastic (differentiation)

M3 – promyelocytic

M4 – myelomonocytic

M5 – monoblastic

M6 – erythroleukaemic

M7 – megakaryoblastic.

- Immunophenotyping useful in diagnosis of M0, 4, 5, 6 and 7 (see p540).
- Cytogenetics important in detecting translocations and deletions.
  - t(15;17) in M3
  - t(8;21) in M2
  - inv(16) in M4Eo, are all associated with better prognosis.
  - monosomy 7 and multiple breakages are poor prognosis.

Clinical features

- Acute presentation common; often critically ill.
- Common symptoms include malaise, sweats, anaemic symptoms (breathlessness, faintness and palpitations).
- Infections – particularly chest, mouth, perianal, skin (Staph, *Pseudomonas*, HSV, *Candida*).
- Bleeding, purpura, menorrhagia and bleeding nose, gums, rectal, retina (especially M3 – DIC), and gum and skin infiltration (M4, M5).
- Leucostatic signs eg hypoxia, retinal haemorrhage, or diffuse pulmonary shadowing.

Investigations and diagnosis

- FBC and blood film.
- Bone marrow aspirate and biopsy.
- Total WBC usually ↑↑ with blast cells on film – but may be low.
- Hb and Plts usually ↓.
- Marrow heavily infiltrated with blasts (>30%) – immunophenotyping and karyotyping on blood and marrow allows classification as above.
- Further recommended investigations – see p452.

Emergency treatment

- Seek expert help immediately.
- Cardiovascular and respiratory resuscitation may be needed if septic shock or massive haemorrhage.

- Leucapheresis if peripheral blast count high or signs of leucostasis (retinal haemorrhage, reduced conscious level, diffuse pulmonary shadowing on CXR, or hypoxia).

Supportive treatment
- Give explanation and offer counselling.
- RBC and platelet transfusion support will continue through treatment.
- Start neutropenic regimen (see p460) as prophylaxis.
- Start hydration and allopurinol PO.
- Insert tunnelled central venous catheter (see p480).

Specific treatment
- Enter patient into MRC or other high quality trial if possible. MRC randomised studies in acute leukaemia are based on large patient numbers eg 2000, and on comparison of incremental experimental therapy with best treatment arm from previous trials.
- Treatment protocols are age related; patients >60 only tolerate less intensive treatments and very rarely transplantation.
- Supportive treatment alone is a valid treatment option in the >75 age group or if coexistent serious general medical problems.
- Outline treatment for patients <60 years is 4–5 courses of intensive combination chemotherapy, each lasting 5–10 days with a 2–3 week period of profound myelosuppression.
- Allogeneic or autologous stem cell transplantation are options for younger patients.
- Major complications are infective episodes which may be bacterial (Gram +ve and Gram −ve), fungal (*Candida* and *Aspergillus*), and less commonly viral (esp. HSV, HZV).
- In the longer term, relapse is the main complication.

Prognosis
Great variation with age and risk group. Worst prognostic group is age >60, high WBC, >20% marrow blasts after induction chemotherapy course 1, and CNS disease. Young patients <30 with t(15;17) M3 disease have >80% chance of cure, whereas patients >60 with poor risk cytogenetics have <10% chance of cure. Overall figures for all patients <60 are ~35% chance of cure with chemotherapy alone rising to 45% with additional transplant procedure whereas patients >60 have 15% chance of cure.

Acute lymphoblastic leukaemia

Malignant tumour of haemopoietic precursor cells of the lymphoid lineage probably arising from the marrow in most cases.

Incidence
Commonest malignancy in childhood with the majority of cases in the 2–10 age group (median 3.5 years). Rare leukaemia in adults, ~1 in 70,000 annually, ie ~7 times less common than AML. In adults, there is further slight peak in old age.

Aetiology

Unclear. Known predisposing factors are high dose radiation, eg in Chernobyl survivors, chronic benzene exposure and hereditary predisposition in Down's and Fanconi's syndromes. Chemicals, pollution, viruses, urban/rural population movements, father's radiation exposure, radon levels and proximity to power lines have all been postulated.

Classification – morphological (French-American-British, FAB)

L1	Commonest, small homogeneous blasts, single nucleolus
L2	blasts larger, more pleomorphic and multinucleolate
L3	blasts larger, strongly basophilic and have cytoplasmic vacuoles – associated with B cell phenotype

- Immunophenotyping – lymphocyte maturation markers distinguishes early or null cell ALL from pre-B or common ALL – the most frequent group. <10% are T cell lineage and <5% B cell lineage showing T and B lymphocyte markers respectively.
- Karyotypic analysis – identifies some risk groups of which the presence of the Philadelphia chromosome is poor risk and occurs in 10–20% of cases.

Clinical features – acute, seriously ill presentation is common
- Malaise, sweats, weight loss, anorexia, anaemic symptoms, infections particularly upper and lower respiratory tracts, skin lesions, purpura, nosebleeds, gum bleeding on tooth brushing.
- Signs include widespread lymphadenopathy, mild to moderate splenomegaly, hepatomegaly and orchidomegaly.
- Leucostatic signs (eg diffuse pulmonary shadowing, hypoxia and retinal haemorrhage).
- SVC obstruction may occur with mediastinal nodes.
- CNS signs include altered consciousness, cranial nerve palsies especially of facial VII nerve, sensory disturbances and meningism.

Investigations and diagnosis
- FBC and blood film, bone marrow aspirate and biopsy.
- Total WBC usually high with blast cells on film but may be low (previously known as aleukaemic leukaemia).
- Hb and platelets often low and clotting may be deranged.
- BM heavily infiltrated with blasts – immunophenotyping and karyotyping on blood and marrow allows classification as above.
- CXR and CT scan needed if B or T cell phenotype for abdominal or mediastinal LNs respectively.
- LP mandatory (note – fundoscopy, CT head scan and platelet transfusion usually required).

Leukaemia and lymphoma

Treatment – emergency
- Seek expert help immediately.
- Cardiovascular and respiratory resuscitation may be needed if septic shock or massive haemorrhage.
- Leucapheresis may be needed if peripheral blast count high or signs of leucostasis (retinal haemorrhage, reduced conscious level, diffuse pulmonary shadowing on CXR or hypoxia).
- LP if meningism (note precautions above).

Supportive treatment
- Provide explanation and offer counselling – the disease label and duration of treatment are often distressing.
- RBC and platelet transfusion support will continue through treatment.
- Start neutropenic regimen (see p460) as prophylaxis against infections.
- Start hydration and allopurinol (see p470 Tumour lysis syndrome).
- Insert tunnelled central venous catheter.

Specific
- Enter patient into MRC or other high quality trial if possible.

Treatment plan
- 2 phase induction chemotherapy to induce remission, *then*
- 2 or 3 intensification blocks of further chemotherapy interspersed with intrathecal methotrexate × 6 ± 3 cycles of IV methotrexate or cranial irradiation as CNS prophylaxis.
- Out-patient based chemotherapy (2 years), known as *maintenance* therapy.
- Transplant options
  - Allogeneic and autologous transplantation largely reserved for children who relapse but considered in first CR adults <60 especially if Philadelphia chromosome positive disease.
  - Major complications are infective episodes which may be bacterial (Gram +ve and Gram –ve), viral (esp. HSV, HZV) and fungal (*Candida* and *Aspergillus*).
- In the longer term, relapse is the main complication.

Prognosis
Childhood ALL now has a cure rate of >70% overall and up to 90% in the best prognostic group ie girls aged 1–10 years with low presenting WBC, no CNS disease and absence of Philadelphia chromosome who achieve CR after first phase induction chemotherapy. This is perhaps the finest example of the achievements of modern intensive, combination chemotherapy. Unfortunately, the adult results are less good. Young patients in the best prognostic group with allogeneic BMT after chemotherapy may have 40% cure rate, but overall for adults <60, the cure rate is <20%.

Chronic myeloid leukaemia

Definition
Malignant tumour of an early haemopoietic progenitor cell. The clonal marker is found in all three lineages – erythroid, myeloid and megakaryocytoid demonstrating its primitive origin.

Incidence
Rare disease with a frequency of 1.25 per 100,000. Rare in children and incidence peak is 40–60 years with slight male excess. Irradiation is only known epidemiological factor.

Classification
Haematologically grouped with the myeloproliferative disorders (p187) with which it shares a number of clinical features. However, it also has certain unique biological properties:

- Characterised in >90% patients by the presence of the Philadelphia chromosome (Ph). Balanced translocation between chromosomes 9 and 22 (t9;22) involving two genes, *bcr* and *abl* that fuse to form a hybrid gene *bcr-abl* on chromosome 22 – produces an aberrant protein, which is a tyrosine kinase. Precise action of new enzyme not clear but appears a necessary, but not sufficient, prerequisite for leukaemogenesis. Interestingly, many patients lacking Ph chromosome by standard karyotypic analysis show the presence of *bcr/abl* fusion gene by molecular analysis.
- 3 phases of the disease – *chronic phase, accelerated phase* and *blast crisis.*
- May present with any phase, most commonly chronic phase.
- Duration of chronic phase varies (3 months to 22 years – median 4.5 years).
- All cases eventually transform to blast crisis.

Clinical symptoms and signs
- Many patients asymptomatic and present as incidental finding on FBC performed for another reason eg routine surgery.
- Fatigue, weight loss, sweating.
- Enlargement of spleen may cause (L) hypochondrial pain, easy satiety and sensation of abdominal fullness.
- Gout, bruising, splenic infarction and occasionally priapism.
- Signs include moderate to large splenomegaly, hepatomegaly.
- Occasional leucostatic signs at presentation.

Diagnosis and investigations
- FBC and blood film shows ↑ WBC, mainly neutrophils and myelocytes plus excess basophils and eosinophils.
- Platelets may be raised and clumped on film.
- ESR and NAP score low in absence of secondary infection.
- LDH and urate levels ↑.
- BM – gross hypercellularity and Ph+ve on chromosomal analysis.
- Blast count rises with blast crisis transition.

Treatment
- Incurable without allogeneic transplantation – option available to few.
- Hydroxyurea is maintenance drug of choice for controlling WBC. Maintenance 1–1.5g PO od. Side-effects: rash, mouth ulcers and diarrhoea.
- IFN-α SC may produce cytogenetic response (reducing % Ph +ve cells).
- All patients on IFN-α have longer survival than those on hydroxyurea.

- 15% may achieve major or complete cytogenetic response (>65% Ph –ve cells). This cohort has greatly improved survival but IFN-α side-effects (malaise, febrile reactions, anorexia and weight loss, depression) may reduce quality of life.
- Sibling-matched allogeneic stem cell transplant is treatment of choice for age <50 unless already have major cytogenetic response, but only 30% will have sibling match.
- MUD allogeneic transplant, if available should be used for <25 age group and considered <40 years but transplant related mortality rises up to 45%.

Complications

- Modest increased infection risk – sometimes atypical organisms.
- Acceleration to blast crisis (80% myeloid, 20% lymphoid).
- Lymphoid blast crisis treatable with modified ALL protocol.
- Myeloid blast crisis usually refractory to conventional chemotherapy.

Prognosis

Overall median survival 5.5 years (range 3 months–22 years). Bad prognostic factors in chronic phase are higher age, larger spleen size, height of WBC, high blast cell percentage in the marrow. Survival improvement with IFN-α not yet quantified. Sibling matched allogeneic transplant (all ages 5 year median survival 60%). MUD transplant (all ages – 5 year median survival 40%). Blast crisis overall median survival – 6 months.

Chronic lymphocytic leukaemia

Commonest adult leukaemia. Predominantly disease of elderly (median age at diagnosis 65 years). ♂:♀ incidence ~2:1. Characterised by peripheral blood lymphocytosis with variable degrees of infiltration of bone marrow, lymph nodes, spleen and liver. 98% are B cell; T cell in 2%.

Aetiology
Incidence rises with increasing age. Small proportion are familial.

Clinical features and presentation

- Often asymptomatic; lymphocytosis (>5.0 × 10^9/l) identified on FBC carried out for unrelated reasons.
- With more advanced disease – lymphadenopathy: painless, often symmetrical, splenic enlargement, hepatomegaly, anaemia, neutropenia and thrombocytopenia (BM infiltration).
- Autoimmune phenomena occur; DAT +ve in 10–20% cases, warm antibody AIHA in <50% these cases. Autoimmune thrombocytopenia in 1–2%.
- Recurrent infection due secondary acquired hypogammaglobulinaemia.
- Weight loss, night sweats, general malaise.

Diagnosis

FBC	Lymphocytosis >5.0 × 10^9/l, anaemia, thrombocytopenia & neutropenia usually absent in early stage CLL; autoimmune haemolysis ± thrombocytopenia (any stage)
Blood film	Lymphocytosis with 'mature' appearance, a percentage of cells are more friable → 'smear' cells
Immunophenotyping	See table
Immunoglobulins	Panhypogammaglobulinaemia commonly present, monoclonal paraprotein in <5% cases
Bone marrow	Lymphocytosis >25% with characteristic immunophenotypic marker pattern
Trephine biopsy	Infiltration is prognostically informative; nodular (favourable) or diffuse (unfavourable)
Lymph node biopsy	Lymphocytic lymphoma
Cytogenetic/molecular	Analysis in ~50% cases show abnormalities including trisomy 12, abnormalities of 13, 14q+ and 11

Clinical assessment

Clinical history & findings – document symptoms, weight, clinical signs of disease, eg lymph node enlargement, splenomegaly.

Imaging – CXR, abdominal USS ± CT scanning useful in identifying mediastinal & retroperitoneal lymphadenopathy.

Other tests – baseline U & E, LFTs, LDH, β2-microglobulin.

Clinical management
- Confirm diagnosis.
- Early cases with lymphocytosis only rarely require BM examination.

Leukaemia and lymphoma

- Patients are classified according to one of the accepted international staging systems which document the status of disease at the time of treatment and are prognostic. The two accepted staging systems are shown.
- Patients with asymptomatic lymphocytosis simply require monitoring.

Rai staging

		Median survival (years)
0	Lymphocytosis alone – low risk	14.5
I	Lymphocytosis, lymphadenopathy – intermediate risk	7.5
II	Lymphocytosis, spleen ± liver enlargement – intermediate risk	7.5
III	Lymphocytosis, anaemia (Hb 11.0 g/dl) – high risk	2.5
IV	Lymphocytosis, thrombocytopenia (platelets <100 x10^9/l not due to autoimmune effects) – high risk	2.5

Binet staging

		Median survival (years)
A	Lymphocytosis <3 areas of lymphadenopathy	14.0
B	Lymphocytosis ≥ 3 areas of lymphadenopathy	5.0
C	Compromised BM function – anaemia, thrombocytopenia + A or B above	2.5

- If evidence of advanced disease perform BM biopsy as part of the staging.
- Chemotherapy reserved for patients with symptomatic or progressive disease, eg disease-related symptoms, doubling of lymphocytosis <6 months, bulky lymphadenopathy, hepatosplenomegaly.
- Advise patients to report infection promptly since immunocompromised ± added effects of hypogammaglobulinaemia.
- IVIg will reduce recurrent infections but no effect on survival.
- Manage symptomatic autoimmune complications with corticosteroids.
- Chlorambucil is standard therapy – low dose continuous form or intermittently until disease stabilised. Long-term exposure increases risk of 2° leukaemia or myelodysplasia. Cyclophosphamide is effective alternative.
- Avoid steroids unless autoimmune complications.
- DXT helpful for persistent or bulky lymphadenopathy; splenic irradiation is sometimes helpful in frail patients unfit for splenectomy.
- Consider splenectomy for patients with massive splenomegaly.
- New therapies, eg purine analogues fludarabine and 2-CDA induce apoptosis in CLL. Response rate is greater and incidence of remission higher but do not appear curative. Currently second line treatment. *Note:* purine analogues cause ↓ circulating CD4+ cells with risk of opportunistic infection.
- PBSCT has been carried out after high dose chemotherapy ± TBI for younger (<55 years) patients who achieve remission with fludarabine. Investigative treatment at present.
- Allografting – limited success in small numbers of younger, symptomatic patients with HLA-matched siblings.

Natural history

Most patients with early stage, asymptomatic CLL die of other, unrelated causes. Infection is major cause of morbidity & mortality in symptomatic patients. Advanced stage patients eventually develop refractory disease. Terminally some refractory patients show prolymphocytic transformation, a minority (<3%) show evidence of high grade lymphomatous change (Richter's syndrome).

Cell markers in chronic lymphoproliferative disorders

Chronic B cell leukaemia and NHL

Marker	CLL	PLL	HCL*	SLVL	FL	PCL
Surface Ig	+	++	++	++	++	−
Cyto Ig	−	−/+	−/++	−/++	−	++
CD5	+	−/+	−	−	−	−
CD22	−/+	++	++	++	++	−
CD19	++	++	++	++	++	−
CD10	−	−/+	−	−	+	−/+
CD38	−	−	−	−	−	+

Mature T cell leukaemias

Marker	T-CLL	T-PLL	ATLL	Sézary
CD2	+	+	+	−
CD3	+	+/−	+	+
CD4	−	+/−	+	+
CD8	+	−/+	−	−
CD5	−	+	+	+
CD7	−/+	++	−	−
CD25	−	−/+	++	−/+

Legend: CLL, chronic lymphocytic leukaemia; PLL, prolymphocytic leukaemia; HCL, hairy cell leukaemia; SLVL, splenic lymphoma with villous lymphocytes; FL, follicular lymphoma; PCL, plasma cell leukaemia; T-CLL, T cell CLL; T-PLL, T cell PLL; ATLL, adult T cell leukaemia/lymphoma; Sézary, Sézary syndrome. *HCL shows typical reactivity with specific HCL markers.

Leukaemia and lymphoma

Large granular lymphocyte leukaemia

Clonal lymphoproliferative disorder, characterised by an increase in LGLs in blood. Heterogeneous disorder – better characterisation with new molecular techniques.

Clinical presentation
- Asymptomatic, large granular lymphocytosis an incidental finding on FBC.
- Recurrent bacterial infections.
- Arthralgia, itching, mouth ulcers
- Splenomegaly recorded in 50% cases. Some patients described as Felty's syndrome.

Laboratory findings
- Hb and platelets usually normal; mild anaemia may be present.
- Mild/moderate lymphocytosis; cells are large with abundant cytoplasm and distinct granules.
- Lymphocytes may type as typical NK cells eg CD3– CD8– CD56+ or as CD3+ CD8+ CD56–.
- Clonal T-cell receptor gene rearrangement, typically $\gamma\delta$ may be present.
- Polyclonal increase in Igs.
- May be +ve autoimmune serology, rheumatoid and antinuclear factors.

Management
Condition is incurable. Those patients in whom a clonal disorder is established by $\gamma\delta$ rearrangements ie a true leukaemia have a more aggressive course. In contrast, patients with polyclonal disease associated with rheumatoid factor and modest neutropenia may run a more benign course. Care is essentially supportive with prompt treatment of infection with appropriate broad spectrum antibiotics. Corticosteroids in modest dosage may improve neutropenia but can predispose to infection, including fungal infections. Chemotherapy generally unrewarding, but pulsed methotrexate may be tried.

Prolymphocytic leukaemia

Clinicopathological variant of CLL with characteristic morphology and clinical features. B-cell and T-cell forms recognised. CLL and PLL are not always easily distinguished since overlap syndromes occur.

Epidemiology

Median age at presentation is ~70 years; $\male:\female$ =2:1. Accounts for ≤8% cases of CLL. B-PLL 75%, T-PLL 25%.

Clinical features

- Constitutional symptoms, weight loss, fatigue, etc.
- Massive splenomegaly, typically >10cm below costal margin.
- Minimal lymphadenopathy in B-PLL, generalised lymphadenopathy commoner in T-PLL.
- Skin lesions seen in 25% T-PLL.

Diagnosis

- High WBC (typically >100 × 10^9/l; commonly >200 × 10^9/l in T-PLL).
- Anaemia, thrombocytopenia usually present.
- Differential shows >90% prolymphocytes.
- Morphology shows large lymphoid cells, abundant cytoplasm (B-PLL mainly), prominent single nucleolus.
- Immunophenotype: *see table p154*.
- Cytogenetics – abnormalities of chromosome 14q in 60%.

Management

Differentiation from CLL ; clinical features, morphology and markers.

Splenectomy symptomatically helpful, 'debulking', follow up with other therapy.

Splenic irradiation – symptomatic relief if unfit for splenectomy.

Combination chemotherapy – CHOP may achieve responses and prolong survival in younger patients.

Single agent chemotherapy

Fludarabine, 2-CDA or deoxycoformicin may produce responses. PLL is typically resistant to chlorambucil.

Natural history

T-PLL carries poor prognosis with median survival 6–7 months. Median survival in B-PLL is 3–4 years.

Hairy cell leukaemia and variant

Low grade B-cell lymphoproliferative disorder. Accounts for 2% of leukaemias with characteristic morphology and typically associated with pancytopenia and splenomegaly. No known aetiological factors. Presents in middle age (>45 years) with ♂:♀=4:1

Clinical features
- Non-specific fatigue, weight loss.
- 15% present with infections, often atypical organisms due to monocytopenia.
- Splenomegaly in 90% (massive in 20–30%), hepatomegaly in ≤50%.
- Lymphadenopathy uncommon.
- Pancytopenia may be an incidental finding.

Laboratory findings
- Pancytopenia on FBC; variable, moderate to severe.
- Circulating 'hairy cells' in low numbers; florid leukaemic features unusual.
- Hairy cells – kidney shaped nuclei, clear cytoplasm and irregular cytoplasmic projections.
- Neutropenia, often <1.0 × 10^9/l; monocytopenia usual.
- Cytochemistry: +ve for Tartrate Resistant Acid Phosphatase (TRAP) in 95%.
- Cell markers: *see table, p154.*
- BM: aspirate often unsuccessful – 'dry tap' due to increased BM fibrosis; trephine shows diagnostic features with focal or diffuse infiltration of HCL, cells have characteristic 'halo' of cytoplasm.

Management
Confirmation of diagnosis may be difficult because of low numbers of circulating leukaemic cells and dry tap on marrow aspiration; trephine histology usually diagnostic; differential diagnosis includes *myelofibrosis* and *other low grade lymphomas.* Asymptomatic cases with minimal haematological upset and splenomegaly do not require chemotherapy and can be observed; many will be non/slowly progressive. Active therapy reserved for symptomatic cases and those with marked pancytopenia or splenomegaly. Therapy choices include splenectomy, chemotherapy or IFN-α. Patients must always be managed supportively and treated promptly for infections. Increased incidence of atypical mycobacterial infections in HCL.

- Splenectomy – formerly treatment of choice; indicated for massive splenomegaly and beneficial in managing severe pancytopenia. Non-curative but will not compromise need for subsequent therapies.
- 2-CDA: purine analogue given as 7-day infusion will produce remission in up to 75% cases; temporarily myelosuppressive and produces period of CD4 suppression. Becoming established as best first line therapy.
- Deoxycoformycin (Pentostatin): purine analogue given as IV bolus every 1–2 weeks, remissions achieved in ~50%; also CD4 suppressive.
- IFN-α achieves a partial response in up to 75% but remissions in <10%; requires ongoing self-administration for 6–24 months. Expensive with significant incidence of side-effects.

Natural history
Hairy cell leukaemia is associated with prolonged survival, with newer agents capable of producing remissions; some patients may achieve long term cure. For

others careful application of available treatments at points of disease relapse/
progression will still allow prolonged, good quality survival.

Hairy cell variant

Describes an entity of HCL where the presenting WBC count is high due to
circulating leukaemic cells. Marrow is aspirated easily and associated neutropenia and monocytopenia are absent. Cells are larger than classical HCL,
nucleus is centrally located with a prominent nucleolus, cells are TRAP +ve.
Membrane phenotype and ultrastructure studies suggest the cells may represent
an intermediate disease between HCL and B-PLL. Response to deoxycoformycin or IFN-α appears poor but chlorambucil appears active in this form,
and the variant carries a good prognosis.

Splenic lymphoma with villous lymphocytes (SLVL)

B-cell lymphoproliferative disorder in which splenomegaly with a moderate lymphocytosis (usually <40 × 10^9/l) represent the main clinical findings. Commoner in ♂ and affects older patients, mean age at diagnosis 72 years.

Clinical & laboratory features

- Non-specific symptoms, eg fatigue.
- Moderate to massive splenomegaly.
- Lymphadenopathy rare.

- Minimal upset of neutrophils and platelets.
- Total WBC not grossly elevated (*cf.* PLL).
- Cell morphology: larger than typical CLL cells, round/oval nuclei, villous cytoplasmic projections at one/both poles of the cells.
- Immunophenotype: *see table p154.*
- BM aspirate may show lymphocytosis with typical marker pattern; biopsy may be normal but usually shows patchy/nodular lymphoid infiltration.
- Spleen histology: characteristic with nodular infiltration.

Prognosis and treatment

Generally follows an indolent course. ≥10% may require no treatment. Splenectomy recommended for bulky organ enlargement (and/or to confirm diagnosis in some cases). Progression after splenectomy may respond to chlorambucil given as for CLL.

Non-Hodgkin's lymphoma

NHL is among top 5 causes of cancer mortality in young adults. Incidence has increased in each of the last five decades.

Epidemiology

Maximal in advanced Western countries. Incidence increases with age. ♂:♀=1.5:1. Families have been described with high incidence among siblings and first degree relatives. Some associated with inherited immunodeficiency syndromes, eg Ataxia-Telangiectasia, Wiskott-Aldrich syndrome, etc. Environmental factors eg chemotherapeutic drugs, immunosuppressive drugs and radiation. Occupational associations – vinyl chloride, rubber, leather production, etc.

Viruses have role in pathogenesis of a number of lymphomas eg African (not sporadic) Burkitt's lymphoma (EBV). ATLL is associated with HTLV-1. AIDS is associated with high incidence of NHL with frequent CNS involvement.

Histopathology and classification

Several classifications eg Rappaport; Kiel; Lukes & Collins. Latest is more biologically orientated – The Revised European American Lymphoma (REAL) Classification.

Clinical features

Reflects a spectrum from *low grade lymphoma* (widely disseminated at diagnosis but follows indolent course) to *high grade lymphomas* (short history of localised rapidly enlarging lymphadenopathy ± constitutional upset). Superficial lymphadenopathy is most common presenting feature of NHL but may present with oropharyngeal involvement (5–10%), autoimmune cytopenias, GIT involvement (15%), CNS involvement (5–10%, esp. high grade NHL) or skin involvement (esp. T-cell lymphomas). Patients with GIT involvement have a higher frequency of oropharyngeal involvement (Waldeyer's ring) and vice versa.

Low grade up to 40% of cases, most common in middle/old age (median age 55 years). Generally indolent, presents with stage III or IV disease in ⅔ patients and frequently involve BM at diagnosis. May present with painless lymphadenopathy at ≥1 sites, effects of BM infiltration or constitutional symptoms. Median survival ~8 years. In ~30% may transform to more aggressive histology often resistant to treatment.

Marginal zone lymphomas take 2 forms: *mucosa-associated lymphoid tissue* (MALT) lymphomas – associated with local invasion at site tumour arises, eg stomach, small bowel, salivary gland or lung; *monocytoid B-cell lymphoma* is associated with Sjögren's syndrome – usually localised to head, neck and parotid gland. Mycosis fungoides is a T-cell lymphoma which presents as localised or generalised plaque or erythroderma associated with lymphadenopathy in 50%; median survival 10 years but prognosis worse with lymphadenopathy or visceral involvement.

Intermediate grade ~50% of cases with diffuse large B-cell NHL the most common histology – presents with stage I or II disease in 50% of patients but disseminated extranodal disease is not uncommon and ⅓ patients have constitutional symptoms. Other subtypes of intermediate grade lymphoma often present with widespread disease and are more likely than the low grade histologies to progress without treatment. Median survival ~3 years.

Leukaemia and lymphoma

REAL classification of lymphoid malignancies

I Indolent lymphomas (low risk)

B cell lineage CLL/small lymphocytic lymphoma ± plasmacytoid differentiation
lymphoplasmacytic lymphoma/immunocytoma/Waldenström's
hairy cell leukaemia
splenic marginal zone lymphoma
marginal zone B-cell lymphoma
extranodal (MALT-B-cell lymphoma)
nodal (monocytoid)
follicle centre lymphoma/follicular, (small cell)-grade I
follicle centre lymphoma/follicular, (mixed small & large cell)-grade II

T cell lineage large granular lymphocytic leukaemia, T & NK cell types
mycosis fungoides/Sézary syndrome
smouldering & chronic adult T-cell leukaemia/lymphoma (HTLV-1+)

II Aggressive lymphomas (intermediate risk)

B cell lineage prolymphocytic leukaemia
plasmacytoma/multiple myeloma
mantle cell lymphoma
follicle centre lymphoma/follicular, (large cell)-grade III
diffuse large B-cell lymphoma (includes immunoblastic & diffuse large &
        centroblastic lymphomas)
primary mediastinal (thymic) large B-cell lymphoma
high grade B-cell lymphoma, Burkitt-like

T cell lineage prolymphocytic leukaemia
peripheral T-cell lymphoma, unspecified
angioimmunoblastic lymphoma
angiocentric lymphoma
intestinal T-cell lymphoma
anaplastic large cell lymphoma (T & null cell type)

III Very aggressive lymphomas (high risk)

B cell lineage precursor B-lymphoblastic lymphoma/leukaemia
Burkitt's lymphoma/B-cell acute leukaemia
plasma cell leukaemia

T cell lineage precursor T-lymphoblastic lymphoma/leukaemia
adult T-cell lymphoma/leukaemia

IV Hodgkin's disease

Mantle cell lymphoma recently defined as a distinct histology with poor therapeutic outcome. Angio-immunoblastic lymphadenopathy is associated with constitutional symptoms, generalised lymphadenopathy, hepatosplenomegaly, skin rash, polyclonal hyperglobulinaemia, DAT+ve haemolytic anaemia and eosinophilia; ⅓ patients progress to immunoblastic lymphoma.

High grade ~10% cases of NHL. Younger patients (>50% of childhood lymphomas), aggressive tumours requiring prompt treatment. B and T-cell lymphoblastic lymphomas share features with ALL. T-cell variety usually associated with thymic mass and a ⅓ of patients present with BM involvement. Blood and CNS involvement common. *Endemic* Burkitt's lymphoma presents in childhood/adolescence with large extranodal tumours in jaw bones or abdominal viscera. *Sporadic* Burkitt's lymphoma often presents with an intra-abdominal mass arising from a Peyer's patch or mesenteric node. Median survival <2 years.

Laboratory features
- Normochromic normocytic anaemia common.
- Leucoerythroblastic film with BM infiltration ± pancytopenia.
- Hypersplenism (occasionally).
- PB may show lymphoma cells: cleaved 'buttock' cells in FL and blasts in high grade disease.
- LFTs abnormal in hepatic infiltration.
- Serum LDH is a useful prognostic factor (see p167).

Low grade – small lymphocytic lymphoma – features similar to CLL with Ig gene rearrangement (see Cell marker table p154 for immunophenotype). Follicular NHL associated with the t(14;18)(q32;q21) (see Cell marker table for immunophenotype). Marginal zone lymphomas are CD5–, CD19+.

Intermediate grade – mantle cell lymphoma has characteristic translocation t(11;14)(q13;q32); cells are CD5+, CD19+, CD20+. Translocations involving 14q and the T cell receptor are frequent in T cell NHL.

High grade – most cases of Burkitt's have translocation involving juxtaposition of *c-myc* oncogene (chromosome 8) with one of the Ig gene loci (heavy chain 75% t(8;14), λ chain 20% t(8;22), κ chain 8% t(8;2)). Endemic cases have ↑ antibody titres to EBV antigens and multiple copies of EBV DNA in the tumour (unusual in sporadic cases).

Staging investigations
- History and examination.
- Histological diagnosis: lymph node biopsy or extranodal mass.
- FBC, plasma viscosity/ESR and blood film.
- U & E, uric acid, LFTs, LDH.
- Bone marrow trephine biopsy.
- Imaging for occult sites of disease: CXR, CT of chest, abdomen and pelvis ± MRI scan, USS, LP, gallium scan.

Staging helps *define prognosis* and to *select appropriate therapy*. Also helps assess response to therapy. The Ann-Arbor staging system developed for Hodgkin's disease is widely used in NHL (see Hodgkin's disease p171).

Prognostic factors
- Histologic grade.
- Performance status.
- Constitutional symptoms.
- Age (better <60 years).

- Extranodal disease (poorer).
- Bulk disease (poorer if >10 cm).
- ↑ serum LDH (poorer if elevated).
- Prior history of low grade disease (in high grade NHL).

International Prognostic Index has been developed using age, stage, the number of extranodal sites of disease, performance status and serum LDH to identify 4 risk groups, low, low/intermediate, intermediate/high and high risk. Index has been validated for all 3 clinical grades as predictor of response to therapy, survival and relapse.

No of risk factors	Risk group	Projected 5 year survival (%)
0	Low	83
1	Low/Intermediate	69
2	Intermediate/High	46
3	High	32

NEJM 1993 **329** 987

Initial therapy

Low-grade NHL

Usually responsive to chemotherapy and radiotherapy. No convincing evidence of a curative therapy for advanced disease.

Localised low-grade NHL Involved field radiotherapy ± chemotherapy may be curative in the minority of patients with localised disease. 5-year disease-free survival >50% may be expected. Recurrence generally outside radiation field.

Advanced low-grade NHL Three approaches used: (1) watch and wait; (2) moderate chemotherapy or radiotherapy; (3) aggressive chemotherapy and radiotherapy.

Watch-and-wait Therapy may not be required for many months/years after the initial diagnosis and patients may have better quality of life and avoid exposure to chemotherapeutic agents. Patients must be monitored closely to prevent or identify promptly insidious complications. Median survival >5 years.

Moderate therapy Generally involves one of the following approaches:
- Chlorambucil (0.1–0.2 mg/kg/d or 0.4–0.6 mg/kg every 2 weeks) or cyclophosphamide (50–150 mg/d PO) as single-agents or in combination with prednisolone: response rates of 50–80%.
- Combination chemotherapy eg CVP or MCP: response rates 80–90%.
- Radiotherapy for treatment of local problems eg cord compression.

Aggressive chemotherapy High CR rates with CHOP-type regimens but continuous pattern of relapse occurs. Overall survival not convincingly improved.

Aggressive radiotherapy TBI or total lymphoid irradiation may achieve very high CR rates with 5-year DFS rates >60%.

Intermediate-grade NHL

Many can be cured by combination chemotherapy or by radiotherapy.

Localised diffuse large cell NHL Radiotherapy may be curative in patients with stage I or IE non-bulky (mass <10 cm) disease without systemic symptoms and occasional II/IIE patients.

Advanced stage intermediate-grade NHL Several chemotherapy regimens shown to have curative potential. CR rates 50% to >80%. Although CR rates to CHOP regimen have been bettered by some multi-agent regimens, long term follow-up has revealed comparable or inferior long term relapse free survival rates with greater treatment related toxicity. A prospective randomised trial comparing CHOP, m-BACOD, ProMACE-CytaBOM, and MACOP-B revealed no significant difference in response rates, time to treatment failure, or survival. Several trials have failed to demonstrate the superiority of any particular chemotherapy regimen for NHL. The CHOP regimen is widely used because of its ease of administration and relative tolerability and some 30% of patients may be cured with this approach. A common approach would be to evaluate response to therapy after 3–4 courses and complete 6 courses if complete remission has been achieved.

High-grade NHL

The use of conventional NHL chemotherapy regimens in lymphoblastic lymphoma has been disappointing. In children markedly improved results with regimens used in ALL (including CNS prophylaxis) when used for treatment of lymphoblastic lymphoma. This has led to a similar approach in adults. Although high complete response rates (up to 95%) and 5 year DFS of up to 45% have been reported, the poor outlook for patients with this condition have led to evaluation of high-dose therapy with autologous or allogeneic BMT early in its management.

High remission rates and long-term DFS have been achieved with several multi-agent chemotherapy regimens eg COMP combined with CNS prophylaxis in children with Burkitt's lymphoma. Protocols that were designed for lymphoblastic lymphoma or ALL are clearly inferior to specific Burkitt's lymphoma protocols. Most trials report 50–75% overall survival rates in childhood Burkitt's lymphoma. The therapy for adults is less well defined.

Salvage therapy

Patients failing to achieve remission with initial therapy have poor prognosis – almost all will die of progressive lymphoma without effective second-line (salvage) therapy.

Conventional chemotherapy – although relatively high CR rates have been reported with several salvage regimens, <10% patients with relapsed or refractory NHL will achieve long-term DFS.

High dose therapy and BMT

High-dose therapy and ABMT have been widely used to treat patients with relapsed or refractory intermediate or high grade NHL. Syngeneic and allogeneic transplants have been used less frequently. A significant proportion of patients can be cured with this approach. Best results are obtained when patients have NHL that is still responsive to conventional dosage therapy and undergo BMT in a state of minimal residual disease.

Hodgkin's disease

Origin of Hodgkin's disease (HD) remains uncertain over 150 years after the first description by Thomas Hodgkin in 1832.

Epidemiology

1% cancer registrations per annum. Annual incidence ~3 per 100,000 in Europe and USA (less common in Japan). Bimodal age incidence – peaks in young adulthood (20–24) and older adulthood (>60) reported. Nodular sclerosing HD is most common subtype in young adults (>75% of cases in this subtype are <40 years). Higher incidence in ♂. Associated with high socio-economic status in childhood and with Caucasian race in the USA. Familial aggregations have been reported. Considerable evidence linking EBV to HD: ↑ risk of HD in individuals with a history of infectious mononucleosis.

Clinical features

- Most common presentation is painless supradiaphragmatic lymph node enlargement
  - may be solitary rubbery cervical gland
  - often involves supraclavicular and axillary glands and other sites
- Lymphadenopathy in HD may wax and wane during observation.
- Spleen involved in ~30%.
- Abdominal lymphadenopathy is unusual without splenic involvement.
- Waldeyer's ring involvement is rare and suggests a diagnosis of NHL.
- Initial mode of spread occurs predictably to contiguous nodal chains. Supradiaphragmatic disease ± intra-abdominal involvement is the rule, and regional disease limited to subdiaphragmatic sites is uncommon.
- Bulky mediastinal and hilar lymphadenopathy may produce local symptoms (eg bronchial compression) or direct extension (eg to lung, pericardium, pleura or rib). Pleural effusions in 20%.
- Extranodal spread may also occur via bloodstream (eg to bone marrow, lung or liver). Presence of disseminated extranodal disease is generally accompanied by generalised lymphadenopathy and splenic involvement.
- ~⅓ patients have ≥1 associated 'B' symptoms at presentation, eg fever, drenching night sweats, weight loss >10% body weight during the previous 6 months. 'B' symptoms correlate with disease extent, bulk and prognosis. Further systemic symptoms associated with HD are generalized pruritus and alcohol-induced lymph node pain.

Histopathology

Histological examination of a lymph node is the diagnostic investigation. Presence of the multinucleate CD30+ Reed-Sternberg cell in association with a heterogeneous population of leucocytes and variable fibrosis is characteristic.

Four subclasses

Nodular sclerosis (NS)	good prognosis stage I-II; young ♀
Lymphocyte predominant (LP)	most favourable prognosis; children
Mixed cellularity (MC)	intermediate prognosis
Lymphocyte depleted (LD)	relatively poor prognosis; elderly

Investigation & staging

- Confirm diagnosis by biopsy (normally lymph node).
- Document 'B' symptoms in history.
- Document extent of nodal involvement by clinical examination, CXR, CT chest, abdomen and pelvis.

- Document bone marrow status by bone marrow trephine biopsy.
- ± biopsy of other suspicious sites.

Ann-Arbor staging system

Stage I   disease confined to a single lymph node site

Stage IE   localised extranodal disease is designated stage (isolated)

Stage II   ≥2 nodal sites confined to one side of the diaphragm

Stage IIE   if associated with regional lymphadenopathy

Stage III   disease confined to lymphatic tissue (including the spleen) on both sides of the diaphragm

Stage IV   involvement outside lymphatic tissue (eg BM, liver or other extranodal sites with widespread lymphoma).

A absence of constitutional symptoms

B if they have fever, weight loss >10% in 6 months or drenching night sweats

Above are used to stage the patient according to Ann-Arbor system which has strong prognostic value. Prognostic factors not reflected in the original Ann-Arbor system which may influence treatment decisions and outcome include: *disease bulk, number of involved nodal regions, distribution of intra-abdominal lymphadenopathy* and *extent of splenic involvement*. The number of involved sites in regional disease is denoted by a subscript (eg stage II_2). The extent of intra-abdominal adenopathy is also defined and denoted by a subscript (stage III_1 represents a patient with spleen or splenic hilar, coeliac, or portal node involvement; stage III_2 represents para-aortic, iliac, inguinal, or mesenteric involvement). Bulky disease (defined as maximum dimension (>10 cm) or by at least one-third mass/thorax ratio) is identifed by the subscript x. Contiguous spread to adjacent extranodal tissues is clearly distinguished from disseminated extra-nodal involvement by the subscript E. Thus a patient with a mediastinal mass might be designated II_X for bulky disease or II_E for extranodal extension of lymph node disease into adjacent tissues with a numerical subscript for the number of nodal sites involved above the diaphragm.

Clinical staging includes the initial biopsy site and all other abnormalities detected by noninvasive methods while pathological staging requires biopsy confirmation of potentially abnormal sites. The primary purpose of staging laparotomy is to determine whether radiation alone can be used for treatment. The indications for staging laparotomy in HD have decreased as a result of the wider application and success of combination chemotherapy. Laparotomy is not required in very favourable subsets of patients with early-stage supradiaphragmatic HD in whom the risk of intra-abdominal disease is <5–10% (eg clinical stage IA disease in the mediastinum; females with clinical stage IA at other supradiaphragmatic sites) or in those for whom initial chemotherapy is indicated (bulk disease best treated with combined modality, clinical stage III_2A, IIIB and IVB).

Other investigations

- FBC may show normochromic, normocytic anaemia, reactive leucocytosis, eosinophilia and/or a reactive mild thrombocytosis

171

- BM may show reactive appearances. Bone marrow involvement is most common in patients with B symptoms, clinical stage III or IV disease, or MCHD or LDHD and in patients with leucopenia or thrombocytopenia.
- Serum alkaline phosphatase may be ↑ either nonspecifically or in association with bone or liver involvement.
- ↑ serum LDH is an indicator of bulky disease.
- Gallium scanning – most useful in the anterior mediastinum to evaluate the response of bulky disease to treatment.

Initial therapy

Aim of treatment is to provide each patient with the best probability of cure while minimising acute and long-term treatment-related morbidity. The long-term survival of patients with early-stage HD is >85% and the overall 5-year survival rate for all patients is >75%.

Extended field radiotherapy

Standard treatment for most patients with stage I–IIA HD and achieves excellent long-term survival with minimal complications. An early-stage patient who has relapsed after radiation therapy alone may be cured with chemotherapy administered at relapse. A subset of patients with stage IIIA disease may be treated in the same manner. Chemotherapy is the standard treatment for most patients with stage IIIA disease and those with advanced disease (IIIB & IV). It is also the treatment of choice for most patients with 'B' symptoms. Combined modality therapy (chemotherapy followed by limited field radiotherapy) is useful for patients with bulky sites of disease but is associated with a higher risk of late neoplasia, cardiac & pulmonary toxicity.

The MOPP regimen was the standard treatment for patients with stage IIIB or IV disease for many years and produced a complete remission rate of 84% and cure in over 50%. Improved failure-free (65% at 5 years) and overall survival can be achieved with alternating monthly MOPP/ABVD or the MOPP/ABV hybrid regimen. The ABVD regimen gives comparable results as initial therapy with lower toxicity. Six to eight cycles of ABVD is the first choice regimen for patients treated outside a clinical trial. Limited-field irradiation to initial sites of bulky disease may be added in selected patients to reduce the risk of recurrence.

Salvage therapy

>50% of patients with early-stage disease relapsing from primary radiotherapy may be cured by ABVD chemotherapy. High-dose chemotherapy (BEAM or CBV) with autologous peripheral blood stem cell transplantation (PBSCT) has become the standard salvage approach for most patients relapsing after initial chemotherapy, producing high complete response rates (up to 80%), durable complete remissions in 50% and low morbidity and mortality in selected patients.

Late complications of chemotherapy

- Treatment-induced sterility is frequently seen in ♂ after treatment with MOPP and MOPP-like regimens regardless of age. The ABVD regimen produces significantly less infertility.
- Premature menopause is more common in older females.
- ABVD + mantle radiotherapy → higher incidence of post-irradiation para-mediastinal fibrosis causing persistent effort dyspnoea.

- Patients cured of HD are at an increased risk of the development of second tumours: acute myeloblastic leukemia is most common (up to 9% between 3-9 years) and is particularly associated with combined modality therapy and MOPP chemotherapy; the risk of solid tumours, notably NHL, is 7% and rises beyond 10 years.

174

Myelodysplasia 5

Myelodysplasia (MDS)

MDS describes a range of acquired clonal disorders of bone marrow. Biologically they are characterised by maturation abnormalities in one or more haemopoietic cell lines. Evidence of clonal abnormality in the form of karyotypic abnormality may be detected in up to 80% cases.

Presentation varies from minor degrees of anaemia to profound pancytopenia; circulating blast cells may be present in small numbers. Bone marrow shows maturation abnormalities with visible blast cell populations but criteria fall short of those of acute leukaemia.

Many myelodysplastic conditions do not progress, some will progress and ultimately become acute myeloid leukaemia.

MDS subtypes
- Refractory anaemia (RA).
- Refractory anaemia with ring sideroblasts (RARS).
- Refractory anaemia with excess blasts (RAEB).
- Refractory anaemia with excess blasts in transformation (RAEB-t).
- Chronic myelomonocytic leukaemia.

Aetiology & pathogenesis
Incidence of MDS increases with age; usually >50 years although juvenile MDS is recognised. Down's syndrome, previous chemotherapy, chemical exposure (eg benzene) or irradiation are recognised risk/predisposing factors.

Cytogenetic analysis of bone marrow is a key part of the diagnostic assessment of MDS. Commoner abnormalities include +8, loss of long arms of 5, 7, 9, 20 or 21, and monosomy 7. Simple or complex abnormalities may be present. Some abnormalities have prognostic significance eg 5q– generally carries a favourable prognosis whereas monosomy 7 indicates a poor prognosis.

Clinical features
- May be asymptomatic with minor degrees of macrocytic anaemia identified on FBC carried out for other reasons, including health screening.
- Symptomatic anaemia.
- Infection (neutropenia and/or impaired granulocyte function).
- Bruising or other haemorrhagic manifestations of thrombocytopenia and/or functionally deficient platelets.
- Constitutional symptoms including weight loss, sweats etc. usually feature of the more 'advanced' subgroups.

Management
Consists of supportive therapy, ie transfusions and prompt treatment of infections, etc. Most MDS patients are elderly and do not respond to chemotherapy. Younger patients with RAEB and RAEB-t should be offered intensive chemotherapy and treated identically to AML. A minority will be eligible for bone marrow allografting.

Specific prognosis and management of each subtype are described below.

FAB classification of MDS

MDS FAB Subtype	Blood	Marrow blasts (%)
RA	Monocytes <1%, Blasts <1%	<5
RARS	Monocytes <1%, Blasts <1%	<5
RAEB	Blasts <5%	5–20
RAEB-t	Blasts–variable	20–30
CMML	Monocytes >1% Blasts <5%	<20

177

Note: >30% marrow blasts indicates progression to AML

FAB classification is exclusively morphological; broadly patients with RA and RARS carry a much more favourable prognosis than those with RAEB and RAEB-t. Progression to AML or death from marrow failure related complications occurs much earlier in these latter groups with median survival generally <12 months. CMML has much more varied prognosis. Presenting Hb, neutrophil and platelet counts, as well as cytogenetic findings within each FAB subgroup provide the most helpful prognostic data for the individual patient.

French-American-British Classification JM Bennett et al 1982 Brit J Haematol 51 189

Refractory anaemia

FAB MDS classification RA. A favourable prognosis MDS.

Features
- Typically presents with mild to moderate anaemia.
- MCV usually raised 100–110fl.
- Variable degree of RBC morphological abnormality, including poikilocytosis and macrocytosis.
- Neutrophils may be normal or ↓.
- Platelets may be normal, ↓ or ↑.
- Other cause of anaemia excluded.
- RBCs – dysplastic maturation in BM; may be dysplastic changes in other cell lines.
- Reticuloendothelial Fe usually normal or ↑; few sideroblasts.
- Marrow cellularity usually normal or ↑ on trephine biopsy.
- Anaemia non-responsive to haematinics.
- Not usually transfusion dependent at presentation but some will become so.

Natural history
Prognosis usually several years (median survival 60 months); <10% may progress to AML.

Management
- Supportive – red cell transfusion. If started in younger ager group consider desferrioxamine (transfusion haemosiderosis).
- Prompt recognition and treatment of infections.

Refractory anaemia with ring sideroblasts

FAB MDS classification RARS. A favourable prognosis MDS.

Features

- Typically presents with mild to moderate anaemia.
- MCV usually raised 100–110fl.
- Variable degree of RBC morphological abnormality; film classically dimorphic with hypochromic and normochromic RBCs; poikilocytosis, macrocytosis and basophilic stippling.
- Neutrophils may be normal or ↓.
- Platelets may be normal, ↓ or ↑.
- Other cause of anaemia excluded.
- RBCs – dysplastic maturation in BM; may be dysplastic changes in other cell lines.
- Reticuloendothelial Fe usually normal or ↑.
- Ringed sideroblasts a feature and should be >15% nucleated cells in BM. Demonstrated by Perls' iron stain of BM aspirate. Ring sideroblasts are normoblastic red cell precursors that have 'blue dot' positivity around the nuclear edge – hence 'ring' sideroblasts.
- Marrow cellularity increased on trephine biopsy.
- Anaemia non-responsive to haematinics; occasional responses to pyridoxine reported.
- Not usually transfusion dependent.

Natural history

Prognosis usually several years (median survival 49 months); <10% may progress to AML.

Refractory anaemia with excess blasts and refractory anaemia with excess blasts in transformation

MDS FAB classifications RAEB and RAEB-t. Describes forms of MDS with moderate to severe degrees of marrow failure with 30–50% showing progression to AML. Distinction between RAEB and RAEB-t is arbitrary and based on marrow blast percentage of <20% for RAEB and 20–29% for RAEB-t (marrow blasts of >30% classified as AML). Overlap between RAEB and RAEB-t as well as RAEB-t and AML, due to limitations in the accuracy of visual differential counting of nucleated marrow cells, which makes precise clinical separation difficult in some cases. Marrow blasts in MDS usually express typical AML phenotype and cytochemistry features – CD13+, CD33+ and myeloperoxidase/Sudan Black positivity.

Presentation

- Moderate to severe anaemia.
- Neutropenia and thrombocytopenia generally present.
- Variable degree of RBC morphological abnormality including macrocytes, stippling, nucleated and dysplastic RBCs.
- Occasional presentation as acquired HbH disease (see p82, 90).
- Atypical maturation features in granulocyte series, eg hypogranular neutrophils, bilobed ('pseudo-Pelger') neutrophils; atypical myeloid precursors ± circulating blasts.
- Marrow cellularity variable–normal, ↑ or ↓.
- Abnormal maturation in all haematopoietic cell lines and detectable blast population on marrow aspirate smears.
- Karyotype abnormalities common, up to 80%; some with prognostic significance, eg monosomy 7 indicative of poor prognosis.

Management

Most patients with RAEB and RAEB-t are >60 years and should be managed supportively with transfusion of RBCs and platelets as clinically indicated. Symptomatic infection should be treated promptly and vigorously with broad spectrum antibiotics, IV if necessary. Median survival 6–12 months. No overall survival gain from additional measures such as low dose cytosine therapy, retinoids or growth factors.

Patients <60 years with MDS showing marrow blasts >30% should be treated as for AML; remissions are achievable in 40–50% using AML chemotherapy schedules. Fit patients in the 60–70 year age group with RAEB and RAEB-t may also be considered for chemotherapy in the absence of adverse karyotypic features. A further minority of much younger MDS patients who achieve remission also appear to benefit from bone marrow allografting.

Long term survival for chemotherapy treated MDS is achievable but rates are lower than for *de novo* presenting AML cases treated similarly.

Chronic myelomonocytic leukaemia (CMML)

Although classified with MDS it has distinctive clinical and biological behaviour.

Clinical features
- Predominantly presents in >60 year age group.
- Many asymptomatic and found on FBC done for other reasons.
- Weight loss, fatigue, night sweats occur in symptomatic patients.
- Other (reactive) causes of monocytosis need to be excluded (see p140).
- Skin and gum infiltration may be seen.
- Splenomegaly and hepatomegaly usually only in cases with symptoms and leucocytosis.
- Monocyte count $>1.0 \times 10^9$/l is diagnostic minimum, but may be much higher.
- Anaemia and leucocytosis variable.
- Platelets usually normal or ↓.
- Marrow typically hypercellular; blasts and promyelocytes <30%.
- Lysozyme raised in serum and urine.
- Hypokalaemia may be present.

Management and prognosis

Asymptomatic cases with near normal haematology apart from a monocytosis of $>1.0 \times 10^9$/l require no intervention and only occasional follow up. Therapy otherwise supportive.

Patients with symptoms organomegaly and/or high WBC may respond to oral chemotherapy with hydroxyurea or etoposide PO.

Natural history

Prognosis for asymptomatic is favourable (several years). For those requiring therapy median survival is 6–12 months. Acute myelomonocytic leukaemia (AMML) develops in ~20%; poorly responsive to intensive chemotherapy.

Myeloproliferative disorders 6

Polycythaemia

A polycythaemic state is suspected by finding a raised haematocrit/packed cell volume (PCV) although polycythaemia is defined as an increase in the total red blood cell mass (RCM). Persistent elevation of PCV >0.48 in an adult ♀ and >0.51 in adult ♂ is abnormal (*note:* PCV can be raised with a normal RCM if the plasma volume is reduced).

Clinical evaluation

Detailed clinical history with attention to detail on smoking habits, alcohol consumption and diuretic therapy. History of pruritus (especially after a warm bath) suggests primary proliferative polycythaemia (PPP). Burning sensation in fingers and toes (erythromelalgia) typical of PPP. Physical examination may identify obvious abnormalities such as gross obesity, hypertension, evidence of obstructive airways disease or cyanotic cardiac conditions. The presence of hepatomegaly or splenomegaly should be assessed. An elevated PCV in the absence of identifiable factors in clinical assessment requires referral for specialist evaluation.

Classification of polycythaemic states

- **Polycythaemia due to autonomous marrow over-activity (PPP)**
  – clonal neoplastic marrow disorder with RBC over-production independent of Epo levels.
- **2° hypoxic polycythaemias (Epo-driven ↑ in RBC production)**
  – chronic obstructive airways disease (COAD)
  – cyanotic congenital heart disease with right → left shunt
  – high altitude dwelling
  – chronic alveolar hypoventilation, eg gross obesity
  – sleep apnoea syndromes
  – altered Hb O_2 affinity or carboxyHb
  – high O_2 affinity Hb.
- **Polycythaemia due to ↑ Epo production.**
  – renal lesions eg polycystic, hypernephroma, post-renal transplantation
  – other rare tumours eg cerebellar haemangioblastoma, uterine leiomyoma.
- **Apparent polycythaemia – normal RCM with ↓ plasma volume**
  – diuretic therapy or dehydration
  – Gaisbock's syndrome (see p192)
  – Smoking, alcohol, hypertension.
- **Idiopathic erythrocytosis**
  Persistent ↑ RCM, no cause found but no clear evidence of myeloproliferative disease or PPP.

Investigation

- FBC: ↑↑ RCC and ↓ or ↔ MCV. Neutrophils and platelets ↑ in PPP (rare in other causes of polycythaemia).
- NAP score: ↑ score usually present in PPP (not diagnostic in isolation).
- Urinalysis.
- Serum U & E.
- LFTs.
- CXR (of value in COAD).
- Abdominal USS (hepatosplenomegaly, renal or pelvic abnormalities).
- Red cell volume studies: patient's red cells incubated with ^{51}Cr label and re-injected. Simultaneously plasma volume measured using ^{131}I labelled albumin. An ↑ RCM >25% of predicted is *diagnostic* of polycythaemia.

Myeloproliferative disorders

- Arterial gases/O_2 saturation (eg chronic hypoxia).
- BM examination: Trephine may be diagnostic. In PPP features include ↑ cellularity, erythroid hyperplasia, and a combination of hyperplasia and dysplasia of megakaryocytes. Increased fibrosis may be present. Finding normal histology does not exclude PPP (but is a more usual finding in secondary polycythaemias).
- Erythropoietin assays: not yet part of routine laboratory investigation.
- Vitamin B_{12} levels are commonly ↑ in PPP due to associated leucocytosis, the raised level reflects increased transcobalamin bound B_{12} transport proteins present in neutrophils.
- Serum ferritin: ↓ or ↔ (esp. PPP) and occasionally overt clinical iron deficiency.
- Serum urate ↑ or ↔.

Summary of diagnostic features

PPP
- ↑ RCM + splenomegaly.
- *Or* ↑ RCM + 2 or more of ↑ WBC, ↑ platelets, ↑ NAP, ↑ B_{12}.

Secondary
- ↑ RCM and underlying cause identified.

Idiopathic erythrocytosis
- ↑ RCM, no underlying cause and no criteria for PPP.

Apparent
- Normal RCM and ↓ plasma cell volume.

Management of PPP

Venesection/phlebotomy: to ↓ Hct and prevent complications (target Hct for ♂ <0.47, ♀ <0.44). Removal of RBCs by venesection is quickest way of reducing red cell mass. 450ml blood (± isovolaemic replacement with 0.9% saline) removed safely from younger adults every 2–3 days (reduce frequency in older patients). If PCV very high venesection may be technically difficult due to extreme viscosity.

Maintenance therapy: venesection alone can be used to maintain the PCV in the normal range. Individual requirements are variable (eg 2 procedures per year – monthly venesection).

Myelosuppressive therapy: hydroxyurea, a ribonucleotide reductase inhibitor, is most commonly used therapy. Onset of myelosuppression with hydroxyurea is rapid, but overdosage quickly corrected by temporary withdrawal. Once Hct reduced, a daily dosage of 10–20mg/kg/d normally sufficient as maintenance therapy.

Radioactive phosphorus (^{32}P): long established treatment for PPP. Produces ↓ in RCM by 6–12 weeks of injection. Up to the age of 65 years myelosuppressive therapy in PPP should be with hydroxyurea, >65 either hydroxyurea or ^{32}P can be considered.

Supportive treatment: maintain adequate fluid intake and avoid dehydration. Give allopurinol to minimise complications of hyperuricaemia. Acute gout is managed in usual manner. Pruritus is a troublesome complication for some patients, unfortunately there is no satisfactory treatment. Sometimes abates when excess myeloproliferation controlled and PCV reduced but may persist despite adequate control of the Hct. Worth trying antihistamines, paracetamol or cimetidine.

Aspirin 75mg daily as antiplatelet therapy is common practice in myeloproliferative conditions.

Surgical procedures relatively contraindicated in active PPP – defer until the PCV is normalised (risk of thrombotic and haemorrhagic complications).

Continued care and follow-up

Patients with PPP and idiopathic erythrocytosis should have long-term haematological follow-up. Measure PCV at least 3 monthly. For patients on cytotoxic therapy with hydroxyurea the FBC should be checked 8–12 weekly. Over time 10–15% of patients with PPP undergo transformation → myelofibrotic phase (or less commonly AML).

Spurious (apparent) polycythaemia

Elevation of Hb and Hct with normal or minimally raised RBC mass and normal or reduced plasma volume defines apparent polycythaemia.

Pseudopolycythaemia, **stress erythrocytosis** and **Gaisbock's syndrome** are synonymous terms for this disorder.

Aetiology
Unclear – some cases may represent extreme ends of normal ranges for red cell and plasma volumes, but in most there are associated features of obesity, cigarette smoking and hypertension present singly or in combination. Haemoconcentration from dehydration or diuretic therapy should be excluded.

Investigation
- Should be undertaken as appropriate for suspected polycythaemia but, by definition, fails to reveal any other abnormality.

- Bone marrow biopsy is normal when carried out.

Management
- Involves dealing with reversible associated features, ie weight reduction, cessation of smoking and control of ↑ BP. Correction of these factors will result in spontaneous improvement.
- Venesection is not standard management; however, it is suggested that patients with PCV levels chronically >0.54 should be considered for venesection.

Natural history and treatment
- Not clear. Retrospective analysis appears to suggest an increased incidence of vaso-occlusive episodes which may relate to associated risk factors in the lifestyle of the patients under observation (rather than the raised PCV).
- Low dose aspirin (75mg/d) advisable for patients with overt thrombotic risks.
- No role for myelosuppressive therapy.
- While many patients improve with the measures specified, follow up should continue at 4–6 monthly intervals on those with persistent elevation of Hct. Some may correct spontaneously. In a minority another form of poly-cythaemia may become apparent.

Pearson TC Blood Rev 1991 5 205

Myeloproliferative disorders

Essential (1°) thrombocythaemia (ET)

One of the myeloproliferative disorders. Clonal stem cell disorder–all haematopoietic cell lines are affected (predominant abnormality expressed in megakaryocytes and manifest as persistent elevation of platelet count). Main incidence is 50–70 years; identified with increasing frequency at all ages due to increased availability of platelet count as part of automated FBC.

Clinical features
- Diagnosis often by routine blood testing – many patients asymptomatic.
- Clinical presentation may be with thrombotic and/or haemorrhagic symptoms/signs.
- Haemorrhagic symptoms include ease of bruising, mucosal or GIT bleeding or unexplained/prolonged bleeding after trauma/surgery.
- Thrombotic manifestations – arterial > venous, eg MI, CVA.
- Erythromelalgia (burning discomfort in hands or feet) due to digital microvascular occlusion, a common symptom in ET.
- Splenic atrophy – recognised complication from repeat microvascular infarction.
- Splenomegaly in <40% and less common than in other myeloproliferative disorders.

Diagnostic and laboratory features
- ↑↑ platelet count; persistently >500 × 10^9/l may be as high as 5000 × 10^9/l in severe cases.
- Other causes of thrombocytosis excluded.
- Hb normal or ↓. MCV ↔or ↓ due to chronic blood loss.
- WBC normal, ↓ or ↑.
- Blood film: thrombocytosis, variable shapes and sizes (platelet anisocytosis), giant platelets and platelet clumps; basophilia may be present; variable degree of RBC abnormality, may be changes of hyposplenism.
- Automated FBC may give erroneous data in severe cases as giant platelets may be counted as RBCs.
- Marrow aspirate – not reliable diagnostically; may show ↑ platelet clumps, atypical megakaryocytes including micromegakaryocytes and other maturation abnormalities. Marrow trephine biopsy – megakaryocytes ↑, with clustering, dysplasia and atypical nuclear ploidy. Other elements may show abnormal distribution and maturation abnormalities. Reticulin ↑ or normal. Marrow cellularity ↑ or normal.
- Bleeding time normal or ↑ in ~20%; platelet aggregometry studies not clinically helpful or diagnostic.
- Karyotype – no recognised diagnostic abnormalities but may show 20q– or occasionally Ph chromosome.

No single diagnostic test exists for ET – diagnosis rests on summation of clinical and laboratory findings and exclusion of other causes, eg identifying a Ph chromosome indicates a variant presentation of CML. Mild forms of ET can be very difficult diagnostically to differentiate from reactive thrombocytosis even on marrow histology. Thrombocytosis may occur in other myeloproliferative disorders especially PRV.

Myeloproliferative disorders

Management

- Aim to reduce the risks and incidence of bleeding and thrombotic complications. With normalisation of platelet count haemorrhagic and thrombotic risks are greatly reduced. Need to balance these with potential short and long term risks of specific antiplatelet aggregating therapy (eg aspirin) and cytotoxic therapy.

- Antiplatelet aggregation therapy with aspirin 75–300mg/d recommended if definite thrombotic events have occurred, there is considered to be a major risk of thrombosis when platelets >1000 × 10^9/l. Will relieve erythromelalgia. Caution advised with haemorrhagic complications or history of peptic ulceration. H_2-antagonist or proton pump inhibitors may be needed. Dipyridamole alternative agent for those unable to tolerate aspirin.

- Cytotoxic/cytoreductive therapy – hydroxyurea is treatment of choice; dose 10–30 mg/kg/d. Alkylating agent therapy with busulphan effective (*but risk of myelotoxicity and ↑ leukaemic transformation*). Anagrelide used in US, about to undergo clinical study in UK.

- ^{32}P is active in ET; reserved for >75yrs and those unable to comply with simple oral therapy.

- IFN-α active in ET but expense, subcutaneous administration and side effects render it unsuitable for routine use; may be considered to manage ET in pregnancy.

- Asymptomatic patients with no apparent risk factors for thrombosis, who are <60 years with platelets <800–1000 × 10^9/l may be best left off therapy except, possibly, low dose aspirin.

- Supportive measures such as RBC transfusion are infrequently required in ET.

- Surgical procedures may require specific antithrombotic strategies, eg heparin. Thrombotic risks lessened if platelet count normal.

Natural history

ET generally has an indolent course. However, increased risk of leukaemic transformation over 10–20 years which may be enhanced by cytotoxic therapy. The need for therapy has to be individualised taking this into account balanced against independent thrombotic risks (eg cigarette smoking, family history), FBC results, co-morbidity and age. Evidence of other myeloproliferative disease phenotypes including myelofibrosis may occur in some individuals and will require to be managed appropriately.

Other causes of thrombocytosis

Platelet counts of $>450 \times 10^9/l$ occur as a reactive phenomenon and may be seen in

- Chronic inflammatory states, eg collagen disorders.
- Chronic infection.
- Malignancy, eg underlying carcinoma.
- Chronic blood loss and iron deficiency.
- Rebound in response to haematinics and/or chemotherapy.
- Following surgery, especially splenectomy.
- Any severely ill patient on ITU.

Raised platelet count in clonal haematological disorders occurs in PRV, CML, MF and also in MDS.

In reactive thrombocytosis platelets are usually $<1000 \times 10^9/l$ but levels of $1500 \times 10^9/l$ may occur. Platelet morphology usually normal but differentiation from ET relies on full clinical evaluation. No specific treatment is required for reactive thrombocytosis. Short term anticoagulant or antiplatelet therapy is advised for marked thrombocytosis in the immediate post-splenectomy period.

Myelofibrosis

Myelofibrosis (*syn.* agnogenic myeloid metaplasia) is a clonal neoplastic disorder of all haematopoietic cell lines with associated marrow fibrosis and varying degrees of splenomegaly ± extramedullary haematopoiesis, which is mostly ineffective. It represents a distinct clinical form of the myeloproliferative diseases.

Aetiology & pathology

Occurs mainly in middle aged and elderly, median age of 60 years, ♂ = ♀. May evolve from PRV or ET. Minority may follow previous chemotherapy or radiotherapy. Myelofibrosis is a disorder with intense fibrosis of the marrow which may progress to thick collagen bands (especially type III collagen) giving the characteristic increase in reticulin. Extramedullary haemopoiesis may be seen in spleen and/or liver – occasionally other locations, e.g. lymph nodes and serosal surfaces. Haemopoietic cells are clonal, fibrosis is reactive and not derived from the same clone.

Clinical presentation

- ≤25% may be asymptomatic, mild FBC abnormalities identified or splenomegaly found on clinical examination.
- General symptomatology – fatigue, weight loss, night sweats, etc.
- Local symptoms – abdominal discomfort and/or dyspepsia from splenic enlargement.
- Symptoms and signs of marrow failure (cytopenias, infections, bleeding – *see below*).
- Splenomegaly – moderate to massive enlargement; variable hepatomegaly, very few cases (<10%) lack measurable splenic enlargement.

Diagnostic features

- Hb usually ↓ or normal.
- WBC ↓, normal or ↑ (rarely >100 × 10^9/l).
- Platelets usually ↓ or normal; occasionally ↑.
- Blood film shows leucoerythroblastic anaemia (nucleated red cells, immature WBC) with tear drop cells.
- Bone marrow aspirate usually unsuccessful ('dry tap').
- Marrow trephine biopsy shows variable amounts of normal haemopoiesis with moderate to marked ↑ in reticulin; dysplasia of maturation usual, especially megakaryocytes.
- Cytogenetic abnormalities in ~50%.
- Urate typically ↑.

Differential diagnosis

- CML – Ph chromosome does not occur in myelofibrosis. Myelofibrosis can overlap with other myeloproliferative disorders. Presenting features can be similar to hairy cell leukaemia.
- Metastatic cancer in marrow, especially breast, prostate and thyroid, can give similar FBC features but without splenomegaly. Metastatic carcinoma cells are apparent on marrow biopsy and/or aspirate.

Management and prognosis

Myelofibrosis is incurable except by allogeneic marrow transplant, suitable only for patients <40 years with sibling matched donor. Median survival for symptomatic cases is probably ~5 years, the more marked the degree of marrow failure or symptomatology the poorer the prognosis. Many patients survive >10 years.

Myeloproliferative disorders

- Observation is all that is required for asymptomatic cases with minimal FBC abnormalities and splenic enlargement.
- Supportive treatment of anaemia with regular blood transfusion for those who develop anaemic symptoms; treatment is on the basis of symptoms as opposed to a specific Hb level. Only those with symptomatic anaemia should receive RBC transfusion.
- Allopurinol to treat/prevent hyperuricaemia.
- Splenectomy indicated for massive splenomegaly, excessive blood transfusion requirements, constitutional symptoms (weight loss and night sweats).
- Radiotherapy – to reduce splenic size and discomfort in those unfit for splenectomy; treatment of extramedullary infiltrates.
- Chemotherapy – hydroxyurea may be used to treat leucocytosis and to reduce splenic enlargement.
- Corticosteroids – sometimes used to improve Hb and ameliorate constitutional symptoms.

Other therapies without evidence of consistent benefit include androgenic steroids and erythropoietin in attempts to improve anaemia. Allogeneic bone marrow transplantation has been carried out successfully in a very few younger, symptomatic cases.

Death in symptomatic cases usually due to infection and haemorrhage. Around 5–10% transform to AML which is refractory to intensive chemotherapy. Asymptomatic cases will usually die from other unrelated causes.

.

Plasma cell disorders 7

Monoclonal gammopathy of undetermined significance

Disorders characterised by production of paraprotein include *monoclonal gammopathy of undetermined significance* (MGUS – also called *benign monoclonal gammopathy*, BMG), *multiple myeloma* (MM) and *Waldenström's macroglobulinaemia* (WM). Paraprotein may also be a feature of amyloidosis, CLL, and occasionally NHL.

MGUS describes the presence of a monoclonal paraprotein of serum Ig in absence of clinicopathological evidence of MM, WM, amyloidosis or NHL. Found in 1% of the population >60 years of age, increasing to 3% >70 years. Blacks > whites. Typically asymptomatic and often incidental finding. No abnormal physical findings. Associated lymphadenopathy or splenomegaly with an IgM paraprotein suggests a diagnosis of Waldenström's macroglobulinaenia. Lack of progression on follow up with demonstration of no other evidence of progressive plasma cell or B cell lymphoproliferative malignancy are the basic diagnostic criteria for a diagnosis.

Assessment

Serum protein electrophoresis with immunoelectrophoresis and immunofixation are used to identify and quantitate Ig and paraprotein levels.

Features

- IgG is commonest (50%) > IgA (20–25%) > IgM (10%).
- IgG paraprotein <30g/l; IgA paraprotein <20g/l.
- IgD, IgE and free light chains are much rarer.
- Idiopathic Bence-Jones proteinuria is a form of BMG.
- Biclonal gammopathy also occurs where two M-protein are identified.
- Normal Ig subtypes commonly present in normal quantities (*cf.* myeloma – they are ↓).
- β_2-microglobulin levels are normal (unless renal impairment).
- Bone marrow: no malignant infiltration with plasma cells or lymphocytes although cell marker analysis may suggest the presence of a small population of monoclonal plasma cells or B-cells. <10% plasma cells in BM.
- No anaemia, hypercalcaemia or renal impairment.
- Renal function and serum Ca^{2+} are normal.
- Radiology: no evidence of lytic lesions; osteoporosis is not a clinical effect of MGUS but may co-exist from other causes, eg post menopausal females.
- *Stable M protein and other parameters on prolonged observation.*

Treatment

No treatment required. If all staging investigations are negative patients can be reassured that the condition is benign but long term follow up is required. No specific features at initial presentation that predict those who will progress – clinical re-evaluation at 6–12 monthly intervals recommended.

Follow up studies

- 50% patients die of other (unrelated) causes.
- 25% patients do not progress to symptomatic MM or WM, some may show a ↑ in paraprotein levels.
- 25% develop myeloma or Waldenström's over 20–25 year period.
- 10% develop myeloma or Waldenström's within 8 years follow-up.

Plasma cell disorders

Criteria for a diagnosis of MGUS
- No unexplained symptoms suggestive of myeloma.
- Serum M protein <30g/1.
- <10% plasma cells in bone marrow.
- Little or no urine M protein.
- No bone lesions.
- No anaemia, hypercalcaemia or renal impairment.
- Stable M protein and other parameters on prolonged observation.

Kyle RA 1997 Monoclonal gammopathy of undetermined significance and solitary plasmacytoma. Hematology Oncology Clinics of North America 11, 71.

Smouldering myeloma

Smouldering myeloma, indolent myeloma or *equivocal myelomatosis* describe situations in which diagnostic criteria for myeloma are met (specifically, >10% plasma cells in BM or IgG paraprotein >30g/l or IgA paraprotein >20g/l) but with no clinical evidence of progression or of severe complications associated with myeloma. This group is important to recognise clinically because there is *no* survival gain in giving chemotherapy before progressive or symptomatic disease develops. Clinical stability may persist for months or years and careful clinical follow up is required. Survival is the same as for newly diagnosed myeloma from the time chemotherapy is started.

Features

- Absence of symptoms or physical signs attributable to myeloma.
- Performance status of >50%.
- Pre-transfusion haemoglobin >10g/dl.
- Post-rehydration creatinine <130μmol/l.
- Normal serum Ca^{2+}.
- BM plasmacytosis >10% but normally <25%.
- Radiology should be normal.
- β2 microglobulin levels normal or minimally raised.
- Plasma cell labelling index (when measured) <1%.
- *Stable M protein and other parameters on prolonged observation.*

Management

Chemotherapy is *not* indicated for these patients until there is evidence of clinical progression. Median survival following chemotherapy is 3–4 years, ie identical to that of *de novo* symptomatic myeloma.

Criteria for the diagnosis of smouldering myeloma
- No unexplained symptoms suggestive of myeloma.
- Serum M protein >30g/l.
- ≥10% plasma cells in bone marrow.
- Little or no urine M protein (<500mg/24h).
- No bone lesions.
- No anaemia, hypercalcaemia or renal impairment.
- Stable M protein and other parameters on prolonged observation.

Multiple myeloma

Pathophysiology

Multiple myeloma (*syn.* myelomatosis) is a B-cell lymphoid malignancy characterised by malignant clonal proliferation and accumulation of plasma cells that secrete *paraprotein* (monoclonal intact Ig, κ or λ light chains); normal Ig production is impaired (hypogammaglobulinaemia). <1% cases are *non-secretory*.

Epidemiology

3 per 100,000 per annum, 2500 new cases/year in UK; median age at diagnosis 60–65 years; <2% are <40 years. Incidence twice as high in Afro-Caribbeans than Caucasians and lower in Asians. Most cases present *de novo* but minority arise from BMG or MGUS.

Diagnosis & assessment

Clinical effects – wide spectrum: from asymptomatic paraproteinaemia (~20%) to rapidly progressive illness with compromised BM and renal function with extensive, destructive bony disease.

Diagnosis – demonstrate monoclonal paraprotein with infiltration of the marrow. At presentation, most patients have evidence of skeletal involvement (eg osteoporosis or lytic lesions).

Infection – common at presentation (functional hypogammaglobulinaemia ± neutropenia).

Skeletal disease – In many symptomatic patients generalised bone pain and osteoporosis will be present at diagnosis. There may be loss of height and vertebral fractures in addition to the typical osteolytic lesions in up to 70% of patients.

Bone marrow suppression – from infiltration of marrow by plasma cells. Also causes leucopenia and thrombocytopenia. Associated renal impairment in some cases may worsen anaemia.

Hyperviscosity – associated with IgA myeloma or very high IgG paraproteins.

Hypercalcaemia – usually associated with extensive bone disease.

Renal impairment – may be present in 20–25% due to dehydration and/or hypercalcaemia and for most will be reversible with hydration. Irreversible renal damage from light chain deposition occurs in a small percentage and is not ameliorated by chemotherapy and hydration.

> ### Minimal diagnostic criteria for myeloma
> - >10% plasma cells in BM or plasmacytoma on biopsy.
> - Clinical features of myeloma.
> - Plus at least one of: – serum M protein (IgG >30g/l, IgA >20g/l)
>   – urine M protein (BJP)
>   – osteolytic lesions on skeletal survey

Other – occasionally presents as neurological emergency due to plasmacytom deposits causing spinal compression.

Clinical assessment involves staging to assess tumour mass and evaluate likely associated complicating features, eg renal impairment. Medical Research Council trials have shown that Hb, blood urea after hydration, and performance status give reliable prognostic information. Durie & Salmon system remains the standard system of staging – assigns patients to low, intermediate or high tumour mass. Level of β2-microglobulin (surrogate marker for proliferative index), a peptide component of the class 1 HLA complex, forms one of the most important prognostic indicators in myeloma (high levels of β2-microglobulin are associated with poor prognosis). Levels need correction for renal impairment. A high proliferative index of plasma cells at presentation is an adverse prognostic feature. High levels of IL-6 or C-reactive are also associated with poor prognosis.

A useful and simple prognostic index is obtained using the β2-microglobulin and CRP (or β2-microglobulin and IL-6):

  if both are elevated the patient is *high* risk (median survival 6 months)
  if either is elevated the patient is *intermediate* risk (median survival 27 months)
  if none is elevated the patient is *low* risk (54 months median survival)

Bataille R, Boccadoro M, Klein B *et al.* 1992 Blood **80** 733

Durie & Salmon staging system

Stage 1	**Low mass**
	Hb >10g/dl
	Serum Ca^{2+} <3.0 mmol/l
	No myeloma changes on skeletal X-rays
	Low myeloma protein: IgG <50g/l; IgA <30g/l
	Bence-Jones protein <4g/24h
Stage 2	**Intermediate mass** – fits neither stage 1 nor 3
Stage 3	**High mass**
	Hb <8.5g/dl
	Serum Ca^{2+} >3.0 mmol/l
	High myeloma protein: Ig G >50g/l; IgA >30g/l
	Bence-Jones protein >12g/24h

Features of poor prognosis at diagnosis

- Low haemoglobin (<8.5g/dl).
- Hypercalcaemia.
- Advanced lytic bone lesions.
- High M protein production rates (IgG >70g/l; IgA >50g/l; BJP >12g/24h).
- Abnormal renal function.
- High % bone marrow plasma cells.
- Plasmablast morphology.
- Circulating plasma cells in peripheral blood.
- High β2-microglobulin (>6mg/ml).
- High plasma cell labelling index.
- Low serum albumin (<30g/l).
- High C-reactive protein.
- High serum IL-6.

Investigation

- Height, weight and performance status. Note location/severity of bony pain.
- FBC, ESR/plasma viscosity (typically ↑ but may be ↔ in light chain or non-secretory disease).
- Urea, creatinine, electrolytes, serum Ca^{2+}, LFTs (alkaline phosphatase is usually ↔ or minimally raised in myeloma despite significant bony disease).
- Urinalysis for Bence-Jones protein with quantitation; check for albuminuria (eg nephrotic syndrome due to amyloid/myeloma kidney).
- Igs; electrophoresis and immunofixation to identify and quantify paraprotein (serum and urine).
- BM aspiration ± biopsy; identify plasma cell infiltration; immunophenotype will show clonality (CD38+, CD56±, CD19−).
- Radiology – skeletal survey to include pelvis, femora and lateral views of spine. CT or MRI scanning are not helpful *routinely* unless evaluating potential or actual spinal compression.

Management

Initial management – good supportive measures are essential

Patients frequently require sedation, analgesia, correction of hypercalcaemia, treatment of renal impairment and treatment of infection. Local radiotherapy for severe bone pain may be required before chemotherapy. Plasma exchange may be required for symptomatic hyperviscosity.

Conventional chemotherapy

For patients >70 years there are no convincing data to suggest alternatives to regular pulses of oral melphalan ± prednisolone given 4–6 weekly to stabilise the disease and achieve 'plateau phase', after which patients are left off treatment until disease progression occurs. Survival is *not* increased by continued chemotherapy and morbidity from infection and secondary myelodysplasia may be increased. For younger myeloma patients combination chemotherapy including the use of nitrosoureas and anthracyclines probably produces better survival than oral melphalan ± prednisolone.

High dose chemotherapy & rescue with marrow or stem cell transplantation – Identification that high doses of dexamethasone with infusion of vincristine and adriamycin (VAD) produced remarkable responses in relapsed/refractory disease led to studies involving this combination as front-line approach. Response is more rapid and the degrees of responsiveness are greater, but this therapy does not produce any increase in survival. More complex to administer (requires central line). Following this therapy up with high dose chemotherapy using melphalan ± rescue with peripheral blood stem cells or bone marrow will produce periods of long-term disease control and may improve survival. Allogeneic BMT has been carried out in myeloma, and a small number of patients appear to benefit but toxicity is high and the approach is not applicable to the majority of myeloma patients.

IFN-α – Data suggest that plateau can be prolonged for up to 6 months by IFN-α maintenance therapy, but survival does *not* appear to be increased.

Bisphosphonates – Conventional chemotherapy has little impact on the progression of bony disease. Bisphosphonates inhibit bone reabsorption and have been shown to reduce the rate of progression of bony disease.

Relapsed and refractory disease – All patients with myeloma will ultimately develop disease progression and ultimately become refractory. While a small number may be offered a high dose chemotherapy approach, the

majority will be managed with conventional therapy. Patients who relapse after achieving plateau are likely to achieve a second plateau with melphalan or simple combination treatments. The VAD approach will produce a high response rate but the survival may not be different to that using high dose pulses of dexamethasone alone.

Radiotherapy – Helpful in palliating symptoms of advanced bony disease. Also useful for localised areas of bone pain early in the disorder that do not respond well to chemotherapy.

Complication	Contributing factor	Management
Infection	Hypogammaglobulinaemia Neutropenia Reduced mobility Chemotherapy High dose steroids	Patient and GP education Antibiotics (oral/intravenous) Prophylactic measures – cotrimoxazole, antifungals, IVIg
Bone pain/fractures	Lytic lesions Osteoporosis	Analgesia–simple analgesics, NSAIDs, fentanyl patches, opiates Orthopaedic management Local DXT Chemotherapy (will ↓ bone pain)
Hypercalcaemia	Resorption of Ca^{2+} from bones (osteoclast-activating factors)	IV/oral rehydration, 3–4L/24h Loop diuretics Bisphosphonates IV clodronate or pamidronate Corticosteroids Chemotherapy
Renal	Dehydration Hypercalcaemia Hyperviscosity Myeloma kidney Amyloid	Hydration (>3–4L/24h) Consider dialysis Chemotherapy Renal transplant (selected cases)
Hyperviscosity	High paraprotein levels Polymerising Ig molecules (IgG, IgA, IgM)	Hydration Plasma exchange Chemotherapy
Spinal compression	Spinal deposits/infiltration Vertebral collapse	Diagnosis by MRI or CT scan Dexamethasone Local DXT Neurosurgical/Orthopaedic intervention if necessary
Neuropathy	Light chain neurological damage	Plasma exchange Chemotherapy
Anaemia	Marrow infiltration Haemodilution Chemotherapy effects (short term) Renal impairment	Treatment of contributory factors Blood transfusion (care: hyperviscosity) Erythropoietin

R Bataille & J Harousseau NEJM 1997 **336** 1657

Waldenström's macroglobulinaemia and IgM paraproteinaemia

Low-grade B-cell lymphoplasmacytic malignancy with circulating monoclonal IgM paraprotein. IgM paraprotein is not absolutely specific for WM – isolated IgM paraproteinaemia occurs in absence of evidence of lymphoproliferative disease and in MGUS. Seen in association with other forms of low grade lymphoma and rarely true IgM myeloma occurs. Peak incidence of WM is 6th–7th decades. No other known aetiological factors.

Diagnosis

- Demonstrate clonal IgM paraprotein; may be ↓ normal levels of IgG and IgA.
- FBC – normochromic, normocytic anaemia in ≥80%; circulating lymphoplasmacytic cells may be present on film; WBC and platelets normal.
- ESR/plasma viscosity ↑; ESR commonly >100mm/h.
- BM aspirate usually ↑ cellularity with lymphocyte or lymphoplasmacytic infiltration. Trephine also cellular with diffuse and/or focal infiltration by lymphoplasmacytic lymphoma.
- Cell surface markers: +ve for B-cell markers (CD19, CD20 etc.); variable degree of surface Ig expression; CD5 & CD10 expression occur.
- Absence of bony changes or involvement as seen in myeloma.

Clinical features

Non-specific complaints, fatigue, lethargy, weight loss. Bruising and bleeding episodes, eg epistaxis, associated with hyperviscosity. Splenomegaly, hepatomegaly and lymphadenopathy may be present. Hyperviscosity syndrome (viscosity >4cP) may be present in ~20% (visual disturbance, impaired concentration, haemorrhagic manifestations, dilatation and ↑ tortuosity of retinal vessels with haemorrhages and exudates in more severe cases). Absence of bony changes or pain which otherwise would suggest a plasma cell dyscrasia. Renal involvement and amyloid occur infrequently in WM although elevation of urea may be present at diagnosis it will correct with hydration and chemotherapy.

Management

- Confirm diagnosis.
- Hydration.
- Correct hyperviscosity
  - avoid RBC transfusion on basis of low Hb (plasma volume is ↑ and anaemia protects against hyperviscosity effects of macroglobulinaemia)
  - venesection/manual plasmapheresis may be done in an emergency otherwise plasma exchange. Rarely regular plasma exchange is needed in addition to chemotherapy to avoid chronic hyperviscosity problems.
- Chemotherapy
  - chlorambucil or cyclophosphamide (alkylating agents)
  - fludarabine and 2-CDA are effective second line therapies for early or multiply relapsed WM patients.

Natural history

Runs an indolent course. Treat progression/relapse >18 months from last course of chemotherapy with alkylating agents. Incurable with median survival (symptomatic patients) ~5 years. Asymptomatic patients may be observed without therapy until symptoms develop or IgM levels start to rise and risks of hyperviscosity develop. No role for aggressive combination chemotherapy in WM.

Amyloidosis

Describes a range of disorders characterised by extracellular deposition of fibrillar protein. Clinical features determined by site of amyloid deposition; commoner locations for amyloid involvement along with clinical manifestations include

Renal	Nephrotic syndrome, renal failure
Liver, spleen	Organ enlargement
Gastrointestinal tract	Malabsorption, macroglossia
Heart	Cardiomegaly, cardiac failure
Skin	Purpura, papular or nodular lesions
CNS	Peripheral neuropathy, carpal tunnel syndrome

Pathology

Some forms of amyloid are reactive; the amyloid fibrils derive from acute phase serum protein-A.

AA amyloid arises as a long term complication of chronic inflammatory or infective states. Treatment of the amyloid involves supportive management of the affected impaired organ system(s). If the underlying chronic infection or inflammatory source can be treated then there may be regression of the amyloid; most amyloid is not reversible.

In AL amyloid the fibrils are derived from monoclonal Ig light chains; it is a rare form of plasma cell dyscrasia. Investigation of peripheral blood, urine and marrow usually will demonstrate hypogammaglobulinaemia ± evidence of circulating light chains, urinary Bence-Jones protein and a clonal plasma cell population in marrow. Occasionally AL amyloid may be the only manifestation of the dyscrasia. AL amyloid may also occur as a long term complication of myeloma in up to 15% cases. Cardiac, renal and neuropathic manifestations are more usual with this form of amyloid.

Diagnosis & management

Histology from suspected organ stained with Congo Red will identify amyloid; immunohistochemistry should be done to differentiate AA, AL or other types of amyloid. AL amyloid patients should be assessed as for myeloma.

Management

Predominantly supportive. Melphalan ± prednisolone given as for myeloma may reduce formation of amyloid and allow some improvement in organ function. A small minority of patients with renal disease have benefited from renal transplantation. Prognosis in amyloid is 1–4 years with renal or cardiac failure principal causes of death.

Bone marrow and blood stem cell transplantation

Transplantation is the reconstitution of the full haemopoietic system by transfer of pluripotent cells in the BM – stem cells. Usually requires prior ablation of the patient's own marrow and immune system (in the allogeneic setting) by intensive chemotherapy or chemoradiotherapy. The most appropriate generic term for the procedure is *haemopoietic transplantation* although stem cell transplantation is now probably the most commonly used term. Stem cell transplants may be *allogeneic* transplant (another individual acts as donor eg sibling or normal volunteer) or *autologous* transplant (patient acts as his/her own source of stem cells). Stem cells may be obtained from the bone marrow (BMT) or obtained from peripheral blood after BM stimulation known as peripheral blood stem cell transplants (PBSCT) or peripheral blood precursor cell transplants (PBPCT). All are infused IV.

Aims of transplantation Elimination of underlying disease with restoration of haemopoietic and immune function.

Graft procurement for BMT, bone marrow is obtained by puncture of the iliac crests under general anaesthesia, a procedure known as harvesting. BM is aspirated directly from the marrow cavity using marrow biopsy needles. 1L marrow may be required to provide sufficient stem cells for transplant. Well tolerated requiring only simple analgesia post-operatively. Serious complications are extremely rare (see p226). PBSCT is gradually replacing BMT. Stem cells are effluxed into the peripheral blood (known as mobilisation) by single agent chemotherapy, combination chemotherapy, or a haemopoietic growth factor e.g. granulocyte colony stimulating factor (G-CSF) or combinations of these (see p228). When stem cells have appeared in the blood, the individual is connected to a cell separation machine. Blood is drawn off, spun in a centrifuge and stem cells are collected while the remaining blood elements are returned to the patient. The procedure takes between 2-4 hours and is well tolerated, no general anaesthesia is required, engraftment is more rapid with earlier hospital discharge post-transplant and the procedure is cheaper.

Transplant procedure – recipient is treated with high dose chemo/radiotherapy (termed *conditioning*, destroys recipient BM). On the day after the end of this treatment, BM or PBSC are infused IV (allogeneic or autologous). After a period of severe myelosuppression (7–25d), engraftment occurs with production of WBCs, platelets and RBCs. Unlike autologous transplantation, immunosuppression is required following allogeneic transplantation to prevent GvHD and rejection.

Early complications of the transplant procedure

Chemoradiotherapy	Nausea/vomiting, reversible alopecia, fatigue, dry skin, mucositis
	VOD (see p250)
Infection	Bacterial (Gram –ve and +ve)
	Viral–HZV, CMV (particularly pneumonitis)
	Fungal – *Candida, Aspergillus, Mucor*
	Atypical organisms–Pneumocystis (PCP), *Toxoplasma, Mycoplasma, Legionella*

Graft versus host disease (GvHD)

May occur in allograft recipients due to immunological disparity between donor and recipient.

Late complications of transplantation

- Infertility (both sexes).
- Hypothyroidism.
- Secondary malignancy.
- Late sepsis due to hyposplenism.
- Cataracts (where TBI used).
- Psychological disturbance.

Follow up and post-transplant surveillance

Life-long supervision required due to the nature of the disease and the transplant treatment. The particular risks and monitoring required depend on the type of graft and whether TBI was used. Suitable protocols are shown later (p260).

219

Allogeneic bone marrow and blood stem cell transplantation

In allogeneic transplant another individual acts a donor of stem cells (eg sibling or unrelated donor).

Suitability

Profoundly toxic procedure and potential recipients should be in good clinical condition, and <55 years old. Since bone marrow contains B and T lymphocytes, macrophages and antigen presenting cells, it is necessary for donor and recipient to be fully or near fully HLA-matched to prevent life threatening GvHD or rejection. Within the patient's family the greatest chance of full HLA match is with the patient's siblings (small chance of full match with cousins). Average potential recipient in Western countries has ~1:4 chance of having a sibling who is fully HLA-matched. Since this restricts the applicability of allogeneic transplantation, interest has surrounded the use of normal volunteer donors who show a close HLA match to the potential recipient. Achieved by establishment of bone marrow registries to which volunteers agree to be willing to donate marrow eg (in UK) The National Blood Authority and Anthony Nolan panels.

Allogeneic transplantation indications
Conditions for which it is the sole chance of cure
- Primary immunodeficiency syndromes.
- Aplastic anaemia.
- Thalassaemia.
- Sickle cell disease.
- Inborn errors of metabolism.
- Chronic myeloid leukaemia.
- Myelodysplasia.

Conditions where there is probably benefit over conventional treatment
- AML (first or second CR).
- ALL (first or second CR)*.

*Most children with ALL will be cured by standard chemotherapy alone – transplantation is reserved for those who relapse. (cf. Paeds section)

Allogeneic transplant procedure Recipient is treated with high dose chemotherapy or chemoradiotherapy to ablate the marrow and immune system (conditioning). One day after the end of this treatment, BM or PBSC are harvested from donor and transplant performed by infusing the stem cells IV through central line. After period of severe myelosuppression (7–21d), engraftment of the transplanted material occurs. Immunosuppression required to prevent GvHD/rejection. Generally use cyclosporin A/methotrexate combinations, or by depletion of T-cells (using MoAbs).

Mechanism of cure The consistent observation that patients who experience GvHD have lower relapse rates than matched controls has aroused interest in the nature of the phenomenon known as the *graft versus leukaemia (GvL) effect*. Although originally described in leukaemic recipients, it is observable in other underlying conditions and confirms the importance of immunological mechanisms of disease eradication in addition to the myeloablative conditioning regimens.

Early complications of the transplant procedure

Overall transplant related mortality for sibling HLA matched allografts is 15–30%, and for volunteer unrelated donors – may reach 45%. Major categories of complications are summarised in BM and PBSCT section. The severe myelo-suppression following allograft together with immune dysfunction from delayed reconstitution or GvHD predisposes to a wide variety of potentially fatal infections with bacterial (Gram +ve and –ve), viral, fungal and atypical organisms. Both HSV and HZV infections are common – may present with fulminant extensive lesions. Main causes of infective death post-transplant are: CMV pneumonitis and invasive fungal infections with moulds eg *Aspergillus*.

Graft versus host disease (GvHD) Termed *acute* if occurs ≤100d of transplant and *chronic* if >100d. Clinical features, staging, prevention and therapy protocols are discussed in separate sections – see *Acute GvHD, Chronic GvHD, GvHD prophylaxis*.

Other complications

- Endocrine eg infertility (both sexes), early menopause and occasionally hypothyroidism.
- Cataract formation (TBI induced) >12 months post-transplant.
- 2° malignancies (esp. skin).
- EBV associated lymphoma.
- Mild psychological disturbances common (serious psychoses are rare).

Follow up treatment and post-transplant surveillance

Immunosuppression requires careful monitoring to avoid toxicity. Unlike solid organ transplant recipients, lifelong immunosuppression is **not** required and Cyclosporin is usually discontinued at about 6 months post-transplant. Prophylactic prescriptions against Pneumococcal sepsis secondary to hyposplenism, HZV reactivation and PCP infections are required. Despite these complications, most patients return to an active, working life without the need for continuing medication.

Future developments

Molecular HLA gene loci mapping The molecular revolution has resulted in improved DNA characterisation of HLA gene loci – should ensure greater applicability and success of transplants from volunteer unrelated donors.

Umbilical cord blood transplants Umbilical cord blood donation post-delivery shown to be entirely safe for mother and child. Cord blood stem cells are immunologically immature and may be more permissive of HLA donor/recipient mismatches with less risk of GvHD. Clinical trials in children are showing encouraging results.

Autologous bone marrow and blood stem cell transplantation

Patient acts as his/her own source of haemopoietic stem cells. In contrast to allogeneic transplantation, there is minimal immunological disturbance. Stresses on the cardiorespiratory, skin and mucosal systems are similar. Recipients should still be in good clinical condition but age range for some procedures can be extended (eg up to ~70).

Indications Evaluation currently being carried out by a number of studies including randomised control trials in a large number of diseases, particularly in malignancy. Indications divided into those in which there is now *proven benefit*, *probable benefit* or *possible benefit*.

Proven benefit	Relapsed NHL (intermediate and high grade)
	AML (first or second CR)
	Multiple myeloma
Probable benefit	Relapsed Hodgkin's disease
	ALL (first or second CR)
	Relapsed testis cancer
Possible benefit	Disseminated breast cancer
	Disseminated lung cancers
	Other solid tumours
	Severe autoimmune disease

Autologous transplant procedure The recipient, in disease remission, undergoes BM or PBSC harvest. Haemopoietic stem cells are processed, frozen and stored in liquid N_2 after which recipient commences conditioning. One day post-conditioning, the stem cell product is thawed rapidly and infused IV. Bags are thawed rapidly by transfer directly from liquid N_2 into water at 37–43°C. Product is infused IV rapidly through indwelling central line. There is period of myelosuppression (7–25d) followed by WBC, platelet and RBC engraftment.

Early complications of the transplant procedure Overall transplant related mortality is <5% for PBSCT and <15% for BMT, ie lower than allograft but morbidity from conditioning regimens may still be seen eg nausea from chemoradiotherapy and mucositis from the widespread mucosal damage to GIT. Oral ulceration, buccal desquamation, oesophagitis, gastritis, abdominal pain and diarrhoea may all be features. The spectrum of infective organisms seen is similar to allografts but severity and mortality are ↓.

Late complications of transplantation Single commonest long-term complication is relapse of original underlying disease. Other late complications are similar to allografts, but less frequent and less severe.

Follow up treatment and post-transplant surveillance Regular haematological follow-up is mandatory and psychological support from the transplant team, family and friends is important for readjustment to normal life. Prophylaxis against specific infections is required including Pneumococcus, HZV and PCP. Most patients return to an active, working life without continuing medication.

Investigations for BMT/PBSCT

Haematology
- FBC, reticulocytes, ESR.
- Serum B_{12} and red cell folate, ferritin.
- Blood group, antibody screen and DAT.
- Coagulation screen, PT, APTT, fibrinogen.
- BM aspirate for morphology (cytogenetics if relevant); BM trephine biopsy.

Biochemistry
- U & Es, LFTs.
- Ca^{2+}, phosphate, random glucose.
- LDH.
- TFTs.
- Serum and urine Igs.
- EDTA clearance.

Virology
- Hepatitis BsAg.
- Hepatitis C antibody.
- HIV I and II antibody (*counselling and consent required*).
- CMV IgG and IgM.
- EBV, HSV and VZV IgG.
- Parvovirus B19 titre (allografts only).
- Toxoplasma titre (allografts only).

Immunology
- Autoantibody screen.
- HLA type – (if not known) in case HLA matched platelets are subsequently required.
- HLA and platelet antibody screen (if previously poor increments to platelet transfusions).
- CRP.

Bacteriology
- Baseline blood cultures (peripheral blood and Hickman line).
- Routine admission swabs: throat, central line site.
- MSU, stool cultures.

Cardiology
- ECG.
- Echocardiogram, to include measurement of systolic ejection fraction.

Respiratory
- Lung function tests.

Radiology
- CXR.
- Sinus X-rays.

Cytogenetics
- Blood for donor/recipient polymorphisms (allografts only).

Other
- Consider semen storage.
- Dental opinion if caries/gum disease.
- Psychiatric opinion if previous history.

Bone marrow harvesting

Pre-operative preparations
Important to give advanced notice so that theatre time can be booked if necessary and the virological screening results obtained.

Within 30 days before the harvest procedure, arrange the following virological investigations
1. Hepatitis B Surface Antigen.
2. Hepatitis C Antibody.
3. HIV 1 and 2.
4. VDRL.
5. Spare serum stored.

Admit patient day before harvest. Clerk patient and arrange:
- U & E.
- FBC.
- X match 2–3 units blood (CMV –ve). If harvest is on normal donor – offer autologous blood collection to donor. If declined, arrange for genotyped, CMV negative and irradiated X-matched blood to be available for the donor. A CXR and ECG may also be arranged, if felt clinically appropriate.

Harvest procedure
1. Give heparin 50 units/kg IV at anaesthetic induction.
2. Prepare harvest bag: adding ACD with a dilution factor of 1:10 for the prospective marrow volume; ie 100ml of ACD if expected harvest is ~1L.
3. Heparinise aspirate needles/syringes (0.9% saline containing at least 100U heparin/ml).
4. Begin with posterior superior iliac crests, limiting the number of skin entry points, the aspirate needle should be manoeuvred to collect as much marrow as possible with 5–10ml maximum from each penetration of the bone. Each aspirate should be deposited in a sterile harvest bag and syringe rinsed in the heparinised saline prior to re-use. Gently agitate bag at intervals.
5. Midway through harvest (or 500ml) a bag sample should be sent for FBC to determine the adequacy of the harvest. The final total WBC count should be at least 2×10^8 cells/kg of the recipient for autografts and 3×10^8 cells/kg for allografts.

The volume of marrow required may be calculated as follows:
Total volume required for autograft = $2.0 \times$ Recipient weight (kg)/(bag WBC $\times$ 10)
eg recip. 100kg and bag WBC 20×10^9/l vol. required = $(2.0 \times 100)/(20 \times 10) = 1.0$l
Volume still needed to be harvested = Total volume – volume already taken at time of count + ~10%

Notes
1. The extra 10% compensates for reduced harvesting efficiency and the ACD.
2. The formula works at whatever volume you choose to do the first WBC but is a more accurate prediction at ~500ml.
3. If need to harvest >1L, remember to add additional ACD in the same 1 in 10 ratio.
4. For allograft calculations, substitute 3.0 for 2.0 in the formula.

If yield not adequate from the posterior iliac crests, other sites may be considered (eg anterior superior iliac crests and sternum). Review puncture sites the following morning for signs of local infection or continuing bleeding. For normal donors, offer out-patient follow-up appointment as additional safeguard and provide access to counselling services.

Peripheral blood stem cell mobilisation and harvesting

Properties of stem cells
- Stem cells are defined as the most primitive haemopoietic precursor cell.
- Unique property is capability of both infinite self-renewal and differentiation to form all the mature cells of the haemopoietic and immune systems.
- In the resting state almost all stem cells reside in the bone marrow although a tiny minority circulate in peripheral blood.
- Stem cells in the marrow can migrate into the blood after treatment with chemotherapy and/or haemopoietic growth factors.
- Once circulating, they can easily be harvested using a cell separator machine.
- Stem cell levels in peripheral blood can be assessed by CD34 immuno-phenotype analysis.
- More than one day of harvesting may be needed.
- The yield can be assessed for engraftment potential.

Protocols
Mobilisation and harvesting protocols differ between diseases and schedules are still being evaluated and optimised. Many new haemopoietic growth factors are on trial. The following illustrate the principal types of schedule:

1. Mobilisation after standard chemotherapy
- No specific additional stimulus given.
- Harvest times determined by WBC and platelet recovery, and CD34 count.
- Yields variable.

Suitable for
- NHL post DHAP chemotherapy.
- AML post ADE/DAT chemotherapy.
- ALL post high dose methotrexate.

2. Mobilisation with chemotherapy & haemopoietic growth factors
The commonest schedule and the best evaluated. Harvest timing and yields more predictable.

Typical protocol for NHL
Day 0 cyclophosphamide 1.5g/m^2 IVI with Mesna.
Day +1 to Day +7–10 G-CSF 5µg/kg/d SC continued until last day of harvesting.
Harvest Day +7–10 when WBC >2.0 × 10^9/l.

Typical protocol for myeloma
Day 0 cyclophosphamide 4g/m^2 IVI with Mesna.
Day +1 to Day +10–13, G-CSF 5–10µg/kg/d SC.
Harvest Day +10 – 13 when WBC >2.0 × 10^9/l.

Mobilisation with haemopoietic growth factor alone
Suitable for normal volunteers eg allograft donors.
G-CSF 5–10µg/kg/d SC for 4–5d.
Harvest Days 4–5.

Yield evaluation
Common parameters are mononuclear cell counts (MNC); CD34 numbers and haemopoietic colony forming unit assays eg CFU-GM. All are a quantitative or

functional assessment of engraftment potential expressed per kg of recipient weight.

Typical target yields (will vary between labs and mobilisation protocols):

MNC $>3.0 \times 10^8$/kg
CD34 $>2.0 \times 10^6$/kg
CFU-GM $>2.0 \times 10^5$/kg

Microbiological screening for stem cell cryopreservation

This topic has assumed great importance recently for a number of reasons. Firstly, there has been increasing awareness of transmission of agents, particularly viruses that can be transmitted through blood products that may cause significant disease in the recipient. HIV focussed attention initially, then hepatitis C-induced liver disease and now there is concern over other hepatitis viruses, HTLV1 and even the possibility of transmission of variant CJD prions (the putative human counterpart of the BSE agent in cattle). Secondly, following the outbreak of hepatitis B in patients after cryopreserved stem cell infusion, it was demonstrated that viral transmission occurred as a result of common storage in a liquid nitrogen tank which contained one patient's hepatitis BsAg +ve bone marrow.

Combining current national guidelines with standards to be adopted throughout Europe and America, the following tests are likely to be mandatory:

- Hepatitis B surface antigen.
- Hepatitis B surface antibody.
- Hepatitis B core antigen.
- Hepatitis B core antibody.
- Hepatitis C antibody.
- HIV 1 and 2 antibodies.
- HIV 1 and 2 antigen.
- HTLV1 antibody.
- VDRL.
- Additional serum for storage for retrospective analysis.

These results must be available to transplant laboratories *before* cryopreservation. Since many of these patients will be receiving blood products as part of their on-going treatment, they must be performed *within 30 days of cryopreservation* to prevent false –ve antibody tests due to the interval between exposure and sero-conversion. In practice these constraints dictate that samples should be taken between 7 and 30 days prior to cryopreservation.

Patient samples shown to be –ve for all the above infectious agents should have stem cells stored in a dedicated liquid nitrogen freezer conventionally in the liquid phase.

Patient samples shown to be +ve for *any* of the above agents should **be double bagged and stored in a separate liquid nitrogen freezer in the vapour phase** (to reduce transmissibility). Data on all stem cell product samples must be registered in a secure environment on a computerised database with a logical inventory and retrieval system. No material should be imported to the freezers unless a complete negative virological audit storage trail can be demonstrated.

Transplantation

Stem cell transplant conditioning protocols

Conditioning is the treatment the patient undergoes immediately prior to a stem cell transplant. The purpose is to reduce the burden of residual disease; in allo-geneic transplant recipients, it also acts as an immunosuppressant to prevent rejection of the alloreactive graft. There are many different protocols using chemotherapy alone or in combination with Total Body Irradiation (TBI). Unrelated transplants also require further immunosuppression with Total Lymphoid Irradiation (TLI), ALG or anti-T cell monoclonal antibodies.

Details are beyond the scope of this book but examples are:
- **AML** – Allo and Autografts
  – Cyclophosphamide plus TBI *or* Cyclophosphamide plus Busulphan.

- **ALL** – Allo and autografts
  – Cyclophosphamide plus TBI or Etoposide plus TBI.

- **NHL** – autografts
  – BEAM (BCNU, Etoposide, Ara-C and Melphalan).

- **Myeloma** – autografts
  – High dose Melphalan.

Infusion of cryopreserved stem cells

Equipment
1. Dewar containing stem cells in liquid N_2.
2. Water bath heated to 37°C–40°C.
3. Tongs.
4. Protective gloves.
5. Patient's notes.
6. Trolley with: syringes, needles, ampoules of 0.9% saline, blood giving sets, sterile dressing towels, Chlorhexidine spray, bags of 500ml N/Saline, sterile gloves.

Ensure the patient has had procedure and any possible side-effects explained.

Method
1. Write up the stem cell infusion on the blood product infusion chart.
2. 30 mins before reinfusion, ensure water bath is filled and heated to 37°C–40°C and give chlorpheniramine 10mg IV and paracetamol 1g PO.
3. When ready to return the stem cells take the dewar and equipment trolley to the patient's bedside.
4. Check the patient's vital signs.
5. Set up a standard blood giving set with microaggregate filter. Never use additional filters. Prime with 500ml 0.9% saline, connect to the patient and ensure good flow before starting to thaw any cells.
6. Check the water bath is 37°C–40°C and using the protective glove and large tongs remove a bag of cells from liquid nitrogen dewar and place on the trolley. Carefully remove from the outer sleeve and place in water bath and allow one minute. DMSO cryopreservative is very toxic to cells once thawed so it is important to go straight from rapid thaw to infusion.
7. Remove bag of cells from water bath using the tongs, spray with Chlorhexidine and allow to dry. Check patient identification number and DOB with the patient and if correct then connect to the giving set.
8. Cells should be returned as quickly as possible. Each bag contains approximately 100–150ml. Providing the flow is good, start thawing the next bag. Only thaw the next bag if you are able to finish the previous bag within the next minute. Check the patient's details on every bag.
9. Check the patient's observations at 15 minute intervals.
10. If the patient complains of abdominal pain, nausea or feeling faint, slow down the IVI for a short time. If symptoms persist or patient develops chest tightness or wheezing – stop the infusion. O_2 ± nebulised salbutamol may be required. Anaphylaxis rarely occurs.
11. At the end of reinfusion ensure no more bags of stem cells in the dewar and clear away all equipment.
12. Write the infusion details in the patient's notes in red ink.

Special considerations
▶ If the bag splits/leaks *do not reinfuse* – contents will not be sterile. Very rarely, a bag could start to expand rapidly upon thawing if all air not removed from the bag before freezing. A sterile needle may be used to pierce the bag if release of pressure appears essential.

▶▶ *Acute anaphylaxis is very rare but adrenalin (1ml of 1:1000) should be available in the patient's room for SC or IM administration.*

Infusion of fresh non-cryopreserved stem cells

Explain procedure and side effects to patient. In general, bone marrow will be in a larger volume than an apheresis product.

Procedure

1. A medical staff member must be available to start the infusion and stay with the patient for the first 30 minutes.
2. Prime blood giving set *without an in-line filter* with 500ml 0.9% saline and connect to the patient – check there is a good flow.
3. Check BP, pulse and chest auscultation before the infusion.
4. Give paracetamol 1g PO and chlorpheniramine 10mg IV at beginning of infusion.
5. Give stem cells as slowly as possible for the first 15 minutes, then increase the rate to 100ml in 60 minutes. If after 2h the patient is tolerating infusion without problems, increase to 200ml/h until completion.
6. Watch for fluid overload – give diuretic if necessary.
7. Nursing staff should monitor BP and pulse every 15–30 mins.
8. Write infusion details in the patient's notes in red ink.

Complications of stem cell infusion

- Microemboli occasionally cause dyspnoea and cyanosis. O_2 should be available. Slow down or stop the stem cell infusion if dyspnoea.
- Pyrexia, rash and rigors can occur – treat with hydrocortisone IV and chlorpheniramine IV.
- Hypertension may occur (especially if patient fluid overloaded). Usually responds to diuretic.

▶▶ *Acute anaphylaxis is very rare but adrenalin (1ml of 1:1000) should be available in the patient's room for SC or IM administration.*

Blood product support for stem cell transplantation

All cellular blood products, ie red cells and platelets must be **_irradiated_**.

Irradiation

- All cellular blood products given to transplant patients must be irradiated to prevent transfusion associated GvHD due to transfused T lymphocytes.
- Transfusion associated GvHD is usually fatal particularly in allografts. Fatality can sometimes be avoided by immediate administration of anti-lymphocyte globulin or Campath antibody.
- Irradiation protocol is standard 2500 cGy.
- Irradiation starts on the first day of conditioning for the transplant. Policy varies on discontinuation as transfusion associated GvHD can occur even years post-transplant. Safest policy is to continue for life.
- Cell-free blood products, eg FFP, cryoprecipitate or albumin do not need to be irradiated.
- Marrow or blood stem cell transplant itself is of course *never* irradiated.

CMV status of blood products

- CMV itself is not destroyed by irradiation.
- All transplant recipients should ideally receive CMV –ve red cells and platelet transfusions *regardless* of their own CMV status if sufficient CMV –ve blood products available. This is because of good evidence that transfused CMV carried in donor white cells may cause disease post-transplant regardless of the CMV status of the patient. CMV –ve recipients must always have –ve products.
- Should CMV negative platelets not be available at any time, it is acceptable to use unscreened red cells or platelets *provided* they go through an in-line leucodepletion filter. This is because CMV is carried predominantly in white cells which are blocked by the filter. Leucocyte depletion 'at source' is, however, a preferable method of leucocyte depletion to bedside filtration.
- For allograft recipients, additional preventive measures are taken against CMV reactivation (see section on CMV, p254).

Indications for RBC and platelet transfusions

Identical to those for patients undergoing intensive chemotherapy (see protocol for platelet support therapy, p456).

Management of ABO incompatibility

Fortunately in allogeneic transplantation, ABO incompatibility between donor and recipient does not affect the long-term success of the transplant nor the incidence of graft failure or GvHD. However, major ABO incompatibility blood complications will occur unless specific steps are taken to manipulate the graft where donor and recipient are ABO mismatched. Furthermore, additional care must be given post-transplant in providing appropriate ABO matched products.

ABO mismatched definitions

1. **_Major ABO mismatch._** This is where the recipient has anti-A or anti-B antibody to donor ABO antigens eg group O recipients with group A donor.

2. **_Minor ABO mismatch._** This is where the donor has antibodies to recipient ABO antigens, eg group A recipient with group O donor.

Management of major ABO mismatch

Manipulation of donor marrow/stem cells: red cells are removed in the transplant laboratory, by starch sedimentation or Ficoll centrifugation, prior to infusion of the graft.

Choice of red cell and platelet supportive transfusions

- Transfuse packed group O red cells only for all major mismatch donor recipient pairs.
- The choice of platelet group is less critical and may be affected by availability. First, second and third choice groups for platelet transfusions are shown in the table below.

Minor ABO mismatch

Manipulation of donor stem cells: prior to infusion, the product will have been plasma reduced in the transplant laboratory by centrifugation to remove antibody that could be passively transferred. Delayed immune haemolysis, which may be severe and intravascular, can occur after minor ABO mismatch due to active production of antibody by engrafting donor lymphocytes. Maximum haemolysis occurs 9–16 days post-transplant.

239

Choice of red cell and platelet transfusions

Always transfuse packed O red cells, ie the same as in major ABO mismatch. Platelet transfusions first, second and third choice group is shown in the table below.

Choice of ABO group of blood/platelets in ABO mismatch BMT

Donor	Recipient	Red cells	Platelets		
			1st choice	2nd choice	3rd choice
Major ABO					
mismatch					
A	O	O	A	B	O
B	O	O	B	A	O
AB	O	O	A	B	O
A	B	O	B	A*	O*
B	A	O	A	B*	O*
AB	A	O	A	B*	O*
AB	B	O	B	A*	O*
Minor ABO					
mismatch					
O	A	O	A	B*	O*
O	B	O	B	A*	O*
O	AB	O	A*	A*	O*
A	AB	O	A*	B*	O*
B	AB	O	B*	A*	O*

(*Risk of haemolysis but do not withhold)

Rhesus (D) mismatch

Anti D is not a naturally occurring antibody but may be induced by sensitisation with D cells through eg pregnancy or previous incompatible transfusion. Important to screen both recipient and donor serum for the presence of anti D.

- When either donor or recipient serum contains anti D, rhesus D –ve blood products should always be given post transplant. *Note:* in the situation where a rhesus D +ve recipient receives a graft from a donor whose serum contains anti D, immune haemolysis may occur despite plasma reduction of the donor marrow due to active production of donor lymphocyte derived anti-D. Cannot be prevented but is rarely severe.
- Provided neither donor nor recipient have anti-D in the serum, specific pre-transplant manipulation of the product is only required in the situation of rhesus D +ve donor going into rhesus D –ve recipient where red cell depletion is required pre-transplant.
- It will occasionally be necessary to give rhesus D +ve platelet support when rhesus D –ve is preferable simply due to lack of abundant availability of rhesus –ve platelet products.
- If rhesus D +ve platelets *have* to be given, give anti-D 250 iu SC immediately post-transfusion.

GvHD prophylaxis

'Seattle protocol' most commonly used. Alternatives include *in vitro* T cell depletion of graft or *in vivo* T cell depletion with Campath or Anti-Lymphocyte Globulin (ALG). Seattle protocol consists of a combination of stat pulses of IV methotrexate (MTX) with bd infusions of cyclosporin:

Methotrexate MTX (IV bolus) 15mg/m^2 on day +1, then 10mg/m^2 days +3, +6 and +11. Folinic acid rescue 15mg/m^2 IV tds may be given 24 hours after each MTX injection for 24 hours (rescue protocol designed to reduce mucositis).

Dosage reductions – if renal/hepatic impairment ↓ MTX dose as follows:

Creatinine (µmol/l)	MTX dose (%)
<145	100
146–165	50
166–180	25
>180	Omit dose

Bilirubin (µmol/l)	MTX dose (%)
<35	100
36–50	50
51–85	25
>85	Omit dose

Side-effects – although reduced by folinic acid rescue mucositis may remain severe and require IV diamorphine.

Cyclosporin administration – powerful immunosuppressant with profound effects on T-cell suppressor function. Available for IV and oral use.

Intravenous regimen – commence on day −1 at 1.5mg/kg IV bd as IVI in 100ml 0.9% saline/2h. If flushing, nausea or pronounced tremor, slow infusion rate 4–6h/dose. Following loading, on day +3 onwards, adjust cyclosporin dosage based on plasma cyclosporin A level together with renal and hepatic function.

Oral regimen – switch intravenous → oral when patient can tolerate oral medication and is eating (usually day +10 to +20). Dosage on conversion is ~1.5–2.0 × IV dose (still bd).

Monitoring cyclosporin levels

- Cyclosporin is toxic and renal impairment is the most frequent dose limiting toxicity.
- Cyclosporin A levels should be done at least twice weekly.
- Never take blood for cyclosporin A levels from the central catheter through which cyclosporin has been given as cyclosporin sticks to the plastic and falsely high levels will be obtained. One lumen should be marked for cyclosporin administration and another lumen marked for blood levels testing.
- 12 hour pre-dose trough whole blood levels are measured.

Instruct patient to delay the morning cyclosporin until after the blood level has been taken. The optimum blood cyclosporin level is not known. Target range: 100–300ng/ml. Aim towards the top of the therapeutic range in the early post-transplant period and lower part of the range at other times. In practice, the dose is often limited by a rise in serum creatinine. If serum creatinine >130μmol/l – adjust dose. Do not give cyclosporin if serum creatinine >180μmol/l.

Dosage adjustment – cyclosporin has a very long t½ so dosage adjustment similar to warfarin adjustment.

1. To ↓ cyclosporin level omit 1–2 doses and make a 25–50% reduction in ongoing maintenance dose, recheck levels at 48h.
2. To ↑ levels, give 1 additional dose, increase maintenance dose by 25–50%, recheck level in 48h.
3. Monitor renal function and LFTs daily. Check serum calcium and magnesium twice weekly.

Cyclosporin toxicity

- Nephrotoxicity (*see above*). Worse with concurrent use of aminoglycosides, vancomycin and amphotericin.
- Hypertension – often associated with fluid retention and potentiated by steroids. Treat initially with diuretic to baseline weight and then nifedipine if persists. Sub-lingual nifedipine useful where emergency reduction of blood pressure is required.
- Neurological syndromes, esp. grand mal fits (usually if untreated hypertension/fluid retention).
- Anorexia, nausea, vomiting, tremor (almost always occurs – if severe suggests overdosage).
- Hirsutism and gum hypertrophy with prolonged usage.
- Hepatotoxicity – less common than nephrotoxicity. Usually intrahepatic cholestatic picture on LFTs. Potentiated by concurrent drug administration eg macrolide antibiotics, norethisterone and the azole antifungals.
- Hypomagnesaemia commonly occurs. Potentiated by combination with amphotericin. Give 20mmol IVI if levels <0.5μmol/l or if symptoms develop. *Note:* only one orally absorbed preparation of magnesium. For hypomagnesaemia persisting on cyclosporin post-discharge, consider magnesium glycerophosphate tablets qds.

Cyclosporin drug interactions

There are substantial and important drug interactions with cyclosporin:

Drugs that ↑ cyclosporin A levels	Drugs that ↓ cyclosporin levels
Azole antifungals	Rifampicin → Major effect
Digoxin	Phenytoin → Major effect
Macrolide antibiotics, especially	Sulphonamides
Erythromycin	Carbamazepine
Imipenem/Meropenem	
Calcium channel blockers	
Oral contraceptives	

243

Drugs WORSENING cyclosporin nephrotoxicity
- Aminoglycosides.
- Amphotericin B.
- Ciprofloxacin.
- Cotrimoxazole.
- ACE inhibitors.

Note: This is not an exhaustive list. Check cyclosporin levels 48h after any drug addition or cessation.

Acute GvHD

Risk factors for acute GvHD include: older recipients, older donors, ♂ recipient of ♀ marrow (↑ risk with previous donor pregnancies), matched unrelated donors. Defined as GVHD occurring within first 100d post-transplant (usually starts between day 7 and 28 post-transplant). Ranges from mild self-limiting condition → extensive disease (may be fatal). Characterised by fever, rash, LFT abnormality, diarrhoea, engraftment suppression and viral reactivation, particularly CMV.

Classified according to the Seattle system by a staging for each organ involved (skin, liver, gut) and overall clinical grading based on the organ staging.

Skin	Involved in >90% cases. May be mild and unremarkable maculopapular rash (esp. palms of hands and soles of feet, but can affect any part of the body). In more severe cases, erythroderma and extensive desquamation and exfoliation can occur.
Liver	Typical pattern of LFT abnormalities is intrahepatic cholestasis with ↑ bilirubin and alkaline phosphatase (relative sparing of transaminases). Note: this picture often does not discriminate between other causes of post-transplant liver dysfunction (eg drugs, infection – particularly CMV and fungal).
Gut	May occasionally be only organ involved, with nausea, vomiting, diarrhoea. Stool appearance may be highly abnormal with mincemeat or redcurrant jelly stools or green coloration.

Diagnosis

- Perform skin biopsy – but do not delay treatment if strong clinical suspicion.
- Rectal biopsy may be helpful (to distinguish infective from pseudomembranous colitis) but beware risk of bleeding and bacteraemia – perform only if it will alter management.
- Where GI symptoms are predominantly upper GI, gastroscopy with oesophageal, gastric and duodenal biopsies may be helpful (eg to distinguish between CMV and fungal oesophagitis and gastritis). Liver biopsy is hazardous and should only be performed where other convincing diagnostic guides are not available. It should be performed only by the transjugular route by an experienced operator and covered appropriately with blood products.

Staging for each organ involved in GvHD

Stage	Skin	Liver	Gut
1	Rash <25% body	Bilirubin 35–50µmol/l	Diarrhoea <1L/d
2	Rash 25-50% body	Bilirubin 51–100µmol/l	Diarrhoea 1–1.5L/d
3	Rash >50% body	Bilirubin 101–250µmol/l	Diarrhoea >1.5L/d
4	Desquam./bullae	Bilirubin >250µmol/l	Pain or ileus

Overall clinical grading for the patient

	Stage		
Grade	**Skin**	**Liver**	**Gut**
0	0	0	0
I	1–2	0	0
II	1–3	1	1
III	2–3	2–3	2–3
IV	2–4	2–4	2–4

Treatment

General measures – good nutrition and weight maintenance important. TPN may be necessary. IV antibiotics and antifungals often necessary in the absence of neutropenia and signs of infection may be masked by steroids. Continue cyclosporin during acute GvHD ensuring levels are not toxic.

Specific treatment should always be discussed with a senior haemato-oncologist. Now known that mild GvHD confers a GvL effect (see p220) in the patient and mild forms of skin GvHD may require no treatment.

Overall grade

I–II   Begin with prednisolone 1–2mg/kg/d PO. If response, taper dose slowly.

        If no response, consider progressing to high dose methylprednisolone.

II–IV   Give high dose methylprednisolone 20mg/kg/over 1h bd IV for 48h, then ↓ dose by 50% every 48h.

Side effects of methylprednisolone

- Gastritis/peptic ulceration – use proton pump inhibitors rather than H_2 blockers.
- Hyperglycaemia, particularly when TPN in use. May require insulin infusion.
- Hypertension may be potentiated by cyclosporin and by fluid retention – treat with diuretics and nifedipine.
- Insomnia and psychosis.

Failure of response to high dose methylprednisolone

Discuss with senior colleague. Outlook poor. Various empirical possibilities include Campath infusion or ALG.

Chronic GvHD

Occurs between 100–300d post-allogeneic transplant. There may not have been preceding acute GvHD, and acute GVHD may have resolved prior to onset of chronic GvHD. Clinical classification is subdivided into *limited* or *extensive* chronic GvHD. Major clinical features are of debility, weight loss with malabsorption, sclerodermatous reaction due to excessive collagen deposition, severe immunosuppression and features of autoimmune disease.

Limited chronic GvHD – clinical features
- Localised skin involvement <50% total surface.
- Hepatic dysfunction – portal lesions but lacking necrosis, aggressive hepatitis or cirrhosis.
- Other localised involvement of eyes, salivary glands and mouth.

Extensive chronic GvHD – clinical features
- Generalised skin involvement >50% of surface – may include sclerodermatous changes and ulceration.
- Abnormal liver function – histology shows centrilobular changes, chronic aggressive hepatitis, bridging necrosis or cirrhosis.
- Liver dysfunction ± localised skin GvHD with involvement of eyes, salivary glands or oral mucosa on labial biopsy.
- Involvement of any other major organ system.

Treatment
Discuss with a senior member of medical team.

General measures
1. Adequate nutrition, vitamin/calorie supplements may be required and severe cases may require TPN.
2. Pneumococcal prophylaxis must be continued lifelong.
3. Consider restarting conventional prophylactic antifungal and antibacterial agents.
4. CMV surveillance is critical (reactivation is more common).
5. Psychological support may be required to adjust to chronic disability.

Specific treatment
1. Commonest protocol used is the Seattle regimen of prednisolone and cyclosporin A on alternate days. Typically: prednisolone 20–25mg/alternate days with cyclosporin A 100mg bd (minimum 2 months).
2. If response, ↓ cyclosporin dose first *then* steroid – usually require small maintenance dose of steroid.
3. If no response or progression add in azathioprine 1.5 mg/kg/d initially (monitor FBC, renal and liver function).
4. Severe refractory cases may respond to experimental measures such as extracorporeal PUVA therapy, anti-lymphocyte globulin, or thalidomide.

Veno-occlusive disease

Presents clinically early post-transplant (usually within the first 14d). Pathophysiology poorly understood. Risk factors for severe VOD include: intensive conditioning regimens, pre-transplant hepatitis and second transplants. VOD is characterised by a triad of hepatomegaly, jaundice and ascites (resulting in rapid post-transplant weight gain) as a result of this. Commoner in allografts than autografts.

Diagnosis is largely clinical but may be supported by typical findings on Doppler ultrasound study of hepatic arterial and venous flows, or by elevated Plasminogen Activator Inhibitor (PAI 1) levels. However, the only definitive diagnostic investigation is transjugular liver biopsy, the risks of which must be weighed against the importance of the information obtained.

There is no treatment currently universally accepted as effective prophylaxis.

Strategies include
- Heparin 100u/kg/d by continuous IVI.
- LMWH sc od or a prostaglandin E1 (PGE1) infusion.

No universally accepted effective treatment. The key is supportive therapy with management of fluid overload with spironolactone and frusemide while maintaining intravascular volume with albumin or plasma substitute. In severe VOD, infusion of TPA or PGE1 may be considered.

If thrombolysis required
- Ensure no active bleeding is occurring and keep platelets $>20 \times 10^9/l$.
- Give Tissue-type Plasminogen Activator (Altaplase™).
             10mg IV into central line over 30 mins
             then 40mg as IVI over next 60 minutes
             ie total dose of 50 mg over 90 minutes
             (reduce doses proportionally for patients weighing <than 60kg).
- Give daily for 3 days minimum and assess against VOD parameters.

Antifungal therapy

Amphotericin

If a patient is unresponsive to second line antibiotics, and there is a suspicion of possible fungal infection, then standard formulation of amphotericin (Fungisone™) should be started. Given daily with escalating dosage each day: 0.25mg/kg, 0.5mg/kg, 0.75mg/kg, increasing to maximum dosage of 1mg/kg. *Alternatively* a test dose of 1mg may be given IV over 30 mins with observation of the patient for 30 mins (for reactions) followed by 1mg/kg as above. Daily urea and electrolytes are recommended and amiloride 5mg (increasing to 10mg if required) should be prescribed to counteract the frequently accompanying hypokalaemia. Oral K⁺ supplements often required. Serum Mg^{2+} and LFTs should be checked twice weekly. All doses of amphotericin should be preceded by a 0.9% saline preload. 500ml 0.9% saline should be infused as fast as tolerated (usually over 1 hour) – reduces nephrotoxicity and side-effects. Paracetamol 1g PO should be given 30 minutes prior to infusion together with chlorpheniramine 10mg IV. Pethidine 25–30mg IV stat may be given if a troublesome reaction occurs.

Liposomal amphotericin

Suggested indications for prescribing a liposomal or other lipid formulation of amphotericin.
1. Refractory fever >72h on standard amphotericin at 1mg/kg.
2. A rise in the creatinine to >50% baseline levels with standard amphotericin despite optimal hydration.
3. Deteriorating LFTs.
4. Evidence of severe disseminated fungal infection – ie multiple lesions on CXR or CT scan, or any two sites of sinuses, lung, liver, spleen or brain.
5. Patients receiving cyclosporin after an allograft. These patients should receive lipid formulation product if baseline creatinine is >130μmol/l. Otherwise, the indication for lipid formulation product is as in 1–4 above.

Lipid formulation amphotericin products

2 lipid formulations of amphotericin in extensive use – both are expensive. No comparative trial of the two products but efficacy data appear similar. An appropriate protocol is suggested:

Commence either amphotericin B Lipid Complex (Abelcet™) at 2.5mg/kg or liposomal amphotericin (AmBisome™) at 1mg/kg (in practice round up or down to standard vial size to avoid wastage and minimize cost). Follow data sheet instructions carefully, observing for anaphylaxis. The dosage should be increased to a maximum of 5mg/kg Abelcet™ or 3–5mg/kg AmBisome™ in patients who have either a confirmed mycological diagnosis or a fever which does not respond within 72h on the lower dose.

Paracetamol and chlorpheniramine pre-medication cover is advised for Abelcet™ (may also be required for AmBisome™). 0.9% saline preload is not normally required unless renal or liver function deteriorate during treatment. Renal function should be checked on alternate days for the duration of the treatment. Serum Mg^{2+} and LFTs should be checked weekly.

Total duration of treatment difficult to asses. General principles are that therapy should continue for at least 2 weeks and until neutrophil recovery and no signs of progression radiologically.

Note

As with all protocols check local policies since these may differ to those outlined in this handbook.

CMV prophylaxis and treatment

All transplant recipients who are CMV sero-negative should receive CMV –ve blood products. If supplies are available, this is recommended also for CMV sero-positive recipients. Limits risk of CMV blood product transmission regardless of donor/recipient serological status.

CMV surveillance
- All allograft patients and CMV sero-positive autograft recipients should receive CMV surveillance.
- The minimum surveillance required is the DEAFF (detection of early antigen fluorescent foci) test. Should detect CMV antigen in culture by immunofluorescence within 48 hours and virus culture continues for 1–2 weeks. Urine and throat washings are not sent routinely for CMV detection.
- 5 ml EDTA blood should be sent weekly on the above cohort of transplant patients from admission until day 100. Screening of allograft recipients should continue until 1 year post-transplant although the frequency of testing may be reduced in the absence of appropriate symptoms.
- More sensitive tests now available to detect CMV antigen or genome by PCR technology in buffy coat of EDTA peripheral blood will soon replace DEAFF as standard tests.

CMV prophylaxis
Indicated in allograft patients when either donor or recipient are CMV sero-positive. Not recommended when both donor and recipient are sero-negative, nor for autograft recipients, even if sero-positive.

Suggested protocol
1. Acyclovir 800mg tds IV from day –5 to discharge, then 800mg tds PO for 3 months *plus*
2. IVIg 200mg/kg IV day –1, day +13 and then every 3 weeks until day +100. *Note:* The graft suppression of this dose of acyclovir may sometimes be dose limiting.

Treatment of CMV infection
A +ve CMV identification in buffy coat by either surveillance method should be treated even if the patient is asymptomatic:
- Gancyclovir: 5 mg/kg IV bd for 14 days minimum.
  Side-effects: myelosuppressive, may be abrogated by G-CSF, nephrotoxic.
- Renal function must be monitored and dose reductions implemented according to the BNF.
- Abnormal LFTs may occur.
- Fever, rashes and headaches.
- Alternative – Foscarnet 90 mg/kg IV bd for 14d minimum.
  Administer through a central line as IVI over 2 hours (may be given as a peripheral IVI but should be given concurrently with a fast running litre of 0.9% saline). *Side-effects* – nephrotoxic and hepatotoxic (follow BNF dosage adjustments).

Treatment plan
On a first episode of CMV antigenaemia, start with Gancyclovir. Failure to become CMV antigen –ve by the end of the 2 week course would lead to immediate progression to Foscarnet.

CMV related disease

May cause pneumonitis, oesophagitis, gastritis, hepatitis, retinitis and myelo-suppression. Where CMV antigenaemia accompanied by symptoms/signs of CMV disease IVIg 400mg/kg IV should be administered once a week plus gancyclovir or foscarnet. Broncho-alveolar lavage (BAL) should be performed to establish the presence of CMV locally in the lung.

Post-transplant vaccination programme

General

The subject of re-vaccination post-transplant remains a contentious topic with various protocols followed from different centres. The general principles are that live vaccination is, of course, forbidden, probably for the lifetime of the patient. Secondly, antibody and T-cell responses to vaccination in the first year following transplantation are sub-optimal. In allogeneic transplants, immune reconstitution continues beyond one and up to two years post-transplant. These general considerations have been used to suggest the following policy.

Allogeneic transplants

No immunisations should be given in the presence of acute or chronic GvHD. In the absence of this, proceed as follows:

At 18 months post-transplant

- Diphtheria and tetanus primary course.
- Primary course of *inactivated* polio vaccine.
- Pneumovax II (repeated every 6 years).
- *Haemophilus influenzae* B.
- Meningococcal A and C.
- Influenza vaccine (and yearly thereafter).

The vaccinations should be staggered with only diphtheria and tetanus being allowed concurrently. It would be reasonable to leave a gap of two weeks between each vaccination. Not only may this enhance antibody responses but it will easily identify the culprit if there are any reactions.

Autologous transplants – 1 year post-transplant

- Tetanus booster.
- *Inactivated* polio vaccine booster.
- Pneumovax II (repeated every 6 years).
- *Haemophilus influenzae* B.
- Meningococcal A and C.
- Influenza vaccine (repeated annually).

Foreign travel

All transplant recipients should take medical advice from their transplant team before travelling abroad.

Post-transplant complications

- Bacterial and fungal infections.
- Pneumonitis.
- CMV reactivation.
- Veno-occlusive disease (VOD) – *see p250*.

Allografts only

- Acute GvHD (see p246).
- Chronic GvHD (see p248).

Longer term effects

- **Endocrine** – hypothyroidism may occur post-transplant. Check TFTs at 3 monthly intervals→1 year
- **Respiratory** – check lung function tests at 6 months and one year if TBI has been given
- **Skin** – advise about sun protection (following TBI avoid the sun). If exposure is unavoidable, total sun block factor 15 or higher is essential for at least one year.
- **Fertility** – most patients will be infertile after transplant (almost invariably if TBI given). Since this cannot be absolutely guaranteed, contraceptive precautions should be taken until the confirmatory tests have been performed ♂ – check sperm counts at 3 and 6 months post-transplant. Zero motile sperm on both samples confirms infertility. ♀ – check FSH, LH and oestradiol at 3 months. FSH and LH levels should be high and oestradiol levels low if no ovulation is occurring.
- **Menopause** – women may have an early menopause due to the treatment and may experience symptoms such as hot flushes, dry skin, dryness of the vagina and loss of libido. Most women should have hormone replacement therapy (Prempak C 1.25 initially starting as soon as early menopause is confirmed) and counselled about HRT problems
- **Cataracts** – patients who have had TBI are at risk of developing cataracts. Refer for Ophthalmological assessment at one year post BMT.
- **Immunisations** at 12–24 months post-transplant (see p256).

Discharge and follow-up

Criteria for discharge
Blood counts should ideally be: Hb >10.0g/dl (but may require transfusion), neutrophils >1.0 × 10^9/l, platelets >25 × 10^9/l, and patients should be able to maintain a fluid intake of 2–3L/d, tolerating diet and oral medications particularly in allografts on cyclosporin. Should be apyrexial and no longer losing weight.

Counsel patients
1. Possible need for blood/platelets.
2. Adherence to neutropenic diet.
3. Check temperature bd and report immediately if febrile.
4. Fatigue post-transplant in irradiated patients due to the late TBI effect usually 6–10 weeks post transplant.
5. Risk of HZV (explain the early symptoms).
6. To continue with mouth care.
7. To report any new symptoms.

Blood tests – twice weekly
- FBC, reticulocytes and blood film.
- Biochemistry including LFTs.
- CyA levels pre-dose (EDTA sample) – allografts only.

Once a week
- Magnesium.
- CRP.
- Clotting screen.
- CMV screening test e.g DEAFF – allografts and seropositive autograft recipients only.
- Stool culture – allografts only unless relevant symptoms.

Drugs
1. *Cyclosporin* capsules–allografts only.
2. *Acyclovir* prophylaxis against HZV 400mg qds PO for minimum of 3 months in non-TBI patients and 6 months in TBI autografts and all allografts. Allografts may be on 800mg tds if Acyclovir chosen for CMV prophylaxis. Consider low dose 200mg bd maintenance until 1–2 years post-transplant.
3. *Penicillin V* 250mg bd PO should be given to all patients. *Erythromycin* 250mg od PO if penicillin allergic.
4. *Ciprofloxacin* 250mg bd PO if neutrophils <1.0 × 10^9/l.
5. Cotrimoxazole 480mg bd PO Mon, Wed, Fri for 1 year minimum **and** until CD4 count >500. Cotrimoxazole should be started when neutrophils >1.5 × 10^9/l and platelets >60 × 10^9/l. Until then, use nebulised pentamidine 300mg every 3 weeks.
6. Itraconazole – allografts only.
7. Nystatin mouth care.
8. Folic acid 5mg bd until full engraftment.
9. Sanatogen Gold™ multivitamins 1/d may be advisable while gaining weight.
10. Antiemetics PRN.

On each day ward unit visit check for
- Fever.
- Nausea and vomiting.
- Diarrhoea.

- Bleeding.
- Rashes.
- Fatigue.
- Dyspnoea.
- Pain.
- Weight loss.
- Jaundice.
- Mucositis.
- Skin surveillance needed to observe for signs of acute and chronic GvHD, HSV, HZV and drug related problems.
- Hickman line infections are common post-transplant. If any signs of infection and fever, line cultures and exit site swab should be taken. Remove line as soon as infusional support no longer needed.

Haemostasis and thrombosis 9

Coagulation disorders – a clinical approach

Bleeding problems present a considerable challenge. Presentation is from simple easy bruising – a common problem – to catastrophic post-traumatic bleeding. Laboratory investigation of a bleeding patient may be difficult. *Acquired disorders are much more common than inherited ones.*

Causes of bleeding eg surgical, trauma, non-accidental injury, coagulation disorders, platelet dysfunction, vascular disorders.

Clinical features History, presenting complaint. Is this an isolated symptom? Type of bleeding eg mucocutaneous, easy bruising, spontaneous, post-traumatic. Duration and time of onset – ?recent, or present in childhood. Menstrual and obstetrical history are important.

Systemic enquiry Do symptoms suggest a systemic disorder, bone marrow failure, infection, liver disease, renal disease?

Past medical history Previous episode, recurrent – ?ITP, congenital disorder. Exposure to trauma, surgery, dental extraction, or pregnancies.

Family history First degree relatives. Pattern of inheritance (eg autosomal, sex-linked). If family history is negative this could be a new mutation.

Drugs Thrombocytopenia (see p310), platelet dysfunction (see p304); not always obvious – aspirin, warfarin. Inhibitors, drug reaction – allergic purpura.

Physical examination

Signs of systemic disease Septicaemia, anaemia, lymphadenopathy ± hepatosplenomegaly?

Assess bleeding site Check palate and fundi. Could this be self inflicted? Check *size* – petechiae (pin head); purpura (larger ≤1 cm); bruises (ecchymoses) ≥1 cm – *measure them.*

Joints Swelling or other signs of chronic arthritis.

Vascular lesions Purpura – allergic, Henoch-Schönlein (p302), senile, steroid-related, hypergammaglobulinaemic, HHT – capillary dilatations (blanches on pressure), vasculitic lesions, autoimmune disorders, hypersensitivity reactions.

Investigation

- Baseline FBC, film, platelet count, biochemistry screen, ESR, coagulation screen.
- Special tests eg BM for 1° haematological disorders; radiology, USS.
- Family studies.

Summary

Exclude surgical bleeding and test *early* before transfusion compounds the problem. Decide whether platelet or coagulation defect or both? Is it hereditary or acquired?

Treatment

Establish diagnosis and treat as appropriate.

Haemostasis and thrombosis

Classification of coagulation disorders

Coagulation disorders – laboratory approach

Establish whether bleeding is of *recent origin* (suggests acquired) or *longstanding* (congenital), *spontaneous* or *induced by trauma/surgery*, *mucocutaneous* (?platelet defect) or *generalised* (?coagulation defect or ?drug induced).

Laboratory tests
- FBC with platelet count, coagulation screen (PT, APTT, fibrinogen).
- Blood sample should be fresh venous stab if possible; fill to the mark.
- Repeat test if result abnormal before investigating further.
- Check patient not on anticoagulants.

Further investigation

Abnormal platelet count
- Both high and low counts may cause bleeding.
- If isolated ↓ platelets see p310; if ↑ platelets see p308.
- If platelets ↓ and coagulation screen abnormal – could be DIC, liver disease, heparin induced thrombocytopenia, massive blood transfusion, primary blood disease (eg leukaemia, MPD).

Abnormal coagulation result
- Check whether abnormal coagulation result corrects to normal with control plasma 50:50 mix.

▶ PT ↑ APTT normal
Deficiency: ↓ VII.
Causes: early liver disease, vitamin K deficiency, warfarin.

▶ PT ↑ APTT↑
Deficiency: ↓ X, II, V, fibrinogen.
Causes: single or multiple deficiency eg DIC, liver failure, vitamin K deficiency.

▶ PT normal APTT↑
Deficiency: ↓ VIII, IX, XI, XII.
Causes: single or multiple deficiency, haemophilia A or B, von Willebrand's disease, lupus anticoagulant, heparin.

▶ PT normal APTT normal
Deficiency: ↓ XIII.
Causes: as above, mild deficiency of any factor, normal patient, platelet abnormality, LMW heparin.

Further investigation
- Input clinical information.
- Further lab tests.
- DIC – check blood film, platelets, thrombin time, fibrinogen, XDPs/D dimer.
- Vit K deficiency; assay IX, X, II, VII; give vitamin K and repeat 24h later.
- Liver disease – check LFTs; will not correct to normal with vitamin K.
- Isolated factor deficiency – assay as indicated by PT/APTT result.
- Inhibitor-specific LA tests; check ACL; other factor-specific assays.
- Heparin ↑ APTT ratio, PT normal if APTT ratio 1.5–2.5, TT ↑, Reptilase normal.
- Warfarin ↓ vitamin K dependent factors. PIVKA, warfarin levels.
- vWD – vWF related activities, bleeding time.

Haemostasis and thrombosis

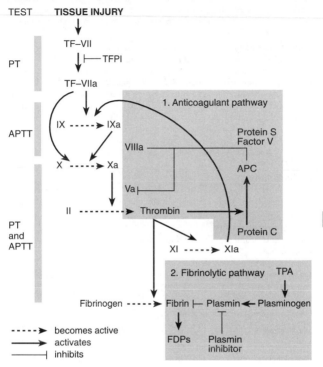

TEST   **TISSUE INJURY**

PT

APTT

PT
and
APTT

----➤ becomes active
——➤ activates
——| inhibits

Blood coagulation system

Tissue injury triggers off a cascade of zymogen-to-protease reactions which amplify resulting in fibrin clot. Many inhibiting factors include Tissue Factor Pathway Inhibitor (TFPI), Antithrombin and Activated Protein C (APC).

Fibrinolytic pathway (see 2.)

Tissue plasminogen activators (TPA) activate plasminogen to plasmin; this breaks down fibrin releasing fibrin degradation products (FDPs, or XDPs when cross linked) into the circulation.

Anticoagulation system (see 1.)

Thrombin binds to a receptor, thrombomodulin (TM) on the surface of endothelial cells. Bound to TM thrombin loses anticoagulant activity and becomes a potent activator of protein C → PC (APC) with co-factors PS and FV, cleaves and inactivates Factors Va and VIIIa.

Haemophilia

Congenital bleeding disorder caused by defective production of a procoagulant protein Factor VIII (haemophilia A) or IX (haemophilia B); sex-linked recessive inheritance. ♀ carry the disease but are rarely symptomatic. Queen Victoria passed the disease on to her great-grandson, Alexis, son of the Tsar, contributing to the fall of Tsarist Russia.

Pathophysiology

Factor VIII activated by thrombin, and IX activated by the TF/Factor VIIa complex, together activate Factor X, leading to the prothrombinase activation of fibrinogen → fibrin (p267). Factor VIII (mw 250,000 daltons) isolated in 1982. Genetic abnormalities include: *rearrangements* within intron 22 in 50%, *point mutations* in 40% and *deletions* in 5%. Linked polymorphisms (ie abnormal DNA markers around the gene) are informative in 85%, and can be used to identify the carrier state in the ♀ but require samples from family members. Factor IX, a vitamin K dependent factor (mw 56,000) isolated in 1982. Genetic defects include gene *deletions, point* and *missense* mutations. ~⅓ have a dysfunctional IX molecule.

Epidemiology

Haemophilia A occurs in 1: 10,000 ♂ in the UK; 6 × more frequent than haemophilia B; in both no family history in ~⅓ cases; no striking racial distribution.

Clinical presentation

Haemophilia A and B – clinically indistinguishable. Symptoms depend on the factor level.

Severe disease (plasma level <2%)	Usually presents in the first years of life with easy bruising and bleeding out of proportion to injury
Moderate disease (2–5% factor level)	Intermediate & variable severity
Mild disease (>5%)	May only present after trauma/surgery in later life
General features	Haemarthrosis; spontaneous bleeding into joints (knees > elbows > ankles > hips > wrists) produce local tingling, pain; later – swelling, limitation of movement, warmth, redness

Bleeds into muscles, spontaneous bleeding into arms, legs, ileopsoas, or any site – may lead to nerve compression, compartment syndrome, muscle contractures – *look for these*. *Haematuria* is common; retroperitoneal and CNS bleeds are life-threatening – but fortunately rare.

Diagnosis

Assess duration, type of bleeding, exposure to previous trauma/surgery and family history. Look for bruising, petechial haemorrhages, early signs of joint damage. Bleeding time ↔. Exclude medical causes of acquired bleeding disorders.

Haemostasis and thrombosis

Laboratory tests
INR ↔; APTT ratio ↑ ~2.5 in severe disease (note: *a normal APTT ratio does not exclude mild disease*). Assay VIII first, then IX. If VIII deficient, exclude von Willebrand's disease at this stage.

Radiology
Acute bleed – USS or CT scan if in doubt. In established disease – chronic synovitis, arthropathy, and other pathological changes seen.

Complications

Chronic arthropathy	Repeated joint bleeds preventable but older haemophiliacs may well have such problems.
Development of Factor VIII inhibitors	Suggested by ↓ response to concentrates; occurs in 18–20% haemophilia A patients following treatment (IX inhibitors are uncommon; <5%).
Transmission of HBV, HCV & HIV	Transmission high prior to the introduction of viral inactivation of concentrates (1985 in the UK). HIV testing (1984–85) identified 60–80% incidence with Factor VIII concentrates. Of ~3000 patients identified at that time, ⅔ have died of AIDS.

HIV management
Prophylaxis against PCP (cotrimoxazole), retroviral inhibition with reverse transcriptase inhibitors, eg *zidovudine, lamivudine*, and recent additions of protease inhibitors, eg *indinovir, sequanivir, retonivir*, have improved prognosis HCV disease has affected ¾ of the patients treated with VIII concentrates before 1985; significant liver damage (chronic aggressive hepatitis, cirrhosis) in 10–25%. Interferon-α is effective in ~10%. New drugs (eg ribavirin) are currently on trial. There is a concern about nvCJD at present.

Management
General Regular medical and haemophilia review and lifelong support are essential. At presentation establish *blood group*, *liver function* and baseline *viral status* (HIV, HCV, HBV, HAV). Vaccinate against HBV & HAV if not immune. Regularly check LFTs, FBC. Avoid aspirin, anti-platelet drugs, and IM injections. Early treatment of bleeding episodes is essential.

Haemophilia A-specific treatment
Mild disease
- Minor bleeds may stop with local pressure.
- Tranexamic acid (15–25mg/kg tds PO) – useful for cuts or dental extraction. Avoid in upper urinary tract bleeds.
- DDAVP (Desmopressin) for minor surgery and bleeds that fail to settle (0.3µg/kg slow IVI/20 min); may also be given SC and by nasal spray. 20 min later take blood sample to check response (if required); plasma level ↑ 3–4 fold. ⅓ do not respond. Response reduced ~30% next time.
- Cryoprecipitate preceded concentrate production as source of Factor VIII, ~75u/bag; comes fresh frozen from donors; *not* virally inactivated and no longer recommended.

Severe disease

- Factor VIII concentrates are cornerstone of management for severe disease and life threatening situations.

Products

- Intermediate purity 8Y (Bio Products Laboratory, BPL), virally inactivated (80°C for 72h); good record of viral safety.

  Monoclonal purified products; <immunogenic but more expensive; recommended for HIV +ve patients. Recombinant Factor VIII, virally safe – the aim for all patients; expensive; recommended for use in children and young patients not previously treated. Principle of treatment: raise Factor VIII to haemostatic level (15–20% for spontaneous bleeds, 40% minor ops; 100% major surgery or life-threatening bleeds).

Formula

1 unit/kg body weight $\uparrow$ plasma concentration by 2%. t½ 8–12h. Spontaneous bleeds usually settle with single treatment. In major surgery provide cover for up to 10d.

Haemophilia B

- General approach: as for haemophilia A – DDAVP and cryoprecipitate of no value.
- Products – high purity Factor IX virally inactivated Replinine 1u/kg body wt raises plasma concentration 1%; t½ 18–24h. PCC no longer used – thrombogenic, contains II, X as well as IX

Special considerations

Antenatal diagnosis

Carriers can be identified in ~85% haemophilia A by simple Factor vWFAg :VIIIC ratio (<1.6 found in carriers); less reliable in haemophilia B. Chorionic villus sample analysis using DNA technology at ~10 weeks' gestation used to identify an affected ♂ child and allow termination of pregnancy; rare nowadays because of improved prognosis. Issue is complex and counselling/testing are usually carried out at specialist centres.

Home treatment Has transformed the life of the haemophiliac. Parents, the local GP, the boy himself from age 6–7 onwards, can be trained to give IV Factor concentrates at home. Central lines for the severe affected young patient.

Prophylaxis eg 3 × weekly injections of concentrate (average dose 15–25u/kg) combined with home treatment.

Specialist support Physiotherapy plays key role in preservation of muscle and joint function and should be available on a daily basis. Combined clinics with orthopaedic surgeons, dental surgeons, hepatologists, paediatricians, HIV physicians, and geneticists are required to give truly comprehensive care.

Natural history

Tragically HIV has had a major effect on the life expectancy of haemophilic patients. The impact of HCV infection and chronic liver disease is still being evaluated. The new generation with optimal treatment should have a normal life expectancy; treatment is expensive, however, and sadly not available for all.

Pediatric Hematology 1996 **43** 709

Other congenital coagulation deficiencies

Pathophysiology

Deficiency of all the coagulation factors is described but with a prevalence of 1–2 per million is rare cf. haemophilia A and B. Autosomal recessive inheritance, the deficiency either due to reduced synthesis (type 1) or production of a variant protein (type 2). All coagulation factors are produced in the liver and their interaction in the coagulation cascade is shown. The t½ of the factors vary and will determine the frequency and ease of treatment. Table summarises these and lists the concentrations required to achieve haemostasis.

	I	II	V	VII	VIII	IX	X	XI	XII	XIII
% to prevent minor bleeds	(g/l) 0.5–1.0	10–15	5–15	5–10	15–20	10–15	5–10	5–15	<10	1
% to treat major surgery/trauma	1	20–40	25	20–40	25	20–25	15–20	15–25	<10	5
t½ (h)	96–144	50–80	24	5–6	12	20–30	25–60	40–84	?	150
Concentrate available?	Y	Y	N	Y	Y	Y	Y	Y	N	Y

Diagnosis

Conditions rarely produce haemarthrosis and commonly present at time of operation. Clinical and laboratory features of the different conditions are listed.

Treatment

Many patients with inherited coagulation deficiencies will not bleed unless exposed to surgery or trauma, and may seldom require treatment. When bleeding arises or cover for surgery is needed, the aim is to achieve a plasma concentrate concentration at least as high as the minimal haemostatic value and make sure it does not drop below this until haemostasis is secure. FFP is a source of all coagulation factors and is the cornerstone of treatment if no concentrate is available (note: not virally inactivated at present and large volumes may be required – so is far from ideal).

Specific conditions

Fibrinogen

Mol wt 340,000. Unlike the other coagulation factors is present in readily measurable amounts in plasma (normal range 2.0–4.0g/l). Produced by liver, it is an acute phase reactive protein and is raised in inflammatory reactions, pregnancy, stress, etc. Converted into fibrin by the action of thrombin and is a key component of a thrombus. Abnormalities of fibrinogen are more often acquired than inherited. Inherited defects are usually quantitative and include heterozygous hypofibrinogenaemia or homozygous (afibrinogenaemia). Qualitative defects – the dysfibrinogenaemias – are inherited as incompletely autosomal dominant traits with >200 reported fibrinogen variants; defective fibrin polymerisation or fibrinopeptide release may occur. Most patients are heterozygous.

Clinical presentation Symptoms of bruising, bleeding usually after trauma or operations will depend on the concentration and are more severe when <0.5g/l. Afibrinogenaemia (fibrinogen <0.2g/l) is a severe disorder with spontaneous bleeding, cerebral and gastrointestinal haemorrhage and haemarthrosis. It may present as haemorrhage in the newborn. Recurrent miscarriages occur. Most patients with dysfibrinogenaemia are heterozygous and bleeding symptoms are usually minor; arterial and venous thrombosis is described.

Diagnosis ↑PT, ↑APTT, ↑thrombin time; in afibrinogenaemia, the blood may be incoagulable and associated platelet abnormalities (thrombocytopenia, platelet functional defect) may be present. Assay methods include the clot weight, a derived fibrinogen given by coagulometers as part of a clotting screen, and the Clauss assay. Acquired hypofibrinogenaemia needs to be excluded (DIC, drug induced, liver disease) and family studies are necessary.

Dysfibrinogenaemia

↑ PT and APTT, thrombin time and Reptilase time; long bleeding time. Confirm diagnosis by demonstrating normal chemical/immunological fibrinogen concentrations with reduced functional properties.

Treatment Fibrinogen has a long t½ (3–5d) with 70–100% recovery and severe deficiency is managed by repeated (twice weekly) prophylactic injections with fibrinogen concentrates (Immuno). Cryoprecipitate, 0.5g/bag/donation, is a good source but is not heat treated; FFP is less effective. Fibrinogen levels should be raised to 0.5–1.0g/l to achieve haemostasis. Prophylaxis during pregnancy to maintain concentrations >0.5g/l may be required to achieve a successful outcome.

273

Factor VII

Vitamin K dependent factor playing a pivotal role in initiating coagulation. The t½ is short. In severe deficiency, bleeding symptoms (similar to haemophilia) occur and spontaneous intracerebral haemorrhage at a young age is reported in up to 20% patients.

Diagnosis ↑PT APTR normal. Assay factor VII to assess severity.

Management Use factor VII concentrate (BPL) 1u/kg body wt ↑plasma conc ~2%. For cerebral bleed give a 50% rise and continue treatment for 10d. Very short half life makes management difficult, requiring IV replacement 3–4 times/24h. If using FFP, give initial IV injection (20ml/kg) and check response.

Factor II prothrombin

Another vitamin K dependent factor. Usually presents as post-op/trauma bleeding.

Diagnosis ↑ PT < ↑APTT. Assay factor II level.

Management Prothrombin Concentrate Complex (PCC) contains II, VII, X (available from BPL); heat-treated. Dose 1u/kg raises concentration 2%. Long metabolic t½. FFP also effective (10–20ml/kg).

Factor V

Not vitamin K dependent. If severe can cause symptoms as for haemophilia.

Diagnosis ↑ PT, ↑ APTT. BT may be prolonged.

Treatment no concentrate; use FFP (20ml/kg) and repeat 12hrly as required.

Factor XI

More common in Ashkenazi Jews (1:10,000) than other groups. Clinically of variable severity, often mild; even low factor levels may not produce symptoms.

Diagnosis PT normal, ↑ APTT. No concentrate available – use FFP 10–20ml/kg. Aim for 50% XI for surgery.

Factor XII

Mr Hageman, the first patient described, had no bleeding problem and died of thrombosis. Haemorrhagic symptoms rare even with low levels. May be a cause of recurrent abortion.

Diagnosis ↑ APTT, PT normal and assay XII. Commonly picked up in asymptomatic patients when an isolated ↑ APTT undergoes investigation.

Treatment rarely necessary.

Factor XIII

Fibrin Stabilising Factor. Characteristically produces delayed post-operative bleeding (6–24h later). APTT & PT both ↔ so will be missed in a bleeding investigation unless specifically looked for by screening test (stability in 5M urea).

Treatment easily achieved with FFP, only very low levels required for haemostasis; t½ is long.

Factor X

Vitamin K dependent. Low levels (2%) associated with severe disease as with haemophilia.

Diagnosis ↑ PT, ↑ APTT .

Treatment PCC available – 1u/kg, aim to ↑ plasma X level to 2% or FFP (10–20ml/kg body wt) and check response. Relatively long t½.

Multiple defects

Rare familial coagulation factor deficiencies described; may be consanguineous parents. Often involves Factor VIII and another Factor (V > IX > VII). Other combinations seen.

Haemophilia 1997 3 63

Haemostasis and thrombosis

von Willebrand's disease (vWD)

Autosomally inherited bleeding disorder due to defective production of von Willebrand factor (vWF); affects both sexes with estimated incidence of 1:5000. First described in 1926 in the Aland Islands, it has a worldwide distribution.

Pathophysiology

vWF, produced in endothelial cells and megakaryocytes, is a large carrier protein consisting of multimers of different molecular weights. The higher molecular weight (HMW) multimers are >2,000,000 daltons and are particularly haemostatically active. vWF has two main functions: (a) it acts as a *carrier protein for factor VIIIC* protecting it from degradation and (b) platelet aggregation and adhesion. vWF acts as a docking agent by combining with receptors in the subendothelium and binding to platelet membrane glycoproteins (Gp)Ib & IIb/IIIa complex. All vWD is caused by mutations at the vWF locus.

>20 subtypes but for simplicity the disease is classified into 3 main types:

- **Type I** – partial quantitative deficiency of vWF (autosomal dominant).
- **Type II** – qualitative deficiency of vWF (autosomal dominant/recessive.)
- **Type III** – almost complete absence of vWF (autosomal recessive).

A secondary classification subdivides Type II into several variant vWD-like disorders; *not* due to genetic mutations at the vWF locus, include pseudo-vWD. Acquired vWD is caused by several underlying conditions (see p293).

Clinical features

Type I is common (70% of cases); type II (A > B) ~25%; type III is rare. Only ⅔ of type I patients are symptomatic. The clinical picture varies markedly. Symptoms may be intermittent and relate to platelet dysfunction eg mucocutaneous bleeding, easy bruising, nose bleeds, prolonged bleeding from cuts, dental extractions, trauma, surgery and menorrhagia. Type IIB causes thrombo cytopenia which may present in pregnancy. Usually the picture is consistent within a family. Factor VIII is seldom low enough to cause the joint bleeds seen in haemophilia except in Type III which is a severe bleeding disorder; parents of an affected child will be asymptomatic.

Laboratory diagnosis

Note vWF is an acute phase protein – increasing with stress, oestrogens, pregnancy neoplasm, thyrotoxicosis etc.

In type I APTT usually ↑, PT and platelets are normal, VIIIC and all vWF functions are moderately ↓, Bleeding time ↑. When mild, the condition may be difficult to diagnose many of the tests being normal including the VIIIC and bleeding time. Repeat testing can give differing results. Family testing is useful.

Haemostasis and thrombosis

Classification of von Willebrand's disease

Type	VIIIC	vWF Ag	vWF activity	RIPA low dose	HMW multimer	BT
I	↓	↓	↓	absent	N	↑
IIA	↓/N	↓/N	↓↓	absent	↓	↑
IIB	↓/N	↓/N	↓/N	N	↓	↑
III	↓	↓	↓	↓	↓	↑
Platelet (pseudo)	N	N	N	N/↑	↓	↑
Normandy	↓	N	N	N	absent	N

Management
- Avoid aspirin and NSAIDs.
- Mild bleeding symptoms – easy bruising, bleeding from cuts may settle with local pressure.
- Tranexamic acid (TXA) is a useful antifibrinolytic drug (15mg/kg body weight PO tds).
- TXA mouthwash 5% is useful for dental work.
- Moderate disease and minor surgery
  - DDAVP
  - Most responders have type I vWD. Avoid in type IIB (may ↓ platelets).
- Major surgery, bleeding symptoms or severe disease
  - Use vWF rich factor VIII concentrate eg intermediate purity VIII eg BPL 8Y, Alphanate, Haemate P.
  - Manage as for severe haemophilia (see p270) but VIII t½ longer in vWD.
  - Adjust according to the VIIIC response; BT may not correct even if the VIIIC >100% but haemostasis will be clinically OK.
    Treat post-op for 7–10 days.
- Pregnancy – VIIIC and vWF ↑ in pregnancy so rarely presents a problem for type I. Postpartum vWF ↓ so watch out for PPH in mod/severely affected women. Give VIII concentrate to maintain levels >30% if clinical problem. In Type IIB ↑ abnormal HMW multimers can cause platelet aggregation and thrombocytopenia. Avoid TXA (thrombotic risk).
- Menorrhagia – may be major problem. TXA for duration of the menstrual period helps some patients. Combined oral contraceptive pill ↑ vWF activities and is useful.

Complications
Some patients have been infected with HCV < HBV < HIV as a result of treatment with concentrates (see p269). Vaccination against HBV and HAV recommended for all patients. Inhibitors arise in <10% treated patients – usually type III disease (see p293 for management).

Natural history
Majority of patients will have type I disease which rarely causes life-threatening bleeds; may have little impact on quality of life/life expectancy. Management with VIII concentrates as for severe haemophilia should enable patients with severe vWD to have reasonable QOL.
Haemophilia 1997 3 (suppl 2) 1

Thrombophilia

Thrombophilia is a familial or acquired disorder of the haemostatic mechanism predisposing to thrombosis which may be venous or arterial. Virchov's Triad remembered by every medical student – slowing of the circulation, vessel damage and alterations in the constituents of the blood – is important in the pathogenesis. Thus prothrombotic changes in the blood are only one of the causes of thrombosis.

Pathogenesis

Arterial thrombosis (myocardial infarction or stroke) is a major cause of death in people over the age of 40 and is usually secondary to underlying arterial disease. Coagulation defects are rarely implicated. Venous thrombosis also is a major cause of morbidity and mortality with an overall annual incidence of <1/1000. Stasis following trauma and surgery is the major aetiological factor as is ↑ age. Up to 40% of people >40 may develop deep vein thrombosis (DVT) following orthopaedic or major abdominal surgery; as many as ⅓ of medical patients in ITU may do so. Many medical conditions ↑ the risk of thrombosis. Before referring patients for thrombophilia tests, look for risk factors:

Arterial thrombosis	Venous thrombosis
Smoking	Malignant disease
Hypertension	Pregnancy/oral contraceptive pill/HRT
Atherosclerosis	Chronic inflammatory bowel disease
Hyperlipidaemia	PNH
Diabetes mellitus	

Clinical features

In many patients with thrombosis an underlying risk factor will be identified; thrombophilia testing will be uninformative and a waste of time and money.

Who should be referred for investigation?

- Arterial thrombosis – patients <30 years, without obvious arterial disease.
- Venous thrombosis
  - patients <40 years with no obvious risk factors
  - unexplained recurrent thrombosis
  - VTE and family history of thrombosis in first degree relatives
  - unusual site eg mesenteric, portal vein thrombosis
  - unexplained neonatal thrombosis
  - recurrent miscarriage (≥3)
  - VTE in pregnancy and the OCP. Incidence of 15/100,000 patients ↑ 30–60 fold with a thrombophilic abnormality.

Laboratory investigation

1. Screen for underlying medical causes.
2. FBC, ESR, LFTs, autoimmune profile, fasting lipids
3. Screen for acquired coagulation defects – PT, APTT, LA /ACL, ↑ fibrinogen.
4. Screen for congenital thrombophilia.
   - First line PC, PS, AT, APCR, FVL in APCR abnormal patients
   - Less established – dysfibrinogenaemia, plasminogen, Factor XII, new tests being developed eg homocysteine, prothrombin variant.

Conclusion

In most patients with thrombosis, contributing factors will be identified by the clinical presentation and by appropriate special investigations. The common acquired thrombophilia defect – the LA/ACL should be routinely sought in patients <40 yr with VTE. Testing for inherited thrombophilia is complex, more expensive and only worthwhile in identified situations listed above. A strong family history of VTE in first degree relatives will increase the chance of identifying such defects.

Inherited thrombophilia

At present 30–50% patients with thrombosis and a positive family history will have a demonstrable thrombophilic abnormality on testing. The frequency of the 4 major factors is set out in table.

Syndrome	Gen population	Patients with 1st VTE	Familial patients with VTE
APCR	3.6–6.0%	20%	10–64%
AT def.	0.02%	1%	4%
PC def.	0.2–0.4%	3%	5%
PS def.	NA	2%	5%

Activated protein C resistance
Described in 1993 by Dahlback and colleagues. This is *the* major thrombophilic abnormality (see above), ~ 0.1% homozygous.

Pathogenesis
APC inactivates membrane bound factor Va through proteolytic cleavage at 3 specific sites in the heavy chain. >90% cases APCR due to mutation in factor V gene, resulting in glutamine→arginine at position 506 (denoted FV:Q506, or Factor V Leiden, FVL). APCR without FVL may be due to other genetic defects not yet identified, or acquired as a result of increased Factor VIII concentration.

Clinical features
VTE is increased 8-fold in heterozygotes and 30-fold in homozygotes. In >90%, DVT with or without PE is the presenting thrombotic event. Most patients with FVL will not develop thrombosis; other risk factors (eg trauma, surgery, OCP, pregnancy) are present in >50% of patients who develop a thrombotic event, and increasing age is a major risk factor. In thrombophilic families, by ~33 years, 40% homozygotes and 20% heterozygotes will have had a thrombotic event (*cf.* 8% FVL –ve). Homozygotes present at an earlier age (average 25 years). A combination of thrombophilic defects increases this risk.

Pregnancy VTE ↑ estimated frequency 0.09%. Acquired APCR due to ↑ Factor VIII levels and other physiological changes. ↑ Recurrent fetal loss in the second trimester.

OCP users have ↑ VTE. The FVL mutation ↑ risk 3-fold; absolute risk ~3/1000 heterozygotes, 3% for homozygotes. Arterial thrombosis – not yet definitely established link as a risk factor for stroke/MI.

Laboratory diagnosis
APCR – initially APTT based; modified tests using Factor V deficient plasma are able to distinguish heterozygotes from homozygotes. The FVL PCR test can be sent by post, is not affected by VIII concentration, OCP and other factors–but costs more than APCR.

Proteins C and S deficiency
Vitamin K dependent factors, these interact to limit activated Factors V and VIII.

Pathogenesis
Less common than APCR, they account for 5–10% of familial thrombosis. Concentrations are ↓ in early life (up to 4 years for PC), following recent

thrombosis, vitamin K deficiency, recent warfarin, in pregnancy (PS) so care must be taken before diagnosing an inherited deficiency. DNA techniques available.

Many patients are asymptomatic and will never have a VTE. Clinically PC and PS deficiency are similar – spontaneous and often recurrent VTE in younger patients including fulminant neonatal purpura in the homozygote (rarely PS). An association with arterial thrombosis is not clearly established. Skin necrosis is reported particularly at the time of warfarin. Increased fetal loss is described.

Antithrombin III (AT) deficiency

AT, the main co-factor of heparin and inhibitor of thrombin, was the first major familial defect described (1965). Epidemiological studies link AT deficiency with arterial thrombosis but this is rare. Clinically the condition is more severe than PC/PS deficiency particularly during pregnancy. Homozygous AT deficiency is very rare, and probably incompatible with life.

Homocysteinaemia

Hyperhomocysteinaemia may be due to genetic defects, vit B_{12} or folate deficiency. A severe form (congenital homocystinuria) is associated with arteriosclerosis, thromboembolic disease and mental retardation. Arterial and venous thrombosis is reported in ~10% patients with mild hyperhomocysteinaemia; may be familial and linked to other thrombophilic defects eg PC deficiency. Treatment with folate, vit B_{12} may ↓ the hyperhomocysteinaemia but the clinical benefit is unproven.

Prothrombin gene mutation

A G→A nucleotide transition at position 20210 in the 3' untranslated region of the prothrombin gene was reported in 1996 and is strongly associated with venous thrombosis. *Incidence:* 18% of selected patient with +ve family history, 6.2% patients with first episode of VTE, and 1% healthy controls have the prothrombin gene mutation which is associated with ↑ prothrombin levels.

Treatment of thrombophilic states

Many factors need to be weighed up when deciding how to manage patients with thrombotic disorders eg the severity of the VTE, other risk factors, and the nature of the thrombophilic defect.

Acute thrombotic event

- Treat appropriately–usually with heparin/warfarin.
  In PC /PS patients make sure heparinisation is adequate – monitor warfarin induction closely to avoid skin necrosis. Patients with AT deficiency may need high heparin doses.
- Duration of anticoagulation following a first event will depend on the severity of the VTE and other risk factors; each patient needs to be individually assessed.

Recurrent thrombosis

- Long-term anticoagulation is usual and at a high INR (3.0–4.5, target 3.5).

Concentrates

AT concentrate has been used in surgical and pregnant patients when response to heparin is inadequate.

PC concentrate (Immuno Ltd) may be used in fulminant neonatal thrombosis.

Prophylaxis

- Anticoagulation is not recommended for asymptomatic patients including pregnancy. For management of pregnant patient with history of VTE, prophylactic heparin has been successful in subsequent pregnancies in women with previous fetal loss.
- High risk situations eg surgery, trauma, should be identified and covered with prophylactic SC heparin. Dose will depend on the thrombotic risk. See p502.
- Patients must be informed of factors that ↑ thrombotic risk and given an information sheet.
- Patients with an identified thrombophilic defect should not be given the OCP or HRT.

Counselling

The knowledge that one or more inherited blood abnormalities which predispose to thrombosis which could be fatal justifiably causes concern. Sympathetic informed handling of the family is required.

Natural history

Complicated. At one end of the spectrum, APCR occurs in 5% of a healthy population and may give rise to no problems throughout life; at the other – PC deficiency causes fatal neonatal purpura fulminans, homozygous AT deficiency is incompatible with life. Thrombophilia has a whole range of clinical problems and new information is accumulating. The patient is best managed in a specialist clinic.

282

Acquired thrombophilia

Lupus anticoagulant
The paradoxically named lupus anticoagulant (LA) is arguably the commonest coagulation abnormality predisposing to thrombosis. It is an IgG /IgM auto-antibody and prolongs phospholipid dependent coagulation tests; bleeding is rare despite the prolonged APTT. The LA and other antiphospholipid anti-bodies (aPL) are found in association with arterial or venous thrombosis and/or recurrent fetal loss, the 'antiphospholipid syndrome', first described by Hughes in 1988.

Pathogenesis
aPL may be idiopathic or secondary when associated with other disorders. The two main aPL are the LA and the anticardiolipin antibody (aCL) occurring together in most cases but also independently. The aCL requires a cofactor, β2-glycoprotein 1 (β2GP1) to bind to cardiolipin. The LA may also bind to β2GP1 and also to prothrombin and can cause hypoprothrombinaemia. The mechanism of thrombosis is not clear; aPL may act against other vitamin K dependent proteins PC and PS, or possibly the autoimmune state may lead to endothelial damage and/or platelet activation.

Acquired thrombophilia due to aPL is a much commoner cause of thrombosis than the congenital defects; the incidence depends on the patient group–eg 18% in young stroke patients, 21% young patients with MI. The LA occurs in 1–2% of the population; most patients will not develop thrombosis.

Diagnosis
Clinical features
The LA was first described in patients with SLE–hence its name. Other under-lying disorders include the lymphoproliferative disorders, HIV, other auto-immune disorders and drugs (eg phenothiazines). The antiphospholipid syndrome (APS) is seen in patients with SLE but is often primary. Thrombosis, the major defining feature, may be arterial (stroke, ocular occlusions, MI, limb thrombosis) or venous (DVT, PE, renal, hepatic and portal veins). Fetal loss may be as high as ~80% in women with aPL.

Other clinical manifestations
- Migraine, visual disturbances.
- Thrombocytopenia.
- Livedo reticularis.
- Heart valve disease.
- Migraine.
- Myelopathy.
- Catastrophic widespread intravascular thrombosis is reported.

Laboratory diagnosis
1. Must double spin or filter to prevent false negative result.
2. Coagulation screen: APTT is usually ↑ and does not correct with normal plasma. Normal result does not rule out the condition. PT usually ↔ unless hypoprothrombinaemia is present.
3. Dilute thromboplastin time.
4. Dilute Russell's viper venom time.
5. Kaolin clotting time: platelet extract or excess phospholipid corrects the abnormal test and is diagnostic.

6. aCL is detected using an immunoassay technique and is quantified.
7. Autoimmune profile: ± ANA ± DNA binding.

Treatment

Asymptomatic patients aPL positive without thrombosis – no specific action; the risk of thrombosis is estimated at <1% per patient year. Low dose aspirin (75mg/d) may be useful but has no proven role in these patients. Educate re preventive measures to reduce risk situations leading to thrombosis. Prophylaxis – may need heparin at the time of surgery, trauma, prolonged immobility.

Antiphospholipid syndrome

Acute thrombotic events Treat as appropriate with heparin/warfarin. Long term anticoagulation is required; a high INR 3.0–4.5; target 3.5 lowers recurrence rate.

Recurrent abortion Subsequent pregnancies have been successfully achieved in women with the antiphospholipid syndrome with combined aspirin and heparin begun as soon as pregnancy is confirmed. Steroids are not much used now.

Prophylactic anticoagulation Would not routinely be given in pregnancy if there is no previous history of abortion/poor fetal development but low-dose aspirin seems logical given the reported high loss. Pregnancy in a woman with aPL and a past history of thrombosis will require prophylactic anticoagulation with aspirin and heparin (see p319).

285

Natural history

The LA may be transient and spontaneous remissions of the APS are reported. Long-term follow up of these patients is indicated since the clinical manifestations can be severe despite long term anticoagulation.

NEJM 1995 **332** 993

Vitamin K deficiency

Pathophysiology
Vitamin K (vit K) is a fat soluble vitamin obtained either by dietary intake (vit K_1) from vegetables and liver, and absorbed in the small gut or produced by bacterial synthesis in the gut and absorbed in the colon (vit K_2). Its essential role in coagulation is as cofactor for the gamma carboxylation of the precursor proteins for factors II, VII, IX, X, protein C and S, all of which are produced in the liver. Until the routine prophylactic administration of vit K, deficiency was common (as high as 1 per 2,500 births) in the neonate, almost exclusively a disease of breast fed babies because ↓ vit K in human breast milk *cf.* formula feeds, and ↓ synthesis in the neonatal gut.

Clinical features
- Dietary deficiency may arise within a few weeks in patients who are not eating well since body stores are limited and the half life of the vitamin is short (days).
- Systemic illness, parenteral nutrition, hepatic or renal failure, hypo-albuminaemia, antibiotics (eg cephalosporins) are compounding factors.
- Haemorrhagic disorder of the newborn.
  Prematurity and maternal intake of anticonvulsants increase the incidence.
  Usually presents in first few days of life with bleeding (eg umbilical stump). Cerebral haemorrhage is rare. A late form seen 3 to 6 months after birth is rare may be due to α-1 antitrypsin deficiency, liver disease, intestinal malabsorption.

Malabsorption
- Disease of the small gut (eg coeliac disease) may lead to clinically manifest vit K deficiency.
- Obstruction of bile flow, either extrahepatic (gallstones, Ca pancreas, or bile ducts) or intrahepatic (liver disease, liver fibrosis) may be associated with overt bleeding or noted on routine coagulation laboratory testing.

Laboratory diagnosis
- Clotting screen shows ↑ PT and ↑ APTT.
- Thrombin time and platelet count are ↔.
- PT is ↑ > APTT, and corrects with normal plasma.
- Further investigation (factor assays, PIVKA levels, vit K concentration) rarely required. A therapeutic trial of vit K will confirm diagnosis, with rapid (± 24h) PT correction.

Treatment

Asymptomatic patients Adult dose vit K 10mg IM/IV; repeat as necessary; can be given by mouth in dietary deficiency.

Neonate prophylaxis 1mg IM 1–3 mg PO. There is some reservation about giving babies vitamin K at birth because of data suggesting it could lead to the development of cancer in later life.

Bleeding patients in addition to vit K as above, give FFP (10–20ml/kg body wt) for immediate replacement of the clotting factors. PCC can be used in life-threatening situations.

Natural history
Response to treatment is good but treatment of the underlying condition is necessary to prevent recurrence.

Haemorrhagic disease of the newborn

Haemorrhagic disease of the newborn is caused by deficiency of the vitamin K dependent factors and is a significant cause of *bleeding* in the neonatal period unless prevented by vitamin K. Two forms described; an *early* classical and a *late* form with different aetiology

Pathophysiology

Classical haemorrhagic disease of the newborn is almost exclusively a disease of breast fed babies; incidence may be as high as 1/2,500 deliveries in the UK. This is a true deficiency; human milk has less vitamin K than formula milk and there is ↓ bacterial synthesis synthesis of vitamin K due to the sterile gut of the newborn. Immaturity of the liver and impaired production of the vitamin K factors may be a contributing factor. The late form ~40–100/million live births also is ↑ in breast fed babies but is mainly due to malabsorption of vitamin K, secondary to cholestasis, or GIT pathology.

Clinical features

- Early haemorrhagic disease of the newborn presents in the first week of life with bleeding – umbilical cord, the skin, post circumcision bleeding is common; ICH is rare. Presents <24h in haemorrhagic disease of the newborn 2° to maternal drug ingestion (anti-epileptic, anti TB).

- Late haemorrhagic disease of the newborn has a peak incidence at 2–6 weeks but can occur up to 6 months of age. Underlying cholestatic disease is often present, biliary atresia, cystic fibrosis, α-1 antitrypsin deficiency and diarrhoea are documented causes. ~½ cases present with ICH.

Diagnosis – laboratory findings

- ↑ PT/APTT – may be markedly prolonged (normal TT, fibrinogen, X/FDPs *cf.* DIC).
- Factor assay (II, VII, IX, X) if in doubt. ↑ PIVKA and ↓ vit K – not routinely available tests.
- Correction of coagulation abnormality in ~24h with parenteral vitamin K confirms diagnosis.

Differential diagnosis

- Exclude other causes of bleeding in the neonatal period.
- Thrombocytopenia – platelets are normal in haemorrhagic disease of the newborn.
- DIC – see above.
- Congenital disorders eg haemophilia.
- Radiological – scan for ICH/internal bleeding as required.

Management

Treatment General support as indicated by clinical presentation. FFP for immediate correction of bleeding. Vitamin K$_1$ 1mg IV/IM will correct PT/APTT to normal for age – takes ~24 h.

Prophylaxis Controversial. 1mg at birth will prevent all early and most delayed vit K deficiency in neonate BUT evidence suggests this is associated with a 2-fold ↑ in ALL/childhood malignancy.

Many SCBU give oral vitamin K (2–3mg) to neonates at routine risk, reserving IM for ↑ risk babies (prems/sick/maternal drugs/birth trauma/LSCS birth).

Further oral vitamin K at intervals recommended for breast-fed babies, to prevent late onset HDN but is difficult to enforce.

Outcome

Treatment with FFP/vitamin K will correct the abnormal coagulation and stop bleeding. In ICH damage done to CNS leads to death or morbidity in ~⅓ cases particularly likely in late onset HDN.

289

Liver disease

Most coagulation factors, including the vitamin K dependent factors, are made exclusively in the liver. Any insult to the liver may cause rapid reduction in their concentration and coagulopathy because of their short half-life. Associated thrombocytopenia is common in established liver disease, increasing the risk of bleeding.

Pathophysiology

Haemostasis is a fine balance between procoagulant and prothrombotic forces. Because of its central role in the production of these factors, coagulation is often disturbed in liver disease. Clotting tests become abnormal early in liver damage and are useful monitors of liver function. The liver functions as a reticuloendothelial organ, clearing activated coagulation factors from the circulation. Impairment of this function sets the scene for DIC which is usually low grade but may be fulminant. Fibrinolysis is decreased in chronic liver disease but is ↑ in liver transplant patients. Dysfibrinogenaemia due to increased sialic acid content of the fibrinogen molecule is described. In obstructive jaundice, impaired bile flow leads to malabsorption of vit K, a fat soluble vitamin. A degree of intrahepatic obstruction secondary to hepatocyte swelling and fibrosis may also have this effect. Thrombocytopenia may be due to portal hypertension, splenic pooling, alcohol, viral infection, drugs, or DIC. Altered platelet function with a prolonged bleeding time may occur.

Clinical features

Most patients with established hepatic dysfunction will have an abnormal coagulation profile but may be asymptomatic. Bleeding becomes a problem when other complications arise such as oesophageal varices, thrombocytopenia, surgery, liver biopsy and infection.

Laboratory diagnosis

Coagulation defect	Laboratory diagnosis	Clinical significance
↓ Vit K dependent factors	PT ↑ >> ↑APTT	PT ratio >4.8 – Poor prognosis
Fibrinogen		
quantitative defect	Fibrinogen assay	↑ infection, neoplasm, obstruction
		↓ severe liver disease
dysfibrinogenaemia	↑thrombin/reptilase time	uncertain; occurs in cirrhosis
Factor VIII	↑, also vWF Ag	seen in acute viral hepatitis
		cirrhosis, hepatic failure
Antithrombin	↓ conc (N=80–120iu/dl)	↓ CLD and liver failure
DIC	↑ PT, APTT , F/XDPs	low grade common in CLD
	↓ fibrinogen, platelets	rarely fulminant

Management

Asymptomatic patients PT (<2.0) does not require treatment other than that directed at the underlying condition. Give vit K (10mg IM) to exclude added vit K deficiency. Complete correction of the PT confirms this diagnosis; partial correction indicates combined hepatocellular dysfunction and vit K deficiency. Further doses of vit K for 1–2d may be given.

Haemostasis and thrombosis

Liver biopsy Aim to get the PT ↓ to ≤1.4 and platelet count >70 × 10^9/l. Check on day of biopsy. Give FFP 10ml/kg (usual starting dose 2u); check PT and repeat FFP dose until PT is satisfactory – not always achieved. Can give PCC eg BPL 9a (II, IX, X); Prothromplex (Immuno; VII, II, IX, X) 12u/kg body weight – not routinely given (?risk of thrombosis, DIC). Platelet transfusion (adult dose = 5 donor units) to ↑ platelets to >70 × 10^9/l if necessary.

Active bleeding Blood transfusion as required. Give vit K, FFP, PCC, platelets as set out for liver biopsy and monitor the response. FFP only temporary correction; repeat 12–24 hourly as indicated. Surgical manoeuvres to control oesophageal bleeding (Sengstaken tube, etc) will be explored. DIC is a feature of fulminant liver failure and after liver surgery and transplantation. Control underlying condition, support with platelet/FFP as required. The use of aprotinin, tranexamic acid, AT concentrates, and heparin has varying success.

Natural history
In fulminant liver failure the coagulopathy may be severe contributing to the mortality. The degree of the hepatocellular failure will be the final denominator determining the outcome.

Acquired anticoagulants

The development of inhibitors against coagulation factors is fortunately uncommon other than antiphospholipid antibodies (see p284). Factor VIII antibodies, either spontaneous or in treated haemophiliacs, are well documented and can be a serious clinical problem. Acquired vWD, inhibitors against other coagulation factors and heparin-like inhibitors are all rare.

Factor VIII inhibitors
Pathophysiology
Spontaneous development of VIII inhibitors in non-haemophiliacs is reported in 1 per million population. Antibody is usually IgG, occasionally IgM or IgA and will neutralise the functional VIII protein. It may be quantitated by different techniques including the Bethesda titre (BU; see below). In 15–20% of haemophilic patients antibodies develop as a result of treatment with concentrates usually within the first 20 (median 9–11) treatment exposures. A familial tendency is noted, inhibitors occurring more often in patients with deletions or mutations within factor VIII gene. The antibody acts against part of the amino-terminal component of the A2 domain or the carboxy-terminal part of the C2 domain of the VIII molecule. Factor IX very rarely (<5%) stimulates inhibitor formation.

Clinical features
Acquired inhibitors develop in the elderly, during pregnancy, in association with autoimmune and malignant disease, various skin disorders (psoriasis, pemphigus, erythema multiforme) infections, drug therapy (penicillin, aminoglycosides, phenothiazines, etc). Patients are usually low responders ie develop low levels of antibody in response to repeated treatment. Symptoms include bleeding (post-operatively this can cause major problems), easy bruising–haemarthrosis is very rare. The mortality is significant, as many as 25% patients with persisting VIII inhibitors will die from bleeding.

In haemophilic patients, inhibitors may be transient and of no clinical significance, being noted incidentally on review. In many, however, an VIII inhibitor will present a major clinical problem. Suspicion is aroused by bleeding that fails to respond to the usual doses of Factor concentrate. Patients may be low (<5BU) or high (>10BU) responders; in the latter, treatment will be difficult.

Laboratory diagnosis
- ↑ APTT with failure to correct with normal plasma.
- Antibody assay – patient's plasma reducing the factor VIII in normal plasma over a 1–2h incubation period. Antibody titres may be reported in BU or New Oxford units (BU stronger = 1.2 × NOU). Check titre against porcine VIII before treatment.

Differential diagnosis of spontaneous inhibitors – need to exclude non-specific inhibitors eg myeloma paraproteins which bind non-specifically to coagulation plasma proteins.

Management of patients with spontaneous inhibitor
- *Asymptomatic* – watch and wait; in some patients the inhibitor goes away (not unusual in pregnancy/puerperium and in the elderly).
- *Mild bleeding* – may respond local pressure, tranexamic acid or DDAVP (see p269).

Haemostasis and thrombosis

- *Severe bleeding* – may be life-threatening. Give steroids (1mg/kg/d); may take weeks to work and VIII replacement will be needed. Human or porcine VIII concentrates are usual first line (50–150 u/kg) repeated 2–4 X/d or given as continuous infusion (1000u/h).
- Monitor lab and clinical response.
- Bypassing agents (FEIBA), rVIIa, high dose IVIg may be tried in resistant/ high titre patients with varying success. The cost of treating these patients is high. Long term immunosuppression may be required.

Management of haemophilic patients with inhibitor

- *Asymptomatic patients* – observation may be all that is necessary. The inhibitor level may gradually subside; avoid treatment with concentrates to limit exposure to the antigen.
- *Mild bleeding* – in low responder/low titre patients large (20–100u/kg) doses of human factor VIII are usually effective. If activity against porcine VIII < human VIII this could be more effective.
- *High responders/high titre patients* – will require porcine/human VIII in large (50–200u/kg) doses or bypassing agents such as FEIBA or recombinant Factor VIIa.
- *Immune tolerance induction* – overcomes the VIII inhibitor in about 80% selected patients. Low dose immune tolerance induction is cost effective and works for low titre inhibitors.
- *High responders* – need high intensity immune tolerance regimes which may take up to 18 months to work (expensive and may fail to work).

293

Acquired vWD

Rare disorder presenting in later life, has a variable bleeding pattern similar to the inherited condition. An associated monoclonal gammopathy/lymphoproliferative disorder is common but the condition may be autoimmune or idiopathic. Bleeding symptoms vary from mild to major eg catastrophic GI haemorrhage requiring frequent blood transfusion.

Laboratory diagnosis

As type 1 congenital vWD. In summary an ↑ APTT which may or may not correct with normal plasma; PT ↔; ↓ VIIIC, vWF antigen, activity RIPA and ↑ bleeding time. *In vitro* evidence of the vWF inhibitor not always demonstrable.

Management

Measures used in the treatment of the hereditary condition (DDAVP, Factor VIII eg BPL 8Y, Haemate-P, cryoprecipitate) are effective. In unresponsive patients, high-dose IVIg (total dose 2g/kg given over 1–5d) is useful; maintenance IVIg may have a role. Platelet transfusions/FFP may help.

Other coagulation inhibitors

Factor IX inhibitors are much less common (<5%) in patients with haemophilia B than A and this is true also of the spontaneously developing IX inhibitors. Treatment is with high doses of Factor IX concentrate and activated PCC as required.

Inhibitors, spontaneous or post treatment, are reported against most other coagulation factors (V, XI and XII, Prothrombin, XI, VII and X); all are very rare. Factor V antibodies may arise in congenitally deficient patients following treatment or spontaneously following antibiotics, infection, blood transfusion. Post-operative cases may develop as a result of exposure to haemostatic agents contaminated with bovine factor V. Most are low titre and transient. Treat with FFP and platelets (a good source of Factor V).

Heparin-like inhibitors are reported in patients with malignant disease, following chemotherapy (eg suramin, mithromycin) and may cause bleeding. Protamine sulphate neutralisation *in vitro* and *in vivo* is a feature of this inhibitor.

Diagnosis
Screening tests (PT, APTT, Thrombin Time) will give abnormal results depending on the factor involved, with failure to correct with normal plasma. Defining the specific factor requires detailed laboratory workup. Exclude acquired deficiencies eg Factor IX deficiency described in Gaucher's Disease and Factor X deficiency in amyloidosis (binding of the abnormal component to the coagulation factors).

Treatment
Reserved for actively bleeding patients since acquired inhibitors may not give rise to symptoms. First line treatment is with FFP but large volumes may be required and efficacy may be limited. Specific concentrates currently available in addition to Factor VIII and IX already described are Prothrombin, Factors X, VII (combined in PCCs), Factors VII, XI and XIII as single agents (see p272). Several are for named patients only. By-passing agents may be given as necessary. Treatment of the underlying condition may cause the inhibitor to disappear.

294

Hay *et al* Blood Coagulation and Fibrinolysis 1996 7 134

Platelet function tests

Platelets play an essential role in arresting bleeding. Following vascular injury they fall out of the circulation, adhere to subendothelial collagen via the docking agent vWF, then stick to each other to form a cohesive mass. Release of internal factors – serotonin, calcium, Platelet factor 4 (PF4), and fibrinogen induces vascular constriction, and coagulation cascade activation. Finally, together with fibrin they form a *thrombus*, plugging the hole in the vessel. Within the platelet prostaglandin synthetic pathway, arachidonic acid forms thromboxane A_2, a potent platelet aggregant and vasoconstrictor. From platelet activation → cessation of bleeding takes 3–5 minutes, *the bleeding time.*

Tests of function
Blood collection needs to be optimal with nontraumatic venepuncture, rapid transport to the lab with storage at room temperature and testing within a maximum of 2–3h.

Tests in use
Platelet count, morphology, adhesion, aggregation, release and bleeding time.

Platelet count
Normal range $150–450 \times 10^9/l$. Adequate function is maintained even when the count is <½ normal level, but progressively deteriorates as it drops. With platelet counts $<20 \times 10^9/l$ there is usually easy bruising, petechial haemorrhages (although more serious bleeding can occur).

Morphology
Large platelets are biochemically more active; ↑ mean platelet volume (MPV>6.5) is associated with less bleeding in patients with severe thrombocytopenia. Reticulated platelets can be counted by new analysers and may prove to be useful in assessing platelet regeneration. Altered platelet size is seen in inherited platelet disorders.

Platelet adhesion
To glass beads now rarely performed in routine lab practice, but useful in vWD diagnosis.

Platelet aggregation
Most useful of the special tests is performed on fresh sample using aggregometer.

Aggregants
- Adenosine 5-diphosphate (ADP) at low and high concentrations. Induces 2 aggregation waves: *primary wave* may disaggregate at low conc. ADP; the *second* is irreversible.
- Collagen has a short lag phase followed by a single wave and is particularly affected by aspirin.
- Ristocetin induced platelet aggregation (RIPA) is carried out at a high (1.2mg/ml) and lower concentrations and is mainly used to diagnose vWD.
- Arachidonic acid.
- Adrenaline, not uncommonly reduced in normal people.

For aggregation patterns in the various platelet disorders see p298.

Platelet release
ELISA or RIA are used to measure the α granule proteins β-thromboglobulin (β-TG) and heparin neutralising activity (HNA). These are sensitive markers of platelet hyperreactivity and beyond the scope of the routine laboratory.

Haemostasis and thrombosis

Practical application of the tests

Main role is in diagnosis of inherited platelet functional defects (see p298). In acquired platelet dysfunction secondary to causes such renal and hepatic disease, DIC, macroglobulinaemia, platelet function is rarely tested.

Drug induced thrombopathy

Many drugs eg aspirin, NSAIDs, corticosteroids, antiplatelet drugs (eg dipyridamole), antibiotics (penicillin, cephalosporins), membrane stabilising agents (β blockers), antihistamines, tricyclic antidepressants, α antagonists, miscellaneous agents (eg heparin, alcohol, dextran) may affect platelet function but tests are rarely performed, the bleeding time being more useful.

Hereditary platelet disorders

All rare. Acquired platelet dysfunction is much more likely to be a cause of bleeding or easy bruising. Two main qualitative defects are found

- **Defective platelet membrane glycoproteins (GPs).**
  GPIIb/IIIa is a receptor for fibrinogen and other adhesive GPs; also affected is GPIb (specific platelet receptor for vWF). Disorders include *Glanzmann's thrombasthenia* (abnormal GPIIb III) and *Bernard Soulier syndrome* (BSS) – abnormal GPIb, a specific receptor for vWF with defective adhesion to blood vessels.
- **Abnormalities of platelet granules ie storage pool deficiency.**
  Either the alpha (α) granules (*gray platelet syndrome*), the dense granules (*May-Hegglin anomaly, Hermansky Pudlak syndrome, Chediak-Higashi syndrome* and the *thrombocytopenia-absent radius (TAR) syndrome,* or both.

Clinical features

Presenting symptoms of inherited platelet dysfunction: mucocutaneous bleeding (skin, nose, gums, gut) with a positive family history (though not always found). All autosomal recessive. Clinically the bleeding symptoms are similar but may be other clinical features to distinguish the syndromes. Carriers asymptomatic. Menorrhagia may be troublesome. Condition is rarely severe. Symptoms may suggest the diagnosis of non-accidental injury in young children. An abnormal BT may be first objective evidence of bleeding disorder.

Laboratory findings

- Long bleeding time.
- Normal platelet count and size (except for BSS).
- Abnormal platelet aggregation with common aggregants (see table).
- Occasionally aggregation is normal.
- Consider aspirin and vWD in the differential diagnosis.

Condition	Platelet		Aggregation with		
	count	size	ADP	Collagen	Ristocetin
Thrombasthenia	N	N	absent	↓	abnormal
Bernard Soulier syndrome	L	↑	N	N	↓
storage pool disease	N	N	abnormal	abnormal	↓/abnormal
Aspirin ingestion	N	N	abnormal	abnormal	N/abnormal
von Willebrand's disease	N	N	N	N	abnormal

Defining abnormality in Glanzmann's thrombasthenia is absent aggregation to both low and high dose ADP. BSS platelets have the same defect as in vWD but they are large. In the gray platelet syndrome, the platelet count is often low and the platelets pale, grey and larger than normal.

Treatment

1. Avoid antiplatelet drugs. Use pressure to control bleeding from minor cuts.
2. Tranexamic acid (TXA, 25mg/kg body wt) 8 hrly for 7–10d for minor surgery and dental work. TXA mouthwash useful to reduce bleeding from dental work.
3. Platelet transfusions are effective in major surgery and severe bleeding.

Haemostasis and thrombosis

Osler-Weber-Rendu syndrome

Definition
Autosomal dominantly inherited disorder characterised by multiple skin telangiectases. Also known as hereditary haemorrhagic telangiectasia. The basic pathology is a developmental structural abnormality of blood vessels. This results in dilatation and convolution of the venules and capillaries which may be present throughout the body. Theses telangiectases are thin-walled and likely to bleed giving rise to recurrent haemorrhage and anaemia.

Incidence
Rare. ♂ = ♀.

Clinical features
- Presentation may not be until later life.
- Facial and buccal mucosa and nail fold telangiectases.
- Iron deficiency common as a result of bleeding from GIT telangiectases.
- Epistaxis – commonest presenting symptom.
- Menorrhagia.
- Prolonged bleeding after dental surgery.

Diagnosis and investigation
- Recognition of typical telangiectases and family history.
- *Beware*, another cause of bleeding may co-exist in a OWR patient.
- FBC and film may show iron deficient picture ie microcytic, hypochromic anaemia, low MCV, raised platelets. Low serum ferritin.
- Angiography of mesenteric circulation in recurrent bleeding.
- ENT examination.

Treatment
- Observation for iron deficiency.
- Iron replacement therapy.
- Consider interventional procedure, eg embolisation (if angiography +ve).
- Oestrogen reduces frequency of bleeding episodes.

Prognosis
Generally a benign chronic disorder provided follow-up as above.

Haemostasis and thrombosis

Henoch-Schönlein purpura

Definition
An immune complex disease characterised by a leucocytoclastic vasculitis. Purpura is *not* of haematological origin.

Incidence and epidemiology
Predominantly affects children aged 2–8 years. Clear preponderance in the winter. Commonly presents 1–3 weeks after upper respiratory tract illness. Various infections, toxins, physical trauma and insect bites, and allergies have all been postulated as triggers of the disease but no clear causation established. May also occur with malignancy.

Clinical features
- Rapid onset usual.
- Classically a palpable purpuric rash over buttocks/legs (extensor surfaces).
- Urticarial plaques and haemorrhagic bullae seen, often bizarrely symmetrical.
- Abdominal pain ?due to mesenteric vasculitis.
- Arthritis, particularly knees and ankles.
- Renal involvement – haematuria ± proteinuria, may lead to either acute or chronic renal failure.

Diagnosis and investigations
- Made by the presence of typical findings above and exclusion of other causes.
- FBC and film normal. Platelet numbers and function are normal. The purpura is not of haematological origin. ESR usually raised.
- Other markers of autoimmune disorders may be present.

Treatment and prognosis
- Spontaneous resolution within a month is commonest outcome in children.
- Long-term sequelae more common in adults eg chronic renal failure.
- Steroids may be of benefit particularly if joint pains are troublesome.

Haemostasis and thrombosis

Acquired disorders of platelet function

Acquired disorders may affect platelet-vessel wall interaction and are among the most common causes of a haemorrhagic tendency. These conditions may be associated with a prolonged bleeding time, abnormal platelet aggregation studies and clinical bleeding or bruising.

Drugs that induce platelet dysfunction

- Aspirin.
- NSAIDs.
- β-lactam antibiotics: penicillins & cephalosporins.
- 'Antiplatelet agents': prostacyclin, dipyridamole.
- Fibrinolytic agents: EACA.
- Heparin.
- Plasma expanders: dextran, hydroxyethyl starch.
- Other drugs: antihistamines, local anaesthetics, β-blockers.
- Food additives: fish oil.

Systemic conditions which affect platelet function

- Renal failure.
- Liver failure.
- Glycogen storage disorders types Ia & Ib.

Conditions causing platelet exhaustion

- Cardiopulmonary bypass surgery.
- DIC.
- Others: valvular heart disease, renal allograft rejection, cavernous haemangioma.

Dysproteinaemias & antiplatelet antibodies

- Multiple myeloma.
- Waldenström's macroglobulinaemia.
- Autoimmune disorders.

Haematological conditions with production of abnormal platelets

- Chronic myeloproliferative disorders.
- Myelodysplasia.
- Leukaemia.

Drugs

Wide range of drugs reported to impair platelet function (most commonly implicated drugs are listed).

Aspirin is commonest cause of clinically significant bleeding, due to irreversible acetylation and inhibition of cyclooxygenase which interferes with formation of thromboxane A_2 in the platelet prostaglandin pathway. Effect on bleeding time occurs within 2h of ingestion of 75mg and lasts up to 4d while the effects on platelet aggregation last up to 10d. Greater effect on the bleeding time and clinical bleeding seen in patients who already have bleeding tendency. Laboratory effects on a normal individual is usually mild and there is marked individual variation in the risk of bleeding.

Effects of aspirin

- Easy bruising, epistaxis, haematomas, haemorrhage after surgery especially in patients with a pre-existing bleeding tendency.

- Prolonged bleeding time.
- Inhibition of platelet release reaction and second wave of platelet aggregation to low concentrations of ADP and collagen.

NSAIDs cause reversible inhibition of cyclooxygenase. Effect on bleeding time and platelet aggregation is brief (only as long as circulating drug present) and less likely to cause clinical bleeding in patients without a prior bleeding disorder. **β-lactam antibiotics** affect platelet function by lipophilic attachment to cell membrane in dose-dependent manner. Do so only after sustained high dosage though effect may last 7–10d after discontinuation. **Antiplatelet agents**, prostacyclin and dipyridamole ↑ cAMP concentration in platelets and inhibit platelet aggregation with little/no effect on bleeding time. A diet rich in **fish oils** (ω-3 fatty acids) can cause mild prolongation of bleeding time. **Ethanol ingestion** can impair *in vitro* platelet function.

Aspirin should be avoided in patients with bleeding tendency. A patient on aspirin should discontinue the drug at least a week prior to a surgical procedure. DDAVP or platelet transfusion should be administered to a patient with severe haemorrhage due to aspirin-induced platelet function defect. In cases with less severe bleeding, discontinuation of the suspected drug is usually effective.

Renal failure Prolongation of bleeding time and clinical bleeding occur in patients with uraemia due to chronic renal failure – the former correlates with the severity of the uraemia. Bleeding time abnormality does not predict risk of haemorrhage. Associated anaemia also contributes to prolongation of bleeding time and correction of anaemia improves the abnormality. Abnormalities of platelet aggregation studies are seen frequently. If haemorrhage occurs in a patient with chronic renal failure, other causes should be excluded before it is attributed to uraemia.

Liver failure Chronic liver disease, most notably cirrhosis, may be associated with platelet function defects which may be due abnormalities in the platelet membrane glycoproteins. Abnormalities in bleeding time and platelet aggregation studies may be improved by infusion of DDAVP. Haemorrhage in a patient with liver disease is usually multifactorial including decreased levels of coagulation factors, dysfibrinogenaemia, thrombocytopenia due to splenic pooling and DIC.

Conditions causing platelet exhaustion A number of conditions have been associated with platelet exhaustion (acquired storage pool defect) in which there is laboratory evidence of *in vivo* platelet activation and decreased platelet aggregation in the pattern of a storage pool defect.

- Cardiopulmonary bypass surgery.
- DIC.
- Valvular heart disease.
- Renal allograft rejection.
- Cavernous haemangioma.
- Aortic aneurysm.
- Transfusion reaction.
- TTP & HUS.

305

Cardiopulmonary bypass surgery Abnormal platelet function and thrombocytopenia are frequently seen in patients subjected to cardiopulmonary bypass surgery. A bleeding time longer than expected for the degree of thrombocytopenia, and impaired aggregation studies *in vitro* occur in proportion to duration of the bypass procedure. Believed due to platelet activation and fragmentation in the extracorporeal loop. Platelet transfusion is required in patients with a prolonged bleeding time and excessive haemorrhage after cardiopulmonary bypass surgery.

DIC Platelet exhaustion due to an acquired storage pool defect may occur in DIC due to *in vivo* platelet stimulation and this may cause abnormal platelet aggregation in *in vitro* tests. However, haemorrhage in DIC is multifactorial (see p422).

Dysproteinaemias Binding of M-proteins to platelet cell membranes in myeloma (particularly IgA) or Waldenström's macroglobulinaemia may result in acquired platelet function defects and less commonly clinical bleeding. Severity of platelet function defect correlates with M-protein concentration. *Note:* haemorrhage is more commonly due to thrombocytopenia or hyperviscosity. Plasmapheresis to remove circulating M-protein may be necessary in bleeding patient in whom the M-protein may be contributory factor through hyperviscosity or impairment of platelet function.

Antiplatelet antibodies Impaired platelet function may be a rare consequence of binding of IgM or IgG molecules to platelet membrane in ITP, SLE and platelet alloimmunisation where the most common result is accelerated platelet destruction and thrombocytopenia. May result in haemorrhagic manifestations at unexpectedly high platelet counts, and in longer than expected bleeding time. If bleeding occurs treatment is that of ITP (see p314).

Haematological disorders

Myeloproliferative disorders Qualitative platelet disorders occur in association with a prolonged bleeding time and clinical bleeding in MPD. Includes abnormal morphology with decreased granules, acquired storage pool defects, abnormalities of platelet glycoproteins, receptors and arachidonic acid metabolism. Haemorrhage (mucocutaneous) occurs in about ⅓ patients with MPD as does thrombosis. Neither bleeding time nor degree of thrombocytosis correlates well with risks of bleeding or thrombosis. An increased whole blood viscosity in patients with polycythaemia is clearly related to risk of haemorrhage. There is widespread belief that lowering an elevated platelet count is associated with a diminished risk in patients with thrombocytosis but no objective evidence. Hydroxyurea is the drug of choice. The role of anagrelide is not yet clear. In patients with polycythaemia rubra vera the haematocrit should be kept below 0.44 (♀) or 0.47 (♂). See p188.

Myelodysplasia & leukaemia Abnormalities of platelet morphology and *in vitro* aggregation occur in these disorders but haemorrhagic problems are commonly due to thrombocytopenia.

Numerical abnormalities of platelets – *thrombocytosis*

Defined as platelet count >450 × 10^9/l. May be secondary (or reactive) to another pathological process or it may be due to a myeloproliferative disorder. It may be associated not only with an increased risk of thrombosis but also with an increased risk of haemorrhage. The former occurs most frequently in patients with polycythaemia rubra vera or post-splenectomy thrombocytosis, the latter most notably with the myeloproliferative disorders.

Causes of reactive thrombocytosis
- Haemorrhage.
- Surgery.
- Trauma.
- Iron deficiency anaemia (see p54).
- Splenectomy (see p494).
- Infection.
- Malignant disease.
- Inflammatory disorders (rheumatoid arthritis, inflammatory bowel disease).

Myeloproliferative disorders associated with thrombocytosis
- Primary (essential) thrombocythaemia (see p194).
- Polycythaemia rubra vera (see p188).
- Chronic myeloid leukaemia (see p150).
- Idiopathic myelofibrosis (see p198).

Management
See relevant sections.

Haemostasis and thrombosis

Numerical abnormalities of platelets – *thrombocytopenia*

Defines a platelet count <150 × 10⁹/l. May be due either to **decreased bone marrow production of platelets** or to **increased destruction or sequestration of platelets** from the circulation (or both). Platelet counts >100 × 10⁹/l are not usually associated with any haemorrhagic problems. As count falls <100 × 10⁹/l there is progressive prolongation of the bleeding time. Purpura, easy bruising and prolonged post-traumatic bleeding are increasingly common as the platelet count falls <50 × 10⁹/l. Although there is no platelet count at which a patient definitely will or will not experience spontaneous haemorrhage the risk is greater in patients with a platelet count <20 × 10⁹/l and increases further in those with a count <10 × 10⁹/l.

Causes of decreased bone marrow production of platelets
- Marrow failure: aplastic anaemia (see p118).
- Marrow infiltration: leukaemias, myelodysplasia, myeloma, myelofibrosis, lymphoma, metastatic carcinoma (see p403).
- Marrow depression: cytotoxic drugs & radiotherapy (see p316), other drugs (eg chloramphenicol).
- Selective megakaryocyte depression: ethanol, drugs (phenylbutazone, co-trimoxazole; penicillamine), chemicals, viral infection (eg HIV, parvovirus).
- Nutritional deficiency: megaloblastic anaemia (see p56–60).
- Hereditary causes (rare): Fanconi's syndrome (see p370), congenital megakaryocytic hypoplasia, absent radii (TAR) syndrome.

Causes of increased destruction of platelets

Immune
- ITP (see p312).
- Associated with other autoimmune states SLE, CLL, lymphoma (see p316).
- Drug-induced: heparin, gold, quinidine, quinine, penicillins, cimetidine, digoxin.
- Infection: HIV, other viruses, malaria (see p328).
- Post-transfusion purpura (see p416).
- Neonatal (isoimmune) purpura (see p354).

Non-immune
- DIC (see p422).
- TTP/HUS (see p438).
- Kasabach-Merritt syndrome.
- Congenital/acquired heart disease.
- Cardiopulmonary bypass (see p306).

Causes of platelet sequestration
- Hypersplenism (see p316).

Causes of dilutional loss of platelets
- Massive transfusion (see p432).
- Exchange transfusion.

Hereditary thrombocytopenia
- Wiskott-Aldrich syndrome, May-Hegglin anomaly, Bernard-Soulier syndrome.

Investigation of thrombocytopenia

- History – drugs, symptoms of viral illness.
- Examination – signs of infection, lymphadenopathy, hepatosplenomegaly.
- FBC – isolated thrombocytopenia or associated disorders.
- Blood film – red cell fragmentation (DIC), WBC differential (atypical lymphocytes/blasts), platelet size (large in ITP and some hereditary conditions),
  platelet clumps (pseudothrombocytopenia).
- Serology – antinuclear antibody, DAT, monospot, antiplatelet antibodies (unreliable), platelet-associated antibodies (unreliable), HIV serology.
- Routine chemistry – renal disease, hepatic disease.
- BM examination – megakaryocyte numbers, marrow disease or infiltration.

Thrombocytopenia due to decreased platelet production

Diagnosis is confirmed on bone marrow examination, and management is essentially that of the underlying condition. Platelet transfusion may be necessary for the treatment of haemorrhage in patients with bone marrow failure and prophylactic platelet transfusion may be necessary if persistent severe thrombocytopenia ($<10 \times 10^9$/l) occurs.

Immune thrombocytopenia

These conditions are due to IgG and IgM antibodies which react with antigenic sites (usually GP IIb/IIIa in ITP, platelet alloantigens in post-transfusion purpura and neonatal isoimmune purpura) on the platelet cell membrane, may fix complement and cause accelerated platelet destruction through phagocytosis by reticulo-endothelial cells in liver and spleen. A compensatory increase in bone marrow megakaryocytopoiesis usually occurs which may occasionally prevent or delay the development of severe thrombocytopenia.

ITP

Usually presents with haemorrhagic manifestations, purpura, epistaxis, menorrhagia or bleeding gums but may occasionally be detected in an asymptomatic adult patient on a routine blood test. Intracranial bleeds occur in <1% (associated with platelet count $<10 \times 10^9$/l). Commonest in young adults ($\female > \male$). The natural history of childhood cases is acute in 90% and usually follows a self-limiting course without treatment. They are often associated with a history of previous viral illness and complete resolution may be expected within three months. In adults a chronic course is usual and spontaneous resolution is rare (<5%).

Diagnosis

The platelet count may be <5 to 100×10^9/l. Platelet size often ↑ on the blood film, reflected in ↑ MPV; represents production of young platelets by the reactive bone marrow. Diagnosis of ITP is confirmed by exclusion of a secondary (other autoimmune or drug-induced cause) or hereditary cause of thrombocytopenia in a patient with a normal physical examination, no splenomegaly and normal bone marrow examination. The demonstration of platelet antibodies or increased platelet associated Ig may be confirmatory but neither positive nor negative results are definitive. A small proportion of patients have associated DAT +ve AIHA (Evan's syndrome), most of whom have an underlying disorder (CLL, lymphoma, SLE).

Treatment of ITP

No need to treat mild compensated ITP ($>50 \times 10^9$/l) unless haemorrhagic manifestations. Keep under regular review and advise urgent FBC if haemorrhagic manifestations. Most children do not require treatment–but those in whom chronic ITP develops are treated in the same way as adults. 90% children eventually recover completely. Aim of therapy of adult ITP is to achieve an improved (preferably normal) platelet count without need for long term maintenance therapy.

Prednisolone
- First-line therapy for most patients.
- Probably ↓ platelet antibody production and interferes with phagocytosis.
- Dose is 1mg/kg/d PO, maintained for at least 3 weeks (therapeutic effect may take 4–6 weeks and a patient should not be regarded as having failed steroid therapy until completing that period of therapy).
- Up to 75% patients will respond but only 15% CR. *Note:* magnitude and speed of response correlates with long term prognosis.
- Once patient has responded, taper prednisolone dose over several months.
- Some patients will maintain an adequate platelet count ($>30 \times 10^9$/l) on discontinuation of steroids or on a low maintenance dose.
- Most adults relapse on tapering the prednisolone dose and require other therapy.

IVIg
- Action: blockade of phagocytes and possible anti-idiotype effect.
- Most ITP patients will have significant platelet rise following administration of 2g/kg over 5d.
- Effect often rapid (within 4d) but usually transient and lasts ~3 weeks (may be prolonged in a minority).
- Increment may be maintained with boosters of 400mg–1g/kg.
- Relatively non-toxic but expensive.
- Useful in patients
  – refractory to other treatments
  – who require an urgent increment for surgery and in pregnancy.

Splenectomy
- The only proven curative therapy for ITP (spleen is major site of platelet destruction). Usual pre- and post-splenectomy care (see p494).
- No reliable test to predict those patients who will benefit.
- Consider for patients
  – who fail to respond to prednisolone
  – requiring prednisolone >10mg/d to maintain acceptable platelet count
  – who have unacceptable side-effects with a lower maintenance dose.
- 60–80% of patients achieve at least a partial response to splenectomy.
- A brisk rise in platelet count in the immediate post-operative period is a good prognostic sign.

Immunosuppressive agents
- Act through inhibition of antibody production.
- Effect takes at least 2 weeks (may be up to 3 months).
- May be useful in patients
  – who have failed to achieve an adequate response to splenectomy
  – in whom splenectomy is contraindicated

- in whom an unacceptably high dose of prednisolone is necessary to maintain a 'safe' platelet count.
- Effective in up to 25% refractory patients.
- Azathioprine is the most widely used agent in the UK (start at 150mg/d). (maintain neutrophil count >1.0×10^9/l and platelet count >30×10^9/l.
- May be used with prednisolone to obtain an acceptable platelet count and minimise the toxicity of each agent.
- Cyclophosphamide and vincristine are alternatives.
- Long term therapy carries risk of serious toxicity including MDS and $2°$ leukaemias with azathioprine and cyclophosphamide.

Danazol
- Effective in ITP.
- May be used as alternative to prednisolone or in combination.
- Normal dose 400–800mg/d for 1–3 months tapering to 50–200mg/d.
- Side-effects: virilisation, weight gain and hepatotoxicity.

Other treatments

Intravenous anti-D (Rho)
- Will produce platelet increment in Rh(D) +ve patients (not splenectomised).
- May have role in the management of children with chronic ITP and HIV-infected patients.
- Mode of action is reticulo-endothelial blockade.
- May cure up to 10% of patients.

High dose dexamethasone
- Eg dexamethasone 20–40mg/d PO for 4 days; repeated 4-weekly.
- May produce a response (less good in patients who have failed splenectomy).

Other causes of thrombocytopenia

ITP in pregnancy
Fetal thrombocytopenia may occur due to placental transfer of IgG anti-platelet antibodies in a pregnant woman with ITP. Risk of intracranial haemorrhage in fetus during delivery is low although thrombocytopenia $<50 \times 10^9/l$ may occur in the fetus in up to 30% of pregnancies in women with previously diagnosed ITP. No good predictor for fetal thrombocytopenia. Differential diagnosis: gestational thrombocytopenia (common); count rarely $<70 \times 10^9/l$. Neonatal count normal. Other causes include pre-eclampsia. Treatment with prednisolone, dexamethasone or IVIg should be administered to the mother with thrombocytopenia severe enough to constitute a haemorrhagic risk to her. Avoid splenectomy – high rate of fetal loss. Severe maternal haemorrhage at delivery is rare but may require platelet transfusion, IVIg and possibly splenectomy. Special antenatal treatment of the fetus is unnecessary but avoid prolonged and complicated labour. Ensure paediatric support at delivery and check neonatal platelet count – monitor for several days (delayed thrombocytopenia). IVIg, prednisolone or exchange transfusion may be required.

Other autoimmune thrombocytopenias
Eg 2° to SLE and lymphoproliferative disorders (esp. low grade NHL and CLL). May present with isolated thrombocytopenia and underlying disorder may only be discovered on further investigation. Often refractory to therapy. Those with lymphoproliferative disorders will require chemotherapy for that condition.

Neonatal alloimmune thrombocytopenia (see p356)

Post-transfusion purpura (see p416)
Rare but life-threatening. Causes severe haemorrhage due to thrombocytopenia ~1 week after transfusion of blood or blood products. Thrombocytopenia may persist for several days. Occurs most commonly in ♀ and is usually due to antibody to the platelet antigen HPA-1a in an individual lacking this (2% of population) who has been previously sensitised (usually by pregnancy).

Hypersplenism
Thrombocytopenia primarily due to platelet pooling in enlarged spleen. If haemorrhagic complications, consider splenectomy if the underlying cause is unknown or if treatment of underlying disorder has been ineffective.

Non-immune thrombocytopenia due to increased destruction
If haemorrhage occurs platelet transfusion is necessary. Patients with platelet counts $>50 \times 10^9/l$ may respond to DDAVP.

Drug-induced thrombocytopenia
Many drugs implicated in idiosyncratic thrombocytopenia, largely through increased destruction – usually immune mechanism. In most cases the patient has been using the drug for several weeks/months and thrombocytopenia is severe ($<20 \times 10^9/l$). Most commonly implicated are heparin, quinine, quinidine, gold, sulphonamides, trimethoprim, penicillins, cephalosporins, cimetidine, ranitidine, diazepam, sodium valproate, phenacitin, rifampicin, PAS, thiazides, frusemide, chlorpropamide, tolbutamide, digoxin, methyldopa. If drug-induced thrombocytopenia suspected, discontinue the offending agent(s). If the patient is bleeding platelet transfusion should be administered. IVIg may be helpful. Thrombocytopenia usually resolves quickly but may persist for a prolonged period notably that due to gold which may be permanent. Implicated drugs should be avoided by that patient in future.

Haemostasis and thrombosis

Anticoagulation in pregnancy and post-partum

Pregnancy is a hypercoagulable state with an ↑ risk of thrombosis throughout and up to 6 weeks post-partum. In addition to ↑ venous stasis secondary to ↑ abdominal pressure and ↓ mobility, physiological prothrombotic changes in coagulation take place – see figure below.

Coagulation changes in normal pregnancy

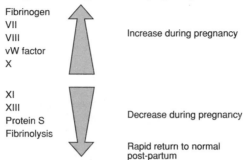

Fibrinogen
VII
VIII
vW factor
X

Increase during pregnancy

XI
XIII
Protein S
Fibrinolysis

Decrease during pregnancy

Rapid return to normal post-partum

Incidence
The risk of venous thromboembolic events (VTE) ↑ 5 fold in normal pregnancy ~0.5–1/1000; fatal PE 10/year in UK is the major cause of maternal death in pregnancy and the puerperium. The risk rises when the pregnancy is complicated (sepsis, prolonged bed rest, advanced maternal age, delivery by LSCS). Previous VTE particularly in pregnancy, inherited/acquired thrombophilia further increase the risk.

Indications for anticoagulation in pregnancy
- Acute VTE presenting in pregnancy.
- Long term anticoagulation for prosthetic heart valves/recurrent VTE.
- Previous VTE, particularly in pregnancy/post-partum.
- Antiphospholipid syndrome (APS).
- Inherited thrombophilia with/without a history of VTE.

General considerations
There are no universally accepted protocols for the management of anticoagulation in pregnancy. There are few controlled studies and much of the information relates to non-pregnant subjects. Both oral anticoagulants and heparin have advantages and disadvantages in pregnancy. The growing use of LMW heparins (LMWH), as yet unlicensed for use in pregnancy, is a significant advance in management.

Warfarin crosses the placenta and is teratogenic in the first trimester. Exposure during weeks 6–12 can cause warfarin embryopathy with nasal hypoplasia, stippled epiphyses and other manifestations. Incidence ranges from <5% to 67% in reported series. Warfarin at any stage of pregnancy is associated with CNS abnormalities and ↑ risk of fetal haemorrhage *in utero* and at delivery.

Haemostasis and thrombosis

Heparin does not cross the placenta and poses no teratogenic or haemorrhagic threat to the fetus. Maternal complications include haemorrhage (severe in <2%), thrombocytopenia (severe in <1%) and osteoporosis, usually asymptomatic and reversible but rare cause of vertebral fractures. SC LMWH, not yet licensed in pregnancy, have been used in many centres for years. Growing evidence suggests they are safe and may have ↓ complications *cf.* unfractionated (UF) heparin.

Treatment of VTE presenting in pregnancy
- Heparin 5–7d
  either monitored IV UF heparin; aim for APTT ratio 1.5-2.0
  or therapeutic SC LMWH based on body wt (*see BNF*)
  then monitored therapeutic SC 12 hrly UF heparin or LMWH OD
- Warfarin can be given weeks 12–36 if there are difficulties with heparin.
- Heparin requirements vary as pregnancy advances so adjust dose as necessary.
- Continue heparin until delivery; *omit heparin during labour.*
- Recommence heparin after delivery and start warfarin if desired.
- Continue treatment for 6 weeks post-partum; stop heparin once INR in therapeutic range.

Prophylaxis of thromboembolism in pregnancy

High risk women – on long term warfarin for prosthetic heart valves
Rarely practical to switch to heparin before pregnancy is commenced. Women must be advised of the risk to the fetus and to report pregnancy as soon as it is confirmed and be switched to heparin immediately.
- Starting dose: UF heparin SC 15–20,000 iu 12hrly.
- Adjust 24–48h later; aim for midpoint APTT ratio 1.5–2.5/Anti-Xa 0.3–0.7u/ml; monitor alternate days until stable then every 2 weeks.
- Continue heparin if possible throughout pregnancy.
- *If problems* – warfarin from 12–36 wks; INR 2.5-3.5; target 3.0; UF heparin after 36 wks.
- At delivery omit heparin; same night give heparin and warfarin. Stop heparin when INR in therapeutic range.

Other high risk women – previous VTE and other risk factors
eg VTE in pregnancy (recurrence rate 10-15%), APS, thrombophilia
- While there is agreement that prophylaxis is needed for these women the intensity and time of starting is not defined by clinical studies and will vary in different centres.

Unless a previous VTE was earlier start at 20 weeks gestation with
- Either fixed dose UF heparin 10,000 iu SC bd or LMWH high risk prophylactic dose SC OD (kinder and perhaps safer).
- Continue until 6 weeks post-partum.
- APS give 75mg aspirin throughout + heparin as above; if previous fetal loss, start heparin prophylaxis as soon fetal viability confirmed.

Low risk women
One VTE, not in pregnancy, no other risk factor; thrombophilia no VTE
- Either observe in pregnancy; consider low dose heparin for 6 weeks post-partum.
- Or give low dose prophylaxis with UF heparin 5000 iu bd/LMWH od in last trimester and 6 weeks post-partum.
- Other at-risk women eg LSCS with obesity (>wt 96kg), ↑ age (>35yr) give prophylactic low dose SC heparin until fully mobile.
- In hereditary thrombophilia no VTE but with prior fetal loss give aspirin/heparin as for APS.

Special notes
Monitor platelet count in first week of heparin, and at 4 weekly intervals. Epidural anaesthesia safe on prophylactic heparin; avoid if ↑ APTT ratio. Breast feeding is safe in warfarin and heparin treatment.

Conclusion
There is an urgent need for controlled trials to establish the appropriate level of anticoagulation in pregnancy. It is likely that the superiority of LMWH over UF heparin both for therapy and prophylaxis will be proven. Currently many centres use LMWH for all women except those with prosthetic heart valves because of ease of administration and ↓ risk of complications.

NEJM 1996 335 108

Immunodeficiency 10

Primary immunodeficiency syndromes

Incidence – rare.

Classification according to whether defect affects B-cells, T-cells, a combination of B and T-cells, or neutrophils.

B cell

- *X-linked hypogammaglobulinaemia* – recessive inheritance, presents a few months from birth with recurrent infections. Patients have no tonsils and low or absent IgG, IgA, and IgM. Treatment is with regular infusions of IVIg.
- *Common variable hypogammaglobulinaemia* – non-inherited, onset often only in adult life, presents with bronchiectasis, malabsorption, low IgG, IgA and IgM. Treatment is with regular infusions of IVIg.
- *IgA subclass deficiency* – relatively benign, may have anti-IgA antibodies in serum which can cause urticarial and anaphylactic reactions to blood product infusions.

T cell

- *DiGeorge syndrome* – non-inherited, associated with other severe abnormalities of CVS and CNS, absent thymus and T cells. Treatment unsatisfactory due to the multiple defects.

Combined

- *Severe combined immunodeficiency syndrome (SCID)* – autosomal recessive group of syndromes, very severe due to low B cells, T cells and NK cells. Some are due to adenine deaminase (ADA) deficiency. Famous as the first human disease to be successfully treated by gene therapy. Lymphocytes transfected with the normal ADA gene were shown to restore ADA activity and lymphocyte function but the effect was transient and the procedure needs to be repeated ~every month. HLA sibling matched BMT is the only permanent chance of cure.
- *Ataxia telangiectasia* – autosomal recessive, presents with chest infections, cerebellar ataxia and oral telangiectases. Patients have thymic hypoplasia and low B cells. Treatment is with HLA sibling matched BMT if available but may not fully restore normal phenotype.
- *Wiskott-Aldrich syndrome* – autosomal recessive, patients have low immunoglobulins, T cells and platelets and present with infections and bleeding. Treatment is with HLA sibling matched BMT if available.

Neutrophil abnormalities

- *Chronic granulomatous disease* – X-linked recessive, presents with bacterial infections of skin, lung and GIT. Neutrophil function defect is the only abnormality. Treatment is with HLA sibling matched BMT if available.
- *Chediak-Higashi syndrome* – presents with infections and bleeding due to neutropenia and thrombocytopenia. Associated with albinism. Treatment is with HLA sibling matched BMT if available.

Acquired immune deficiencies

May be classified according to the nature of the cellular immune defect.

Hypogammaglobulinaemia due to B lymphocyte abnormalities

Causes
CLL and other lymphoproliferative disorders, myeloma, nephrotic syndrome.

Clinical features
Bacterial infections – recurrent chest infections (may lead to bronchiectasis), sinus, skin and urinary tract infections common.

Treatment
- May improve with treatment of the underlying disease.
- IVIg should not be used routinely.
- Patients with severe hypogammaglobulinaemia and recurrent infections may be considered for IVIg replacement therapy – give 200mg/kg every 4 weeks.

T lymphocyte abnormalities

Reduced numbers: HIV infection, post-chemotherapy particularly high dose steroids, ALG, cyclophosphamide and purine analogues eg fludarabine and 2-CDA, post-stem cell transplantation esp. allogeneic.

Reduced function: Lymphoproliferative disorders, Hodgkin's disease, immunosuppressive agents eg cyclosporin and steroids, burns, uraemia.

Clinical features: Increased risk of viral, fungal and atypical infections. HSV, HZV, CMV, EBV, *Candida, Aspergillus, Mycoplasma*, PCP, Toxoplasmosis, TB and atypical Mycobacteria.

Treatment: Treat specific infection where possible. Consider prophylaxis against HZV, CMV, PCP and *Candida* in high risk groups eg post-allogeneic stem cell transplant.

B and T lymphocyte abnormalities

Causes CLL, post-radiotherapy, severe malnutrition.

Clinical features and treatment

As above.

Neutrophil abnormalities

Reduced numbers: See Neutropenia.

Reduced function: eg myelodysplasia.

Clinical features Bacterial and fungal sepsis.

Treatment Treat specific infections and consider prophylaxis.

HIV infection and AIDS

Infection with HIV-1 or HIV-2 produces a large number of haematological effects and can simulate a number of haematological conditions during both the latent pre-clinical phase and once clinical syndrome of AIDS has developed. HIV infection divided into four stages.

Stage 1: primary infection
Entry of HIV-1 or HIV-2 through a mucosal surface after sexual contact, direct inoculation into the bloodstream by contaminated blood products, or IV drug abuse is followed by a transient febrile illness up to 6 weeks later. Associated with oral ulceration, pharyngitis, and lymphadenopathy. Photophobia, meningism, myalgia, prostration, encephalopathy and meningitis may occur. FBC may show lymphopenia or lymphocytosis often with atypical lymphocytes, neutropenia, thrombocytopenia or pancytopenia. Major differential diagnoses are acute viral meningitis and infectious mononucleosis. False +ve IM serology may occur. Specific IgM then IgG antibody to HIV appears 4–12 weeks after infection and routine tests for HIV may be –ve for up to 3 months. However the virus is detectable in plasma and CSF from infected individuals during this period and the patient is highly infectious.

Stage 2: pre-clinical HIV infection
Although viral titres fall in the circulation at this time there is significant and persistent virus replication within lymph nodes and spleen. The clinically latent period may last 8–10 years and circulating CD4 T cell count remains normal for most of this period. However there is a delayed, gradual but progressive fall in CD4 T-lymphocytes in most patients, who may remain asymptomatic for a prolonged period despite modest lymphopenia. A number of minor skin problems are characteristic of the end of the latent phase: eg seborrhoeic dermatitis.

A patient with latent HIV infection may have isolated thrombocytopenia on routine blood testing. This is due to an immune mechanism and may be confused with ITP as there is frequently ↑ platelet associated immunoglobulin.

Stage 3: clinical symptomatology
Marked by onset of symptoms, rising titre of circulating virus and decline in circulating CD4 T-cell count to 0.2–$0.5 \times 10^9/l$. Wide variation in individual patient's rate of progression at this stage. A number of minor opportunistic infections are common: oral/genital candida, herpes zoster, oral leukoplakia. Lethargy, PUO and weight loss occur frequently. Significant lymphopenia (CD4 $<0.4 \times 10^9/l$) invariably present when opportunistic infection occurs. Persistent generalised lymphadenopathy is a condition in which lymphadenopathy >1cm at ≥2 extra-inguinal sites persists for >3 months and is a prodrome to severe immunodeficiency, opportunistic infection and neoplasia.

Stage 4: AIDS
AIDS is now defined as the presence of a +ve HIV antibody test associated with a CD4 lymphocyte count $<0.2 \times 10^9/l$ rather than by the development of a specific opportunistic infection or neoplastic complication. This final stage of HIV infection is associated with a marked reduction in CD4 T-cells, severe life-threatening opportunistic infection, neoplasia and neurological degeneration. Severity of these complications usually reflects the degree of immunodeficiency as measured by the CD4 T-cell count. However there is evidence that

prophylactic therapy reduces the incidence of complications and newer antiviral therapies slow the progression of this stage.

Haematological features of HIV infection

- Lymphopenia – CD4 lymphopenia may be masked by CD8 lymphocytosis in Stage 2; improved by antiviral therapy.
- Neutropenia – marrow suppression by virus or therapy; splenic sequestration.
- Anaemia normocytic/macrocytic due to suppression of marrow by virus or therapy, microangiopathic in TTP, haemolysis, haemorrhage.
- Thrombocytopenia – suppression of marrow by virus or therapy, immune destruction (may respond to antiviral therapy), infection, TTP or splenic sequestration.
- Bone marrow suppression – direct HIV effect, complication of AZT, d4T, gancyclovir, trimethoprim or amphotericin B therapy.
- Bone marrow infiltration – by NHL, Hodgkin's disease, granulomas due to *M tuberculosis* & atypical mycobacteria, disseminated fungal disease.

Complications of HIV infection

Opportunistic infections

1. Fungal

- *Pneumocystis carinii* — pneumonia
- *Candida albicans* — oro-oesophageal
- *Aspergillus fumigatus* — pneumonia
- *Histoplasma capsulatum* — disseminated
- *Cryptococcus neoformans* — meningo-encephalitis, pneumonia

2. Mycobacterial

- *M. avium-intracellulare* — disseminated, intestinal
- *M. tuberculosis* — pulmonary, intestinal

3. Parasitic

- *Cryptosporidium* — hepatobiliary, intestinal
- *Isospora* — colon, hepatobiliary
- *Toxoplasma gondii* — multiple abscesses in CNS; ocular, lymphatic

4. Viral

- Cytomegalovirus — retinal, hepatic, intestinal, CNS
- Herpes zoster — mucocutaneous
- Herpes simplex — mucocutaneous
- JC virus — CNS

5. Bacterial

- Haemophilus influenzae
- Streptococcus pneumoniae

Neoplasia

- AIDS-related Kaposi's sarcoma   20–30% of patients; multiple skin lesions; later lymph nodes, mucous membranes and visceral organs ?role of HHV8
- NHL   up to 10%; 65% diffuse large B-cell, 30% Burkitt-like; extranodal esp. small bowel & CNS; primary effusion lymphomas; aggressive.
  ?role of EBV(100% +ve in 1° CNS NHL)

- Cervical carcinoma
- Anal carcinoma
- Hodgkin's disease   Advanced stage, extranodal sites.

Direct effects of HIV infection

- Bone marrow suppression   Dysplastic appearance; pancytopenia
- Small bowel enteropathy   Malabsorption syndrome
- CNS   Dementia, myelopathy, neuropathy.

HIV infection – therapy

1. Infection prophylaxis

Fluconazole/itraconazole	Oro-oesophageal candidiasis ± crypto-coccal meningitis
Trimethoprim	*Pneumocystis carinii*, ± ocular/CNS toxo-plasmosis
Dapsone/nebulised pentamidine	*Pneumocystis carinii*
Rifabutin/azithromycin/ clarithromycin	*M. avium-intracellulare*
Acyclovir	HSV and HZV
?Gancyclovir	CMV

2. Antiviral therapy

▶*Nucleoside* class of viral reverse transcriptase inhibitors have been widely used both as single agents and in combination: zidovudine (AZT), didanosine (ddI), zalcitabine (ddC), stavudine (d4T), and lamuvidine (3TC). Specific therapy is followed within hours by rapid clearance of virions from the circulation and subsequently by reappearance of circulating T-cells and a rising count over several days. Viral resistance develops with time, especially to single agent treatment. Combination of 3TC + AZT produces marked suppression of virus replication for over 1–2 years.

▶*Protease inhibitors* interfere with virus assembly and have dramatic effects on viral load: saquinavir, ritonavir, indinavir.

▶*Triple therapy* using two nucleosides plus a protease inhibitor is currently recommended for all patients with stage 3 and 4 disease.

3. Treatment of complications

● *Oro-oesophageal candidiasis*	Systemic fluconazole or amphotericin then lifelong prophylaxis.
● *Pneumocystis pneumonia*	High dose co-trimoxazole or pentamidine then lifelong prophylaxis.
● *Tuberculosis*	Multi-agent therapy (drug resistance common) ± lifelong isoniazid prophylaxis.
● *Fungal pneumonia*	Amphotericin B then lifelong prophylaxis.
● *CMV pneumonitis/retinitis*	Gancyclovir/foscarnet then lifelong prophylaxis.
● *CNS Toxoplasmosis*	Pyrimethamine then lifelong prophylaxis.
● *Cryptococcal meningitis*	Amphotericin/fluconazole.
● *AIDS-related Kaposi's sarcoma*	Limited disease: local DXT, cryotherapy, intra-lesional vincristine, interferon-α; advanced disease: combination chemo-therapy eg adriamycin, bleomycin & vincristine (ABV), liposomal daunoru-bicin or paclitaxel.
● *Non-Hodgkin's lymphoma*	Poor prognosis; combination chemo-therapy (often standard regimens at reduced dosage due to toxicity) 50% response, median survival <9 mos; CNS lymphoma particularly poor prognosis; palliative dexamethasone DXT.

Neonatal anaemia

Intrauterine conditions require a state of polycythaemia. Congenital anaemia is present with cord blood Hb <14.0gd/l. In the healthy infant, Hb drops rapidly after birth (see *Normal ranges*) and by end of the neonatal period (4 weeks in a term baby), the mean Hb may be as low as 10.0g/dl. With ↑ RBC destruction, there is a concomitant ↑ in serum bilirubin. Thus complex changes occur in this period making distinction between physiology and pathology difficult.

Pathophysiology

In normal full term babies, red cell production ↓ in the first 2–3 months of life. RBC survival shortens; reticulocytes and erythropoietin production ↓; iron, folate and vit B$_{12}$ stores are normal. Anaemia in the neonate may be due either to *impaired production* of RBCs or to *increased destruction* or *loss*.

Impaired production	Increased loss/destruction	
Anaemia of prematurity	Haemorrhage; birth trauma, occult loss, iatrogenic	
Infection	Haemolytic anaemia	
Congenital conditions	*Non-immune*	*Immune*
DBA	Infection	Rh/ABO HDN
Fanconi anaemia	Congenital RBC abn.	Maternal autoimm. disease
	Other eg drugs, MAHA	

Blood loss during delivery is common, in ~1% severe enough to produce anaemia. Infection is also a significant cause of anaemia; primary haematological disorders are rare. Anaemia in premature infant is almost invariably present, induced and multifactorial. Jaundice is present in 90% healthy infants making interpretation of a raised bilirubin (*see p348*) a critical piece of the jigsaw when investigating an anaemic neonate.

Clinical features

History may make the diagnosis. Check events at time of delivery, past obstetrical history, maternal and family history, non-specific symptoms – lethargy, reluctance to feed, failure to thrive – all may indicate anaemia.

Physical examination

General

Is the baby sick?

Pallor – not a reliable sign of anaemia

differentiate acute anaemia from asphyxia

acute blood loss

    BP ↓

    tachycardia

    rapid respiration

    not cyanosed

    not jaundiced

asphyxia

    laboured breathing

    cyanosis

bradycardia

response to O$_2$

Hb not ↓

Jaundice

Haemorrhagic

?Bruising

Haematoma

Petechial-? ↓ platelets or DIC

Splenomegaly

Infection

Fever may be absent in sick child

Paediatric haematology

Laboratory tests
- FBC and reticulocytes.
- MCV and RBC morphology, bilirubin and Kleihauer
  Interpret as follows:
    - reticulocyte count   ↓ – hypoplastic
                                       ↑ – haemolysis, blood loss
    - Kleihauer if +ve suggests fetomaternal bleed (quantitate amount)
    - Bilirubin ↑ (unconjugated)
    - check DAT   +ve in immune haemolytic anaemia
                                    –ve in other haemolytic anaemia (incl. ABO HDN)
    - Bilirubin ↑ (conjugated/mixed look for hepatobiliary obstruction/
      dysfunction).
- Blood film
  RBC morphology – may be diagnostic eg congenital spherocytosis, other
  RBC membrane disorders, HDN.
- ↓MCV – α thalassaemia syndromes/chronic intrauterine blood loss.
  (*Note:* ↑ *polychromasia, occasional NRBC, spherocytes day1–4 in healthy babies*).
- WBC changes – ?reactive, ?congenital leukaemia.

Further investigation
- Coagulation screen for DIC, TORCH screen/blood culture for infection.
- Special metabolic, serological, haematological (BM in selected cases) and
  other tests as appropriate.
- Radiology: CXR, abdominal USS – ?haematoma, hepatosplenomegaly, etc.

337

Treatment
- Treat the specific cause where this is possible.
- Transfusion as dictated by clinical needs (see p358).
- Avoid unnecessary blood taking.
- Erythropoietin for anaemia of prematurity – *see p350.*
- Hyperbilirubinaemia *see p348 for management.*

Follow up
Iron replacement for the premature infant (see p358).

Outcome
Will depend on the aetiology of the neonatal anaemia. The common causes of
anaemia – blood loss, infection, prematurity are responsive to treatment and the
outlook good.

Haemolytic anaemia in the neonatal period

Jaundice and haemolysis occurs in ~10% of newborns and is usually not associated with anaemia. When present, the common cause in Caucasian populations, is isoimmune HDN secondary to feto-maternal blood group incompatibility. In other ethnic groups G6PD deficiency and congenital infection are major causes.

Pathophysiology

Physiological haemolysis occurs soon after birth and there is a marked drop in the Hb and RBC count in the first weeks of life. The RBC half life is reduced (to 60–70d), even more so in the premature neonate (35–50d). Neonatal RBCs are more susceptible to oxidative stress and there is altered RBC enzyme activity compared to adult RBC and reticulocytes. Thus pathological haemolysis occurs in the neonatal period more than any other time.

Causes of haemolytic anaemia

Haemolysis may be due to intrinsic defects of the RBC which are usually congenital (see p340) or to acquired extracorpuscular factors (see p342) which may be immune or non-immune as shown below.

Congenital RBC defects

Membrane defects
    congenital spherocytosis
    congenital elliptocytosis
Enzyme defects
    G6PD, PK, other enzyme deficiencies
Haemoglobinopathies
    α thalassaemia
    Other rare abnormal haemoglobins

Acquired RBC defects

Immune
    Rh/ABO and other HDN
Non-immune
    Infections
    Metabolic disorders
    Drugs – Heinz body haemolysis
    Physical agents – eg heat
    MAHA

Clinical features

- Jaundice may be clinically obvious at birth or soon after (distinguishing it from the common physiological anaemia which occurs >48h after birth particularly difficult in premature babies). Dark urine noted.
- Anaemia may be severe depending on cause.
- Infections are common cause of hyperbilirubinaemia (see p348) with specific clinical findings. *In utero* infections (TORCH) do not usually cause severe jaundice *cf.* post-natal bacterial sepsis where jaundice may be striking and associated with MAHA.
- Splenomegaly at birth indicates a prenatal event; when noted later it may be secondary to splenic clearance of damaged RBC and is non-specific.
- Kernicterus is the major complication of neonatal hyperbilirubinaemia.
- Family history and drug history may be informative.

Laboratory diagnosis

- ↑ unconjugated bilirubin with anaemia is *hallmark* of haemolytic anaemia.
- ↑ reticulocytes (haptoglobins are less reliable in the newborn).
- Blood film – may show RBC abnormalities eg spherocytes, elliptocytes.
- DAT, if +ve suggests immune haemolysis; –ve does not rule this out eg ABO HDN.

- Heinz body test—positive in drug-induced haemolysis, G6PD deficiency, etc.
- Intravascular haemolysis—look for haemoglobinuria/haemoglobinaemia.
- Specific tests to confirm congenital RBC defects (see p340).
- Serological tests for congenital infection.

Management

1. Important to establish the diagnosis (underlying process often complex and multiple factors present).
2. Supportive measures—fluids, antibiotics, treatment of underlying cause.
3. Transfusion if anaemia becomes symptomatic or severe.
4. Hyperbilirubinaemia—phototherapy, exchange transfusion as required (see p348).

Outcome

With supportive treatment, and with growing maturity of the liver, the condition may resolve even though an intrinsic RBC defect persists. The outlook for severe haemolytic anaemia such as Rh HDN is good in specialist centres and mortality and morbidity from HA in the neonate is rare. Follow up is important to establish the nature of congenital RBC defects.

Haemolytic anaemia in the newborn – congenital RBC defects

Acquired defects of the RBC in the newborn–*see p342*. Specific problems when congenital RBC defects of membrane, enzymes and Hb arise in the neonatal period are presented here.

Pathophysiology

The neonate is uniquely disadvantaged when it comes to handling pathological haemolysis because of ↑ RBC destruction, hepatic immaturity and altered enzyme activity. Thus congenital defects of the RBC commonly present in the newborn *except* for defects involving the β globin chain (eg SCD, β thalassaemia) which become clinically manifest weeks/months after birth but can be diagnosed *in utero*/neonate if suspected. HS is the commonest congenital haemolytic anaemia in Caucasian populations; ~½ present in the neonatal period. Worldwide, G6PD deficiency occurs in 3% population; neonatal presentation is common in Mediterranean and Canton peoples. α thalassaemia (4 gene deletion) is incompatible with life, causing hydrops fetalis, and may present as HbH disease (deletion of 3 α genes) in neonate.

Hereditary RBC defects in neonatal haemolytic anaemia

- **Membrane defects**
  - Hereditary spherocytosis, hereditary elliptocytosis, stomatocytosis/pyropoikilocytosis/acanthocytosis).
- **Haemoglobin defects**
  - αδβ thalassaemia
  - unstable haemoglobins (eg Hb Köln, Hb Zurich).
- **Enzyme defects**
  - glycolytic pathway; pyruvate kinase and other enzyme deficiencies
  - hexose-monophosphate shunt; G6PD deficiency, other enzymes.

Clinical features

Congenital haemolytic anaemia with hyperbilirubinaemia, dark urine, ± hepatosplenomegaly. In many a +ve family history is found.

Laboratory investigation

- Exclude acquired disorders, DCT and other tests (see p342).
- RBC morphology is one key to diagnosis and further investigation.
- Further tests for suspected
  - membrane defect (osmotic fragility, autohaemolysis)
  - Hb defect; Hb electrophoresis, sickle test, etc
  - enzyme defect; Heinz body prep, screening tests for specific enzymes, etc.
- Heinz body test +ve
  - drug or chemical induced in neonate without hereditary defect
  - enzyme deficiency eg G6PD, others
  - unstable Hb
  - α thalassaemia.

Management see p348

Outcome

Clinically significant in neonatal period, most conditions will improve in the first weeks of life as the infant matures.

Haemolytic anaemia in the newborn – acquired RBC defects

These may be either *immune* or *non-immune*. Main cause of the latter will be underlying infection either acquired *in utero* or in the days following delivery. Drug/chemically induced haemolysis in the newborn is rare.

Pathophysiology

Neonatal RBCs have ↑ sensitivity to oxidative stress due to altered enzyme activity, and are more liable to be destroyed by altered physical conditions, mechanical factors, toxins, drugs than adult RBC. Infection acquired *in utero* when haemolysis usually mild, or post-natally is a common cause of haemolytic anaemia. The mechanism is multifactorial and includes ↑ reticuloendothelial activity, microangiopathic damage. Drug induced haemolysis and Heinz body formation is noted transiently in normal RBCs as a result of chemical/drug toxicity but is much more often seen when there is an underlying RBC defect such as G6PD deficiency.

Acquired RBC defects causing congenital haemolytic anaemia
- Infection
  - congenital eg TORCH (toxoplasmosis, rubella, CMV, herpes simplex)
  - post-natal eg viral, Coxsackie B, bacterial eg gram –ve infection.
- Microangiopathic – 2° severe infections ± DIC.
- Drug or chemically-induced.
- Vitamin E deficiency.
- Infantile pyknocytosis.
- Metabolic disease eg galactosaemia, osteopetrosis.

Clinical features

Congenital infections All rare with adequate antenatal care. Most infants with herpes simplex will be symptomatic with DIC and hepatic dysfunction – haemolysis is not a major finding. Haemolytic anaemia is also mild in CMV and rubella infections but ~½ infants with toxoplasmosis will be anaemic (may be severe).

Postnatal infections Severe viral, bacterial and protozoal (remember malaria in endemic regions) – congenital haemolytic anaemia may be severe and of rapid onset.

MAHA 2° to toxic damage to the endothelium is rare in the neonate and is mainly a laboratory diagnosis in infants where clinical factors suggest the diagnosis (eg severe infections, burns, severe asphyxia, shock, thrombosis). These infants are sick and there may be clinical signs of DIC.

Drugs/chemical exposure are more likely to cause Heinz body haemolysis in premature babies or those with G6PD deficiency, etc. Incriminating agents include sulphonamides, chloramphenicol, mothballs, aniline dyes, maternal intake of diuretics and in the past, water soluble vitamin K analogues. Vitamin E (a potent antioxidant) has a number of RBC stabilising activities. Deficiency is more often seen in premature infants, following O_2 therapy and intake of diets rich in polyunsaturated fatty acids. Clinical findings include haemolysis, oedema and CNS signs. Acanthocytosis/pyknocytosis of the RBC is characteristic.

Infantile pyknocytosis

Indicates the diagnostic feature of this acquired disorder. Haemolysis with increased numbers (>6–50%) of pyknocytes (irregularly contracted RBCs with multiple projections) in the peripheral blood. Cause unknown. Anaemia may be severe and present at birth, and is most striking at ~3 weeks (Hb ↓ 5g/dl reported). Exchange transfusion occasionally required but the condition spontaneously remits by ~3 months.

Metabolic disorders – rare.

Laboratory investigation

Criteria set out on p340 will establish the diagnosis of haemolytic anaemia. A +ve DAT points to an immune process – probably Rh/ABO disease. If non-immune, further tests to look for a congenital abnormality.

The diagnosis may be made by

- Peripheral blood findings.
- Heinz body positive – ?chemical/drug induced haemolysis.
- RBC enzyme screen to exclude G6PD, PK deficiency, etc.
- Hb electrophoresis to exclude Hb defects.

Often no definitive cause is found and the HA will be presumed 2° to underlying systemic illness.

Management

1. General supportive measures as for hyperbilirubinaemia (see p348).
2. Treatment of specific conditions
   - haemolytic disease of the newborn – see p344.
   - neonatal infection as appropriate
   - exchange transfusion almost never needed.

343

Outlook

Prognosis is that of the underlying condition. Anaemia will usually respond as the condition is brought under control.

Haemolytic disease of the newborn (HDN)

Arises when there is blood group incompatibility between mother and fetus. Maternal Abs produced against fetal RBC antigens cross the placenta and destroy fetal RBCs. Maternal immunisation with Rhesus (Rh) D immunoglobulin (anti-D) introduced in the late 1960s transformed the outlook. Despite this, HDN due to anti-D and other red cell antibodies (eg anti-c, anti-Kell) remains a significant cause of fetal morbidity.

Pathogenesis

Placental transfer of fetal cells → the maternal circulation is maximal at delivery; the condition does not usually present in the firstborn (▶ *ABO incompatibility is an exception*). Previous maternal transfusion, abortion, amniocentesis, chorionic villus sampling (CVS), obstetric manipulations, can cause antibody formation. Maternal IgG crosses placenta, reacts with Ag +ve fetal RBCs.

Rh HDN

Classically presents as jaundice in first 24h of life.

Mild HDN may go unnoticed and presents as persistent hyperbilirubinaemia or late anaemia weeks after birth.

Severe HDN may result in a macerated fetus, fresh stillbirth or severely anaemic, grossly oedematous infant (hydrops fetalis) with hepatosplenomegaly 2° to compensatory extramedullary haemopoiesis *in utero*.

Kernicterus Neurological damage secondary to bilirubin deposition in the brain, depends on a number of factors including the unconjugated bilirubin level, maturity of the baby, the use of interacting drugs.

Diagnosis

Rh HDN is the commonest cause of neonatal immune haemolysis; routine antenatal screening should identify most cases prior to delivery allowing appropriate action.

In suspected case at delivery *cord blood* is tested for

- ABO and Rh (D) group.
- Presence of maternal antibody on fetal RBCs by DAT.
- Hb and blood film (spherocytes, increased polychromasia, NRBCs).
- Serum bilirubin (↑).

Maternal blood is tested for

- ABO and Rh (D) group.
- Serum antibodies against fetal cells (by *Indirect* anti-globulin test, IAGT).
- Antibody titre.
- Kleihauer test – detects and quantitates fetal RBCs in maternal circulation.

Diagnostic findings include

- DAT +ve haemolytic anaemia ± spherocytosis in the infant.
- Maternal anti-D, or other anti Rh antibody eg anti-c (IAGT +ve).

ABO HDN

Theoretically should occur more frequently since ~1 in 4/5 babies and mothers are ABO incompatible. Group O mothers may have naturally occurring IgG anti-A or B and with a boost to this during pregnancy haemolysis can occur.

Clinical features

First pregnancies are not exempt, but condition is usually mild. Presentation is later than with Rh HDN (2–4d, but may be weeks after birth).

Diagnosis

May be difficult – DAT not always +ve, anti-A and B occur naturally.

Antibody studies maternal high titre anti-A/B almost always in a group O mother cord-blood/infant's serum – an inappropriate antibody (eg anti-A in a group A baby).

Other blood group antibodies

Can produce severe HDN eg anti-Kell in particular. Serological testing will establish diagnosis. Maternal autoimmune haemolytic anaemia may produce a similar picture to alloimmune HDN. Usually the diagnosis will have been made antenatally. Severity in infant varies depending on maternal condition.

Management – prevention

Routine antenatal maternal ABO and Rh D grouping and antibody testing carried out at booking visit (~12–16 weeks).

If antibody positive repeat at intervals to check the antibody titre.

If antibody negative repeat at ~28 weeks gestation. Establish if paternal red cells (heterozygous, homozygous or negative for the specific Ag).

Anti-D prophylaxis

- 250 iu IM prior to delivery to Rh D negative women without antibodies to cover any intrauterine manoeuvre, miscarriage, etc.
- After delivery, a standard dose of 500iu anti-D within 72h unless baby is known to be Rh (D) –ve.
- If Kleihauer test result shows a bleed of >4ml give further anti-D.

Treatment of affected fetus – before delivery

Treatment depends on past obstetric history, the nature and titre of the antibody, paternal expression of the antigen, also cord blood sampling *in utero*. If heterozygous the fetal genotype can be established by CVS, fetal blood sampling and PCR.

Examination of the amniotic fluid to assess the degree of hyperbilirubinaemia is indicated with a poor past history (exchange transfusion or stillbirth in previous baby) and high titre (1:8–1:64) of an antibody likely to cause severe HDN (eg anti-D,-c or Kell). The amniotic fluid bilirubin at optical density 450μm dictates treatment according to the Liley chart.

Options include intrauterine transfusion (IUT) if fetus is not deemed mature enough for delivery (check lung maturity on phospholipid levels) *or* induction of labour if it is. Intensive maternal plasmapheresis according to the protocols of the specialist unit. Advances in management of very premature babies are such that nowadays IUT rarely performed.

After delivery

- Full paediatric support – metabolic, nutritional and respiratory.
- Treat anaemia *(note:* cord blood anaemia if Hb <14.0g/dl) by simple transfusion, if unconjugated hyperbilirubinaemia not a problem.

- Exchange transfusion with *Rh (D) neg* and *group specific blood* if possible for:
  - a severely affected hydropic anaemic baby
  - hyperbilirubinaemia (bilirubin level at or near 20mg or rapidly rising level eg>1mg per hour) in first few days of life
  - signs suggesting kernicterus – exchange transfusion may have to be repeated.
- Phototherapy to reduce the bilirubin level.
- Follow up required – late anaemia can be severe particularly if ET has not been carried out.

Outcome

With modern techniques, the outlook is good even for severely affected infants.

BMJ 1997 **315** 1480

Hyperbilirubinaemia

Bilirubin results from the breakdown of haem, in >75% this is Hb haem. Bilirubin may be unconjugated water insoluble prehepatic (a mark of excessive RBC breakdown) or conjugated soluble post-hepatic (↑ in cholestasis). Unconjugated bilirubin ↑ in most neonates and is usually physiological; conjugated hyperbilirubinaemia, on the other hand, is almost always pathological.

Pathophysiology

Physiological jaundice is defined as a temporary inefficient excretion of bilirubin which results in jaundice in full-term infants between the 2nd and 8th day of life. Occurs in ~90% of healthy neonates. Hepatic immaturity and ↑ RBC breakdown overloads the neonate's ability to handle the bilirubin which is mainly unconjugated. The bilirubin is rarely >100μmol/l. Reaches a maximum day 4–7 and usually ↓ to normal by day 10. In premature neonates it may be higher and take longer to settle. HDN due to blood group incompatibility accounts for ~10% cases of hyperbilirubinaemia and about ¾ cases requiring exchange transfusion.

Causes of hyperbilirubinaemia

Unconjugated	Conjugated
Physiological jaundice	Mechanical obstruction
Haemolytic anaemia	Bile duct abnormalities
Haematoma	eg atresia, cysts, etc
Polycythaemia	Hepatocellular disorders
Biochemical defects	Hepatitis, infection, metabolic, etc

Clinical features

- Clinical jaundice in the first 24h life is always pathological.
- Presenting after this, the jaundice may/not be pathological – usually not. Inadequate food/fluid intake with dehydration can aggravate the physiological ↑ bilirubin. A higher concentration is acceptable for the full-term breast-fed baby (serum bilirubin 240μmol/l) than bottle fed baby (190μmol/l).
- Jaundice in an active healthy infant is likely to be physiological.
- In a sick infant the underlying cause of the jaundice may be clinically obvious – eg infection, anaemia, shock, asphyxia, haemorrhage (may be occult).
- Physical examination – hepatosplenomegaly is pathological.
- Maternal history (drugs, known condition) and family history may help.

Laboratory investigation

- FBC, reticulocyte count and film – ?haemolytic anaemia.
- LFTs and bilirubin – ?conjugated or unconjugated
  - *unconjugated hyperbilirubinaemia*
    - DCT, maternal and neonatal blood group serology
    - Infection evaluation including TORCH
    - Thyroid function
    - Reducing substances
  - *conjugated hyperbilirubinaemia*
    - abdominal USS, liver pathology, choledochal cyst, biliary atresia.
- Further investigation as determined by results and clinical picture.

Management

- General – adequate hydration, nutrition, other supportive measures treat underlying cause – antibiotics, metabolic disturbances. haemolytic anaemia – blood transfusion.
- Specific – phototherapy (light source with wave length between 400–500 mm) effective in treating most causes of unconjugated hyperbilirubinaemia. ▶ Contraindicated in conjugated hyperbilirubinaemia.
- Exchange transfusion – the indications are complex. Main indication is severe haemolytic anaemia and is used in full-term infants when the bilirubin is >340µmol/l and at a lower concentration in premature infants.
- Hyperbilirubinaemia due to mechanical obstruction may need surgery.

Outcome

In most infants hyperbilirubinaemia resolves by 2 weeks. When pathology has been excluded the commonest cause of prolonged hyperbilirubinaemia persisting beyond this period is breastfeeding. In ~⅓ healthy breast-fed infants the bilirubin is still significantly ↑ at day 21. Kernicterus is not a complication but the condition causes concern before it spontaneously remits.

Anaemia of prematurity

Anaemia is an almost invariable finding in the premature infant. By week 3–4 of life the Hb may be ↓ 7.0g/dl in untreated infants. In a study of very low birth weight infants (750–1499g) 75% required blood transfusion. A number of factors are causal.

Pathogenesis
- Bone marrow hypoplasia – RBC production and survival are reduced.
- Reticulocytes ↓ in the neonate.
- Epo production falls in the first few weeks.
- Iatrogenic – eg multiple blood sampling (depletes the RBC mass and Fe stores – by 4 weeks the premature baby may have had its total blood volume removed).

Clinical features
The increased O_2 and metabolic demand of the premature baby makes them less able to tolerate ↓ Hb. Over 50% infants <30 weeks gestation develop tachycardia, tachypnoea, feeding difficulties ↓ activity when anaemic. High HbF level and ↑ O_2 affinity exaggerates the hypoxia.

Laboratory diagnosis
The Hb and Hct concentrations seen at different gestational ages are shown in *Normal ranges*. The anaemia of prematurity is seldom severe, usually being treated early. Ferritin, normal at birth, rapidly ↑ over the first next few weeks because of ↓ erythropoiesis, then ↓ as RBC production switches on.

Complications
Intraventricular haemorrhage, retinopathy of prematurity, and infection are serious complications in the premature baby. There is no evidence that these are related to the presence of the anaemia. Blood transfusion carries a risk of transmission of viral infections (eg CMV in ~10% transfused neonates given CMV +ve blood).

Treatment
- Delayed cord clamping increases Fe stores.
- Close monitoring of blood sampling is important.
- Transfusion indications will vary in neonatal units – decide on clinical grounds eg symptomatic anaemic infants, particularly if ventilated. The following are guidelines only:
  – prems <2 wk with Hb <14.0g/dl, Hct <40%
  – prems >2 wk, Hb <11.0g/dl, Hct <32%.
- A rising reticulocyte count in some centres is used to withhold transfusion.
- Some studies have shown better weight gain in transfused infants (not confirmed by others).
- Fe supplementation (2mg/d PO) after first 2 weeks and until iron sufficient.
- Epo – controversial. Theoretical considerations support its use but controlled studies have shown minimal benefit (see p352).

Natural history
Despite the growing safety of blood and its ready availability and convenient packaging to reduce donor exposure, blood transfusion carries definite risks and is to be avoided. It is likely therefore that in affluent societies the use of Epo will increase, despite its limited effect.

BMJ 1993 **306** 172

Erythropoietin

Glycoprotein hormone produced mainly in the kidneys stimulates the differentiation and growth of erythroid progenitor cells and production of erythrocytes. Its use in the anaemia of prematurity is based on the observation that there is a relative deficiency of endogenous Epo despite the development of anaemia and hypoxia. In the 1980s the gene for Epo was cloned and reliable sensitive radioimmunoassays developed which quantitated Epo concentrations in a variety of conditions. Normal plasma range is 10–20u/L.

Indications for Epo

Chronic renal failure is the best established use of Epo but its use is extending (largely to avoid blood transfusion transmission of infection).

The main indications

Anaemia of renal failure   Anaemia of prematurity
Anaemia of chronic disease   Autologous blood donation
Renal failure

Failure to produce Epo is a major reason for the severe anaemia of CRF. Transfusion dependency is corrected by Epo. Other benefits include improved well being, growth, energy, cardiac output.

Complications include

Hypertension and iron deficiency.

Dosage and administration

Starting dose 50–100u/kg × 3/week (IP/IV/SC) titrating dose to achieve Hct of 30–33%.

Anaemia of prematurity

Controlled studies have shown some benefit in the anaemia of prematurity with ↓ in transfusion: in US multicentre randomised trial 43% treated cf. 31% control did not need blood; European multicentre trial of infants <34 wks gestation 25% treated cf. 4% controls by 7 weeks either did not need transfusion or had Hct >32 %. Iron supplements optimised response. Expensive (£150 per completed course) and concern about the side-effects ↑ septicaemia, ↓ weight gain – but is recommended for premature infants <34 wks, weight 750–1500g beginning ~day 3 and for 6 weeks. Dose 250u/kg SC × 3/week.

Anaemia of chronic disease

Controlled studies show ↑ well-being, ↓ transfusion but no effect on disease in:
- Cancer patients anaemic on chemotherapy, particularly cisplatin.
- HIV/AIDS patients where anaemia limits antiretroviral treatment.
- Other conditions eg rheumatoid arthritis; some may benefit.
- Bone marrow failure – little consistent benefit in conditions such as MDS where transfusion dependency is common; of some use in patients with persistent anaemia post BMT.

Autologous transfusion

Epo improves yield of autologous blood in patients undergoing elective surgery with mild anaemia (Hb 11.0-13.0g/dl). Indicated if large volumes (4–5 units) required and short time to collect. Given IV 3 weeks before surgery with iron allowed ~4u collection in 81% cf. 37% controls.

Administration

Two products available in UK (*see BNF*). May be given SC/IV/IP. Dose and route of administration differs depending on condition being treated.

▶ Contraindicated in uncontrolled hypertension.

Conclusion

Epo is of great benefit in CRF. Its use in anaemia due to other causes is growing but further trials needed to define its optimal role.

Neonatal purpura

Purpura, the extravasation of blood into skin and subcutaneous tissues, includes petechiae (minute pinpoint haemorrhages), and ecchymosis (large bruises >1cm in dia). Being born is a major trauma and prolonged labour can result in purpura over presenting parts *despite* normal platelets and coagulation profile. When the purpuric manifestations extend beyond this an underlying cause should be sought.

Pathophysiology

The causes of neonatal purpura are set out in the flow chart below; secondary thrombocytopenia is the main cause. Increased platelet destruction is the common mechanism here and may be *immune* or *non-immune*. Platelet survival is ↓, MPV ↑ and megakaryocytes present in the bone marrow. ↑ platelet associated IgG (PAIgG) is common in sick infants with severe thrombocytopenia, not related to maternal ITP. Severe neonatal thrombocytopenia is rare (platelet count <20 × 10^9/l occurs in 4/10,000 neonates), but is common in sick neonates in ITU (platelets <50 × 10^9/l in ~20%).

Clinical features

- Varies depending on cause.
- In sick children, thrombocytopenia comes on rapidly in first few days of life, causes include birth asphyxia, respiratory distress syndrome, infection, DIC.
- Maternal history – check if known ITP, past history, family history, delivery details.
- If maternal platelet count ↓ could be ITP, drug induced, maternal illness eg toxaemia.

Physical examination

- Is the baby sick? Consider intrauterine infection (TORCH syndrome), ICH, DIC.
- ?hepatosplenomegaly – infection, neoplasia, haemolysis.
- ?congenital abnormalities eg skeletal (?absent radii), microcephaly, cavernous haemangioma.

Laboratory diagnosis

- FBC – thrombocytopenia present? Use flow chart for further investigation.
- Maternal FBC – if thrombocytopenia look for platelet and autoimmune antibodies.
- Neonatal thrombocytopenia – blood film, coagulation screen, TORCH (infection) screen, platelet antibodies as indicated.
- Further tests eg BM if cause not clear
  - ?primary haem disorder
  - ?megakaryocytes present
  - leukaemic or aplastic.
  - don't forget cytogenetic analysis on BM sample
- Radiological tests – if diagnosis unclear exclude underlying thrombosis eg ?catheter related. USS to exclude.

Treatment

Supportive give platelets (i) to bleeding neonate (ii) as prophylaxis to sick premature baby to keep platelet count >30 × 10^9/l to ↓ risk ICH (iii) for surgery/invasive procedures, keep platelet count >50 × 10^9/l.

Specific treat underlying cause – infection, etc.; maternal ITP (see p316); NAIT see p356.

Outcome

Even when severe, thrombocytopenic bleeding can be controlled with platelet transfusions, and permanent morbidity and death are rare. In systematically ill neonates, treatment of the underlying condition ↑ platelets to normal in most by day 10. In maternal ITP neonatal thrombocytopenia usually resolves in 2–3 wks.

The underlying cause of the neonatal purpura will determine the outcome.

Neonatal Purpura – check platelet count

Platelet count NORMAL

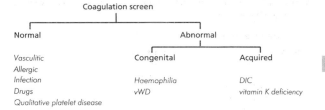

Coagulation screen

Normal — Abnormal

Normal:
Vasculitic
Allergic
Infection
Drugs
Qualitative platelet disease

Congenital
Haemophilia
vWD

Acquired
DIC
vitamin K deficiency

Platelet count LOW

Immune — Non-immune

Immune:
Maternal ITP
Alloimmune TP
Other causes

Congenital
Platelet disorders
Haematological disease
Diamond-Blackfan syn.
Leukaemia

Acquired
DIC
Infection

355

J Pediatr 1986 **108** 749

Neonatal alloimmune thrombocytopenia (NAIT)

Occurs when there is incompatibility between parental and fetal platelet antigens. Maternal antibodies react with neonatal platelets *in utero* causing fetal thrombocytopenia which can be severe, and in some cases life-threatening.

Pathophysiology

In >90% cases the mother will be HPA-1a (old term PLA1) −ve with anti-HPA-1a antibodies against the HPA-1a +ve fetus; only 2% population are HPA-1a −ve (ie homozygous HPA-1b). Incidence of NAIT is 1/1000 pregnancies and accounts for 10–20% cases of neonatal thrombocytopenia.

Clinical features

- Commonly presents in first born infant and recurs in 85–90%.
- Maternal platelet count ↔ with no past history of ITP.
- Bleeding manifestations in 10–20% – most severe within the first few days of life eg umbilical haemorrhage, petechiae, ecchymosis, internal haemorrhage, intracranial haemorrhage (ICH).
- Baby's platelet count ↑ to normal over the next 2–3 weeks as the antibody is cleared.
- Haemorrhage *in utero* with fatal ICH in ~1% cases (neurological symptoms suggest this diagnosis).

Laboratory diagnosis

Neonatal	Maternal
Severe thrombocytopenia	Platelet count normal
platelets <20 × 10^9/l in 50%	Serology
platelets >50 × 10^9/l in only	mother's platelets usually HPA-1a −ve
~10% affected neonates	rarer Ab include anti-HPA-3a, HPA-5b, HLA
Platelet serology unhelpful	mother's serum contains anti-platelet antibody
	(note: antibody titre cannot predict degree of
	thrombocytopenia in fetus in subsequent
	pregnancies)
	Establish parental expression of PL antigen

Management

Acute bleeding neonate give platelets −ve for Ag (usually HPA-1a −ve); use random donor platelets in an emergency. Maternal platelets (irradiated) are a good source. Repeat platelet transfusion PRN. IVIg as for ITP can be used in severe cases (response within days). Close observation (ICH is potentially lethal – screen using USS).

Subsequent pregnancies *in utero* at ~24 wk; cordocentesis, take 1–3ml blood for platelet count and phenotype. If affected, treatment needs to be started immediately.

Options

1. *In utero* CMV −ve platelet transfusions at 2–4 wkly intervals (depending on severity and history). Invasive and technically demanding. Keep platelet count >50 × 10^9/l (platelets ↓ rapidly so frequent follow-up mandatory).

2. Maternal administration of IVIg (1g/kg) weekly from ~24 wk onwards
    Check fetal platelet count ~4 wk later and again near term; 75%
    respond – transfuse platelets if non-responsive. Check cord blood at birth
    and treat as necessary.

Outcome

With aggressive treatment the outcome is good, death *in utero* and ICH occur
rarely. A history of a previous ICH correlates with severe thrombocytopenia in
subsequent pregnancies.

Paediatric transfusion – special considerations in newborn

Babies in SCBU are now amongst the most intensively transfused of our hospital patients. Neonates are more susceptible than adults, to the harmful effects of transfusion.

Small volume transfusions
- To replace blood losses of investigative sampling.
- Alleviate anaemia of prematurity.
- Hb estimation alone is an inadequate assessment.
- Hb reduction with symptoms, eg failure to thrive, support need for transfusion.
- Generally, neonatal Hb <10.5g/dl + symptoms – *transfuse*.
- If neonate requiring O_2 support, aim for Hb 13.0g/dl.

Use of small volume transfusion packs 'Pedipacks' (80ml/pack) from same donor recommended since reduces donor exposure, if multiple transfusions required.

Exchange transfusions
- To prevent kernicterus caused by rapidly using bilirubin.
- Most commonly occur in haemolytic disease of the newborn.

Source of blood
Directed donations (including donations from relatives) cannot be regarded as safer than microbiologically screened volunteer donor blood – therefore not recommended.

Pre-transfusion testing
(Within the first 4 months). Maternal and neonatal samples as shown should be taken and tested as follows:

Maternal samples
1. ABO and Rh group.
2. Antibody screen.

Infant samples
3. ABO and Rh group.
4. DAT.
5. Antibody screen (if maternal sample unavailable).

- Provided no atypical antibodies are present in maternal or infant serum and the DAT on the infant's cells is –ve a conventional cross-match is unnecessary.
- Small volume replacement transfusions can be give repeatedly during the first 4 months of life without further serological testing.
- In practice, transfusion centres may specifically designate a supply of low anti-A, B titre group O Rh (D) –ve blood for use in neonatal transfusions.
- After the first 4 months, compatibility testing should conform to requirements for adults.

Blood component therapy

Special considerations for neonates and children

Albumin 4.5%
No risk of transmitting viral infection. Used at delivery to resuscitate neonates.

FFP
Available in aliquots of 50ml. Must be ABO and Rh compatible. Infused via filter. Main indication – DIC. May need cryoprecipitate also (see p433, 556), if evidence of ↓ fibrinogen (<1.0g/l). No need for CMV screening, or irradiation. Dose: 10–15ml/kg. Check PT and APTT. Repeat as necessary.

Platelets
- Thrombocytopenia more hazardous in neonates.
- Prophylactic therapy if count <30 × 10^9/l.
- One dose (one paediatric platelet concentrate) ~50ml 'fresh' plasma, available either from apheresis or buffy coat derived.
- Check increment 1h later if no clinical response.
- Care with volume overload.
- Must be administered within 2h of receipt on ward.

Neonatal alloimmune thrombocytopenia (NAIT)
- Mortality ~14%.
- If fetus at risk, arrange fetal blood sampling.
- If weekly intrauterine transfusions needed give HPA compatible platelets.
- Need to be CMV –ve, and irradiated.

Granulocytes
- Severely infected neonates may develop profound neutropenia.
- Usually respond to antibiotic therapy.
- Granulocyte transfusions very rarely given.
- Risk of CMV and toxoplasmosis.
- Donor must be antibody negative for these viruses.
- Products must be IRRADIATED.

Note: Evidence is mounting to support use of routine leucodepletion of cellular components, to reduce post-transfusion CMV infection.

Presentation of red cell products

Small volume transfusions
- QUAD packs (SAGM blood).
- Ensure 4 transfusions possible from a single donor.
- ↓ donor exposure in infant needing multiple transfusions.

Exchange transfusions

Age of blood
- Plasma-reduced red cells (Hct 0.50–0.60).
- For small volume transfusions, does not matter. For exchange transfusions – ideally within 5d of collection. (K⁺ levels rise in older blood).

Rate and volume
- Transfusion should not >5h/unit due to risk of bacterial proliferation.
- Volumes of 5ml/kg/h safe.

Special hazards
Main 2 concerns:

GvHD	In congenitally immunodeficient neonates immunocompetent donor T lymphocytes can cause GvHD – rare. Need to irradiate all blood products in these children. Also if first degree relatives used as donors.
CMV infection	Particular risk in low birth weight babies, or immunocompromised children undergoing transplantation. CMV seronegative donations should be used. Alternatively use filter to leucodeplete and eradicate risk.

Also
- Hypocalcaemia – rare now, due to change of additive.
- Citrate toxicity, also rare nowadays due to improvements in additive.
- Rebound hypoglycaemia, induced by high glucose levels of blood transfusion anticoagulants.
- Thrombocytopenia – dilution, DIC.
- Volume overload.
- Haemolytic transfusion reactions in necrotising enterocolitis. This is usually due to the 'T' antigen on baby's RBCs getting exposed due to bacteria entering the blood from diseased gut. Anti 'T' is present in almost all donor plasma.

Polycythaemia in newborn and childhood

As in adults, polycythaemia may be relative or absolute (see p188). The condition is usually secondary. Primary polycythaemia is very rare in children; benign familial erythrocytosis is a autosomal dominant self-limiting condition of unknown aetiology.

Pathophysiology

As discussed on p366, polycythaemia is physiological in the neonatal period with a raised Hct (range 42–60% in cord blood) persisting in the first few weeks of life. Pathological polycythaemia is defined in the neonate as Hct >65% (Hb >22.0g/dl), is uncommon (<5% of all births) and usually due to hypertransfusion or hypoxia.

Causes of polycythaemia in the newborn

- Relative – dehydration, reduced plasma volume.
- Hypertransfusion – delayed cord clamping, maternofetal, twin to twin.
- Hypoxia – placental insufficiency, intrauterine growth retardation.
- Endocrine – congenital adrenal hyperplasia, thyrotoxicosis.
- Maternal disease – toxaemia of pregnancy, DM, heart disease, drugs eg propranolol.
- Miscellaneous – chromosomal abnormalities eg Down's syndrome.

Clinical features

Hyperviscosity may give rise to vomiting, poor feeding, hypotonia, hypoglycaemia, lethargy, irritability and tremulousness. On examination – plethora, cyanosis, jaundice, hepatomegaly. Complications include intracranial haemorrhage, respiratory distress, cardiac failure, necrotising enterocolitis and neonatal thrombosis.

Diagnosis

- Clinical presentation may suggest the diagnosis eg anaemic twin.
- FBC (free flowing venous sample) ↑ neonatal Hct >65%, blood film.
- Hypoglycaemia, hypocalcaemia, unconjugated hyperbilirubinaemia.
- Hb EP ?maternal haemorrhage.
- Radiology; CXR shows ↑ vascularity, infiltrates, cardiomegaly.

Management

- Supportive – IV fluids, close observation for complications.
- Exchange transfusion – partial with FFP/albumin to ↓ Hct<60%.

Vol of exchange (ml) = $\dfrac{\text{Blood vol} \times (\text{observed} - \text{desired Hct})}{\text{observed Hct}}$

Treatment

As required for associated abnormalities.

Outcome

Provided the condition is identified early and appropriate measures taken to reduce the hyperviscosity, the outcome should be good.

Congenital dyserythropoietic anaemias

Group of dyserythropoietic anaemias with several defining abnormalities of unknown etiology. No chromosomal defect is identified and inheritance may be recessive (types I and II) or dominant (type III).

Pathophysiology

Ineffective erythropoiesis (cell death within the BM); RBC survival in PB is not much reduced (III). Abnormal serological and haemolytic characteristics (type II CDA) and membrane abnormalities are described but as yet no defining shared defect.

Type	Bone marrow	Blood findings
I	Megaloblastic intranuclear chromatin bridges	Macrocytic RBC
II	Bi/multinuclearity with pluripolar mitosis	Normocytic RBCs +ve acidified serum (HEMPAS)
III	Giant multinuclearity	Macrocytic

Clinical features

- Age of presentation variable; but usually in older children (>10 yrs).
- Anaemia – in Type I, Hb 8.0–12.0g/dl; Type II (~⅔ CDA) anaemia is more severe, patient often transfusion dependent. Type III (rare) anaemia is mild/moderate.
- Jaundice (2° to intramedullary RBC destruction).
- Gallstones.
- Splenomegaly common.

Laboratory diagnosis

- Peripheral blood – normocytic/macrocytic RBC with anisopoikilocytosis.
- WBC and platelets usually ↔, reticulocytes ↑.
- BM appearance – striking, showing ↑ cellularity.
- Type II known as Hereditary Erythroblastic Multinuclearity with a Positive Acidified Serum (HEMPAS) due to IgM which binds complement.
- Serum Fe ↑ due to ↑ absorption; haemosiderosis occurs.

Differential diagnosis

- CDA variants – not all CDA falls neatly into 3 subtypes on BM findings, serology or clinical features.
- PNH – PAS test is +ve with PNH *and* control serum. In HEMPAS +ve with patient serum.
- Other dyserythropoietic anaemias – eg vitamin B_{12} and folate deficiency.
- Primary/acquired sideroblastic anaemia.

Treatment

Avoid blood transfusion if possible (iron overload) – iron chelation as necessary. Splenectomy not curative but may decrease transfusion requirements. BMT reserved for severe cases. Rare response to vitamin E therapy in Type II CDA.

Natural history

Severity of CDA varies considerably and patient may have good quality of life. Haemosiderosis is a long-term complication which may impact on survival.

Brit J Haem 1997 **98** 785

Red cell aplasia in childhood

Isolated failure of erythropoiesis. Congenital or acquired. Diamond and colleagues described congenital red cell aplasia, the Diamond-Blackfan anaemia (DBA) over 50 years ago. Although rare, the condition needs to be considered in the differential diagnosis of erythroblastopenic anaemia in children.

Pathophysiology of DBA

Hereditary with both autosomal dominant and recessive inheritance. Nature of underlying defect not known. No defining chromosomal abnormality described despite multiple associated developmental abnormalities. Anaemia likely to be due to intrinsic RBC progenitor cell defect rather than one of the micro-environment. ↓ sensitivity of these cells to EPO and other cytokines described.

Clinical features

- Presents in the first year of life: in ⅓ at birth and 90% <6 months of age.
- Developmental abnormalities – low birth weight, abnormal facies with abnormal eyes, webbed neck, malformed thumbs, other skeletal abnormalities, short stature, congenital heart lesions, renal defects in >50% patients.
- Anaemia usually severe and child may be transfusion dependent.
- Susceptibility to infection is not ↑.
- Hepatosplenomegaly absent.
- Family history is +ve in only 10–20% cases.

Laboratory diagnosis

- Hb ↓, reticulocytes ↓, MCV ↑, WBC and platelets are not ↓ (may be ↑).
- Red cells – normal morphology, have ↑ i antigen positivity, ↑ ADA activity.
- HbF ↑, Epo ↑, serum Fe/ferritin ↑.
- BM findings – usually absent erythroid precursors; other cell lines normal.
- Radiological investigation to define other congenital defects.

Differential diagnosis

Distinguish other acquired causes of RBC hypo/aplasia ie:

- Transient erythroblastopenia of childhood (see p372).
  PB and BM findings similar; later presentation, transient, no other defects.
- Drugs, malnutrition, infection.
- Other haemolytic anaemias in hypoplastic phase – with parvovirus B19, delayed recovery in HDN.
- Megaloblastic anaemia in aplastic phase.

Treatment

- Prednisolone 2mg/kg PO in divided doses, slowly ↓ over weeks; ⅔ do well and need low-dose maintenance; ~10% need high dose maintenance; ~30% failure (try high dose methylprednisolone).
- Transfusion dependency (chelation to prevent iron overload). Use CMV –ve leucocyte-depleted packed RBC.
- Splenectomy not helpful (unless hypersplenism).

Natural history

Spontaneous remission in 20% (may last years). Death due to haemosiderosis, complications of steroid therapy, blood transfusion (the rare haematological malignancy is significant). New approaches to treatment including BMT offer better outlook than in the past where median survival was only 31 years. DBA Registry established in 1993 is prospectively gathering new data.

Brit J Haem 1996 **94** 645

Fanconi's anaemia

Characterised by bone marrow failure affecting all 3 cell lines (RBC, WBC and megakaryocytes) and manifest by peripheral blood pancytopenia. As in adults the condition in children is usually acquired and the causes do not differ significantly see p118. The inherited variety—*Fanconi's anaemia*—usually presents in children and will need to be differentiated from other congenital syndromes affecting the bone marrow.

Pathophysiology of Fanconi's anaemia.

Fanconi's anaemia affects cells of the body other than the bone marrow and defects of the cutaneous, musculoskeletal and urogenital systems are reported in ²⁄₃ patients. Striking chromosomal fragility induced chemically in peripheral blood lymphocytes is diagnostic and is associated with defective stem renewal and impaired DNA repair. Delayed presentation (10% present in adult life) and links with chemicals and viral infection suggest that while genetic factors predispose to the condition, other trigger factors lead to the bone marrow failure. The mutation in a FA subtype has been cloned but the biochemical nature of the condition is still unknown.

Clinical features

- Autosomal recessive inheritance—in 10–20% the parents are related.
- Phenotypic expression of the disease varies widely ranging from:
  – aplastic anaemia in a 'normal' individual in adult life to
  – poor growth at birth, multiple congenital defects ± anaemia.
- Aplastic anaemia is often only diagnosed in later childhood (8–9 years).
- Hyperpigmentation, in ¾ with café-au lait spots.
- Congenital abnormalities can affect almost any system—skeletal defects common, >50% in the upper limb especially thumb, abnormal facies.
- Microcephaly ~40% and mental retardation occur.

Diagnosis

Laboratory findings

- Pancytopenia and an empty bone marrow are defining features.
- Bone marrow may be hypoplastic, dyserythropoietic/megaloblastic.
- Anaemia varies in its severity and may be macrocytic (MCV 100–120 fl)
- Chromosomal breaks/rearrangements in cell culture—usually lymphocytes – on stress (mitomycin C/diepoxybutane) are the defining abnormalities, and can be used for antenatal diagnosis.
- Further investigation for systemic congenital abnormalities is indicated.

Differential diagnosis

- Acquired aplastic anaemia (see p118).
- Other congenital conditions with similarities to Fanconi's anaemia.
- Amegakaryocytic thrombocytopenia with absent radii (TAR syndrome) usually diagnosed at birth; no hyperpigmentation; thrombocytopenia but not pancytopenia. Bone marrow lacks megakaryocytes; has adequate WBC/RBC precursors. No chromosomal breaks in cell culture. Better prognosis.
- Dyskeratosis congenita—clinical triad of skin pigmentation, leukoplakia of the mucous membranes, dystrophic nails and in ½ patients severe pancytopenia. Usually sex-linked inheritance ♂ >> ♀. Other congenital and immunological abnormalities described. Bone marrow is hypo/aplastic; chromosome breaks sometimes seen. Premalignant. BMT can be curative.

- Bloom's syndrome – clinically like Fanconi's anaemia with similar congenital defects, chromosomal breaks and a predisposition to leukaemia. Blood picture – no pancytopenia, no bone marrow hypoplasia.
- Shwachman-Diamond syndrome – congenital pancreatic insufficiency; chronic diarrhoea and growth failure, infection. Bone marrow failure not usually trilineage. Isolated neutropenia > thrombocytopenia and anaemia. Bone marrow varies – may be dysplastic/hypo/aplastic. Exclude cystic fibrosis (by normal sweat test).

Treatment

General

Supportive – blood transfusion with iron chelation as required. Treatment of congenital anomalies where possible.

Specific

Combined therapy with steroids (moderate dosage alternate days) and androgens (oxymethalone 2–5mg/kg/d). Most patients respond to treatment but long-term therapy is needed. BMT is indicated for severe non-responsive aplasia.

Outcome

Median survival of treatment responders is ~20 yrs. Unless a BMT is possible, non-responders will have a reduced lifespan (median survival 12 yrs). Leukaemic/malignant transformation occurs in ~1 in 12, usually before age 16.

371

Transient erythroblastopenia of childhood (TEC)

Pathogenesis
Serum and cellular inhibitors of erythropoiesis and defective bone marrow response to stimulating cytokines have been demonstrated. The condition may be idiopathic or secondary to identified factors such as drugs, viral or bacterial infection, malnutrition, or as a complication of a pre-existing congenital haemolytic anaemia. It is not uncommon.

Clinical features
- Boys and girls equally affected: age range 6 months to 4 years.
- Typically a previously well young child presents with symptoms and signs of anaemia often following an infection. Onset is insidious and the child becomes non-specifically unwell.
- Precipitating infections are usually viral (EBV, Parvovirus B19, mumps and others) but may be bacterial, preceding the onset of TEC by some weeks.
- Fever is uncommon; pallor may be striking.
- No lymphadenopathy or hepatosplenomegaly.
- No physical abnormalities.

Laboratory diagnosis
- Normocytic, normochromic anaemia which may be severe (Hb 3.0–8.0g/dl).
- Reticulocytes absent; WBC and platelets usually normal.
- Blood film shows no abnormality.
- Biochemical profile normal.
- BM needed for diagnosis – normocellular picture with absent erythroid precursors. Iron content is normal.
- No karyotypic abnormalities.
- Viral titres may be helpful (see above).
- No other investigation is of diagnostic help.

Differential diagnosis
- Exclude acute blood loss and anaemia of chronic disease.
- Diamond-Blackfan anaemia (see p368). Usually presents within the first 6 months of life and other abnormalities (skeletal malformation, short stature, abnormal facies) are present.
- Look for causes of 2° TEC (drugs, malnutrition, haemolytic anaemia).

Treatment
Blood transfusion should be avoided but may be necessary if symptomatic.

Natural history
Spontaneously remits (if not then it isn't transient) commonly within 4 weeks (may be up to 6 months). Relapse is rare. There are no long-term sequelae or associations.

Paediatric haematology

Haemolytic uraemic syndrome

Characterised by a microangiopathic haemolytic anaemia (MAHA), renal failure and thrombocytopenia. Usually presents in children and is closely related to thrombotic thrombocytopenic purpura (TTP) – a disease of adults.

Pathogenesis

HUS usually occurs in outbreaks (summertime) and in 90% is due to *Escherichia coli* 0157 and other verocytotoxin-producing *E coli*. Food sources of the infection include uncooked/under-cooked meats, hamburgers and poor food hygiene. The verocytotoxin causes endothelial damage, particularly of the renal endothelium, leading to the formation of fibrin-rich microthrombi and MAHA.

Clinical features

- Young children (6months <4 years) are especially prone to the disease.
- Acute onset with a history of preceding diarrhoea/vomiting common.
- Onset of ↓ urine output heralding renal failure occurs days later.
- In ~10% onset is insidious – can be drug (chemotherapy/TBI) induced.
- Other symptoms: anaemia (may be severe), jaundice, bruising, bleeding.
- Neurological symptoms uncommon *cf.* TTP.

Diagnosis

Laboratory findings

- MAHA may be severe.
- Film shows fragmented RBCs/schistocytes/spherocytes.
- Thrombocytopenia common.
- Coagulation tests: PT/APTT – usually normal; fibrinogen and F/XDPs also normal. Reduced large vWF multimers.
- Proteinuria and haematuria.
- Biochemical evidence of renal failure.
- Stool culture may be +ve for *E coli*.

Differential diagnosis

TTP note CNS manifestations; may be spectrum of the same disease, other causes of MAHA see p108.

Complications

- ARF → CRF.
- Microvascular thrombosis and infarction of other organs.

Treatment

- Renal failure – fluid restriction, correct electrolyte imbalance.
- If anuria persists >24h – dialysis as necessary.
- Blood transfusion for anaemia.
- Platelet transfusion rarely needed – may ↑ thrombotic risk.
- Severe persistent disease may require plasmapheresis as for TTP (see p438).
- Specific treatment – none of proven value.

Outcome

Epidemic HUS has a good prognosis, patients usually recover and it rarely recurs. CRF does occur. Insidious onset HUS has a poorer prognosis.

Disorders of leucocytes in children

The main difference between adults and children is the relative and absolute lymphocytosis which continues through the first 4–6 years (see Normal ranges). Alterations in white cell populations are usually acquired with similar causes to those in adults.

Neutrophil disorders

Neutrophilia and neutropenia (see p16) are common; neutrophil dysfunction (see p378) less so.

Neutrophilia

- Physiological (reactive) neutrophilia often present in first 4 days of life.
- Acute infection (bacterial mainly, but also viral, fungal, protozoal, etc).
  In infants/young children the response may be exaggerated resulting in very high white cell counts and 'leukaemoid reaction'. Neutrophils show toxic changes (heavy 'toxic' granulation, vacuolation, Döhle bodies) suggesting the diagnosis.
- Other reactive causes include inflammation, metabolic disorders, haemorrhage, malignancy.
- Drugs – an uncommon cause eg corticosteroids, some poisons eg lead.
- Primary haematological disease eg CML needs to be distinguished from a leukaemoid reaction.

Neutropenia

Usually acquired. Working approach to congenital syndromes is given on p380.

Eosinophilia

See p136.

Basophilia

See p138.

Monocytosis

See p140.

Lymphocytes

Clinicians need to remember that the lymphocyte is the predominant white blood cell in early childhood

Lymphocytosis

- Common finding in acute viral infections in children.
  – Pertussis produces a striking ↑.
- Other causes include infectious mononucleosis, infective hepatitis, CMV, toxoplasmosis.
- Acute infectious lymphocytosis – an uncommon disorder of unknown aetiology, detected often on routine FBC in a child presenting with D & V, URTI, abdominal pain ± fever. Physical examination –ve. Diagnosis rests on a ↑ WBC (40–100 × 10^9/l, predominantly lymphocytes) and exclusion of an infective or malignant disorder. Acute self limiting condition.
- Chronic lymphocytosis; infective causes as seen in adults (TB, Brucellosis, etc).

Lymphopenia

- Lymphocyte count <1 × 10^9/l is common in many infections (viral, TB, etc.).
- Also in HIV and other immunodeficient states eg sex linked agammaglobulinaemia.

Disorders of neutrophil function

Acquired in many clinical situations. Main causes are: postinfective, drugs (steroids, chemotherapy) and systemic disease (malnutrition, diabetes mellitus, rheumatoid arthritis, CRF, sickle cell anaemia) – here the underlying condition will dominate the clinical picture.

Congenital causes rare but several defined syndromes are described particularly in children.

Pathophysiology

Neutrophils produced in BM are released into circulation where they survive for only a few hours. Fundamental role is to kill bacteria. Do this by moving to site of infection drawn there (chemotaxis) by interaction of bacteria with complement and Ig (opsonisation) and engulf them (phagocytosis). Killing is accomplished by H_2O_2 generation, release of lysosomal enzymes, neutrophil degranulation. Several enzyme systems are involved (MPO, cytochrome system, HMP shunt). In the neonate neutrophil function is defective (↓ chemotaxis, phagocytosis, motility) particularly if premature, jaundiced. Killing is normal.

Classification

Disorders of all aspects of neutrophil function are described and there is no consensus as to how best to classify them. All are rare. In several of the best described conditions multiple defects are present.

↓ Chemotaxis	↓ Opsonisation	↓ Killing
Lazy leucocyte syndrome	Complement C_3 deficiency	Chronic granulomatous disease
Hyper IgE syndrome		Chediak-Higashi syndrome ↓
Specific neutrophil granules		MPO deficiency

Clinical features

Lazy leucocyte syndrome Leucocyte adhesion deficiency due to ↓ HMW membrane glycoproteins. Rare. Autosomal recessive. ↑ Recurrent infections often in oral cavity, delayed wound healing. Lab features: ↑ neutrophil count, normal BM, abnormal chemotaxis on Rebuck skin window. Poor prognosis. Treatment – *see below*.

Hyperimmunoglobulin E syndrome Also known as Job's syndrome (see *Old Testament*) because of recurrent staphylococcal abscesses. Autosomal recessive inheritance, particularly red-headed girls. Bacterial/fungal infection, chronic dermatitis. Lab features: ↑ IgE, ↑ eosinophils, +ve Rebuck's window.

Complement deficiency Autosomal recessive inheritance, C_3 deficiency, homozygotes have severe recurrent bacterial infection, particularly encapsulated organisms.

Chronic granulomatous disease (CGD) sex linked ♂:♀ = 7:1; also autosomal incidence 1:750,000 population. Presents in early life but also in adults; carriers asymptomatic. Multiple skin and visceral abscesses, systemic infection (pneumonia, osteitis etc) – bacterial/fungi, lymphadenopathy, hepatosplenomegaly. Lab features: Nitro blue tetrazolium (NBT) test +ve. Outlook grim. Improved by aggressive antibiotic policy and IFN-γ ($50\mu g/m^2$ 3✕/week). Long term prophylaxis.

Chediak-Higashi syndrome Rare, but serious, autosomal recessive disorder. Most will die in childhood. Multiple defects. Partial oculocutaneous albinism, recurrent infection, lymphadenopathy. An accelerated phase occurs in ~85% with lymphocytic infiltration of liver/spleen/nodes/BM, pancytopenia and death. Lab findings: ↓ Hb, ↓ neutrophil count, ↓ platelet count. Characteristic giant greenish grey refractile granules in neutrophils (also lymph inclusions). High dose ascorbic acid IFN-γ tried with varying success.

Myeloperoxidase deficiency Autosomal recessive. Commonest of neutrophil dysfunction conditions (1:2000). Often asymptomatic. Manifest in diabetics. Lab findings: ↓ neutrophil/monocyte peroxidase on histochemical analysis. Good prognosis. Exclude acquired causes (lead poisoning, MDS, AML).

Treatment–basic principles of management
1. Appropriate early antibiotics.
2. Prophylaxis–antibacterial and fungal.
3. G-CSF rarely helpful.
4. BMT offers only good chance of cure in severe disorders.

Outlook
Congenital syndromes are rare and diagnosis of the specific defect difficult. Few haematological/immunological labs are set up to perform the required range of tests. Specialist referral for diagnosis and treatment is indicated and may be able to alter the otherwise grim prognosis in many of these conditions.

Neutropenia in childhood

Neutropenia is common FBC abnormality and may have profound clinical implications with predisposition to infection particularly when neutrophils <0.5 × 10⁹/l. Paradoxically, infection can *cause* neutropenia, particularly in young children.

Pathophysiology

As in adults is more often acquired, has similar causes and is usually 2° to underlying disease – or is idiopathic, immune, or drug-induced. Acquired neutropenia will not be discussed here (see p16). Congenital causes of neutropenia are rare and present in children > adults. Documentation of a previously normal neutrophil count is helpful in distinguishing congenital from acquired causes. Congenital neutropenia is classified on the basis of abnormal or normal phenotype.

Normal phenotype	Abnormal phenotype
Infantile agranulocytosis	Shwachman-Diamond syndrome
Severe congenital neutropenia	Dyskeratosis congenita
Reticular dysgenesis	Cartilage-hair syndrome
Chronic benign neutropenia	Fanconi's anaemia
Cyclic neutropenia	Osteoporosis

Clinical features

All are rare and only a brief outline is provided.

Infantile agranulocytosis (Kostmann's syndrome) Autosomal recessive, presents soon after birth with severe infection (often fatal). Neutrophil count < 0.2 × 10⁹/l. Severe congenital neutropenia occurs with agamma- or dysglobulinaemia.

Reticular dysgenesis Thymic aplasia with ↓ lymphocytes and neutrophils. Presents early in life. Often fatal.

Cyclic neutropenia ~21d cycle lasting 3–6d. Children > adults. Episodes of fever, malaise, mucous membrane ulcers, lymphadenopathy. Improves after puberty. Familial in ⅓.

Chronic benign neutropenia May have autosomal dominant or autosomal recessive family history. Variable severity, often mild with localised infections eg skin. Neutrophils ↓, monocytes ↑.

Osteoporosis, Gaucher's/Niemann-Pick disease – rare causes of neutropenia.

Metabolic disorders May present in the neonatal period with failure to thrive, repeated infections, ↓ neutrophils eg orotic aciduria; megaloblastic BM.

Shwachman-Diamond syndrome Rare autosomal recessive condition characterised by metaphyseal chondroplasia (short stature, hip dysplasia) pancreatic insufficiency with diarrhoea, failure to thrive, intermittent neutropenia and recurrent infection. Diagnosis: ↑ faecal fat, ↓ pancreatic function. Normal sweat test, ↓ neutrophil motility, BM shows ↓ mature myeloid cells.

Dyskeratosis congenita May be sex linked, with pigmented skin, abnormal nails. Neutropenia/pancytopenia and recurrent infections.

Paediatric haematology

Fanconi's anaemia see p370.

Diagnosis/differential diagnosis

Often difficult. Exclude acquired causes. Specific clinical features of congenital syndromes can be diagnostic. Note FBC. Repeat at intervals ?persistent ?cyclical. BM findings eg ↓ mature myeloid cells/maturation arrest are present to a varying degree in all. Non-specific. Cytogenetics rarely helpful except in Fanconi's anaemia.

Treatment

General principles of management common to all. Prevention with good hygiene and care of skin and mucous membranes. Establish bacterial sensitivity and treat infections appropriately. Antibiotic prophylaxis. G-CSF in severe congenital neutropenia (start dose 5μg/kg). BMT may be only chance of survival in some severe congenital conditions. Specific treatment if available eg pancreatic enzymes for Schwachman-Diamond syndrome.

Outcome

Severity of neutropenia is fundamental prognostic finding and will determine the outcome in many of the conditions listed above.

Malignant paediatric haematology: special considerations

Epidemiology

1 in 600 children develops cancer before the age of 15. Annual incidence 1:10,000 ≡ 1200 new cases/year in UK. Pattern of childhood cancers is very different to that seen in adults: carcinomas are rarely seen.

- Leukaemia (~⅓ malignancies): >75% acute lymphoblastic leukaemia, the remainder mainly AML. Chronic leukaemias are rarely seen in childhood.
- Brain tumours are commonest solid malignancy, ~20–25% of cases.
- Embryonal tumours (~15%) seen almost exclusively in children. Include neuroblastoma, nephroblastoma (Wilms' tumour), rhabdomyosarcoma, hepatoblastoma and retinoblastoma.
- Bone tumours – 5% osteosarcoma, Ewing's sarcoma.
- Lymphomas (11% – NHL and Hodgkin's disease).
- Remainder of cases are mainly germ cell and gonadal tumours.

Overall, childhood cancer is more common in boys than girls. Little is known about its aetiology. Although a few cases are attributable to high dose radiation, there is no convincing link to levels of background radiation or electromagnetic fields. Viral infection may contribute to some cases.

Presentation

- Symptoms of BM infiltration: anaemia, bruising, bleeding, bone pain or recurrent infections.
- Other symptoms: pain, swelling, lymphadenopathy.
- Bone pain always a worrying symptom in childhood and should be taken seriously. May be localised and associated with swelling, cause a limp or scoliosis, or generalised reflecting BM involvement.
- Cervical lymphadenopathy usually due to non-malignant causes. Large, non-tender, rubbery/hard fixed nodes, nodes at multiple or atypical sites (supra-clavicular fossae, axillae) more likely to be malignant.

Investigations

Haematological

- FBC & film.
  Leukaemia usually reflected in the blood count: raised or reduced WCC, ± thrombocytopenia & anaemia. Blasts often present. In a small percentage, blood count entirely normal. With other malignancies there may be a low grade anaemia, or no abnormalities at all.
- Coagulation screen.
- BM aspirate & trephine (latter if sample aparticulate), generally needed to confirm diagnosis of leukaemia. In children generally done under GA. Both aspirate & trephine needed in the investigation of marrow involvement with other malignancies, several sites may need to be assessed.

Biochemical

- Full biochemical profile.
- LDH non-specific marker for malignancy.
- Urinary catecholamines for neuroblastoma (easy test to do in unexplained bone pain).
- Tumour markers: αFP, βHCG in hepatoblastoma or germ cell tumours.

Radiological
- CXR for mediastinal mass (mandatory pre-anaesthetic).
- Abdominal USS.
- CT/MRI scan of primary lesion. CT better for showing bony destruction, MRI ideal with soft tissue swellings. CT chest/abdomen may be required for staging. In young children sedation/general anaesthetic usually needed for CT/MRI scans, keep infants still with a feed and appropriate swaddling.

Biopsy
Most solid masses need adequate biopsy for diagnosis under general anaesthetic. Later definitive surgery may be required. Cytogenetics needed in many cases: fresh samples required.

Treatment
- Modalities of treatment are chemotherapy, surgery and radiotherapy.
- Most types of cancer in childhood are chemosensitive: this is mainstay of treatment.
- Multiple agents used to reduce the development of resistance, and side effects on any one organ.
- Most children prefer to have a central line via which chemotherapy can be given and blood tests taken.

A relatively small percentage will need radiotherapy in addition to other treatment. Has major effect on growing tissues. Cranial irradiation avoided in children under 2–3 years due to side effects on the developing brain. Surgery usually required for solid tumours: generally following chemotherapy to reduce tumour bulk to avoid mutilating surgery.

383

Children with suspected malignancy should be referred to a specialist centre for investigation and initial treatment. Thereafter, shared care may be carried out nearer to home at a local hospital. Most children across the country receive treatment as part of a national trial or protocol. This has been happening in increasing numbers since the formation of the UKCCSG (United Kingdom Children's Cancer Study Group) in 1977 and is one of the reasons for the improved outlook for childhood cancers. Overall survival is ~60%.

Long term effects
Estimated 1:900 adults will be the survivors of childhood cancer. Many centres now run long term follow-up clinics. Areas covered include monitoring growth, fertility, side-effects from drugs (eg potential cardiotoxicity) and general well-being. There is a risk of second malignancy developing which varies according to both the primary diagnosis and treatment used.

Aetiology of acute leukaemia

- Congenital syndromes predisposing to acute leukaemia are rare apart from Down's syndrome.
- Most patients with leukaemia do not have apparent predisposing condition.
- Genetic aberrations that cause increased cell proliferation, decreased differentiation or prevent apoptosis may play role in development of acute leukaemia.
- Likely that leukaemia develops as a result of accumulation of a number of somatic mutations in progenitor cells.
- Chromosome translocations may cause gene overexpression or formation of novel fusion gene and point mutations may cause gene activation or inactivation.
- Many translocations associated with leukaemia cause rearrangement of proteins that code for transcriptional regulating factors.

Acute lymphoblastic leukaemia

Aneuploidy as a result of chromosome gains (hyperdiploidy) or losses (hypodiploidy) is frequent in ALL. May be due to frequent recombination events necessary for the generation of idiotype diversity in lymphoid progenitors at Ig and T cell receptor loci. Gene overexpression as a result of chromosome translocation is common in ALL.

Commonly found translocations in ALL

- t(12;21) in ~25% childhood and 3% of adult ALL. Causes fusion of TEL transcription factor to the AML1 transcription factor. Presence of translocation is associated with favourable outcome in children. Other TEL gene on the unrearranged chromosome 12 is almost invariably deleted.

- t(8;14) occurs in 2–5% of childhood ALL. Causes juxtaposition of MYC with the Ig heavy chain locus → aberrant expression of MYC in L3 ALL cells.
- t(9;22) occurs in 4% of childhood and ≤20% of adult ALLs. Produces the Philadelphia chromosome with fusion of the BCR gene (chromosome 22) to the ABL gene (chromosome 9) and production of an aberrant fusion protein (p190) with enhanced tyrosine kinase activity and a potent transforming protein; the translocation is associated with poor prognosis.
- t(1;19) occurs in 5% of childhood ALLs; it produces a fusion protein from the E2A and PBX1 genes which dysregulates transcription and is leukaemogenic in mice.
- t(11;v) occurs in 3% children and 25% infants with ALL. Involves rearrangements of the MLL gene with a range of fusion partners producing an aberrant transcription factor.

Acute myeloblastic (myeloid) leukaemia

Chromosomal anomalies occur frequently in *de novo* AML in children and young adults. Differ from the anomalies found in AML in the elderly, AML 2° to MDS and AML 2° to cancer chemotherapy where anomalies seen in MDS are frequent (−5, del(5q), −7, del(7q), +8 and other complex abnormalities). Two most frequently encountered anomalies in AML, t(8;21) and inv(16) account for ~30% of the karyotypic abnormalities found in AML and result in the disruption of a single transcription factor complex: *AML1–CBFβ*.

The most frequent anomalies found in de novo AML include

- **t(15;17)** in 100% of patients with retinoic acid responsive acute promyelocytic leukaemia (FAB M3). Involves *PML* gene on chromosome 15 and the *RARα* gene on 17 producing two fusion genes; the RARα protein is a transcription factor and the der(15) *RARα/PML* product appears critical to leukaemogenesis.

- **t(8;21)** – up to 15% cases of AML (mainly FAB M1/M2). Involves *AML1* gene on chromosome 21 and *ETO* gene on 8 producing novel chimeric *AML1/ETO* gene. Fusion product may induce transformation through interaction with genes normally regulated by AML1.

- **inv(16)** occurs in 15% of AML. Associated with FAB type M4Eo. Results in rearrangement of *CBFβ* gene into a myosin heavy chain gene producing a *CBFβ/MYH11* chimeric gene; the normal CBFβ product interacts with the AML1 protein to increase its binding affinity to DNA; the abnormal fusion product may transform the cell through altered activity on target genes normally regulated by AML1.

MDS in childhood

A juvenile myelodysplastic syndrome occurs in association with monosomy 7. Occurs most frequently in males, has median age <1 year and is associated with hepatosplenomegaly and facial rash. A number of cases have occurred in siblings. Blood and bone marrow appearances are those of RAEB or CMML. A high proportion develop AML within 2 years.

MDS may occur in children in the absence of monosomy 7 – usually takes the form of RAEB or RAEB-t. Other forms of sideroblastic anaemia and megaloblastic anaemia are important differential diagnoses. Most patients present with anaemia and or thrombocytopenia and a rapidly progressive course is common. RAEB and RAEB-t have high rate of progression to AML which, as in adults, is often poorly responsive to therapy. BMT is the treatment of choice in these cases.

385

Genetic conditions predisposing to childhood AML

- Down's syndrome.
- Fanconi syndrome (see p370).
- Bloom syndrome.
- Ataxia-telangiectasia (see p324).
- Kostmann's syndrome.
- Diamond-Blackfan syndrome (see p368).
- Shwachman-Diamond syndrome.
- Klinefelter syndrome.
- Turner syndrome.
- Neurofibromastosis.
- Incontinentia pigmenti.

Down's syndrome – risk of developing acute leukaemia is increased 20–30×. Usually AML (esp. megakaryoblastic AML – M7) or common pre-B ALL. Response to therapy of patients with Down's syndrome and AML is better than average.

A transient myeloproliferative disorder associated with leucocytosis and blasts in the peripheral blood may occur in the neonatal period in up to ⅓ infants with

Down' syndrome. Also occurs in trisomy 21 mosaicism. May be associated with hepatosplenomegaly and skin infiltration. Blasts have morphology and phenotype of megakaryoblastic AML and chromosomal abnormalities may be found in BM. Progressive marrow failure does not develop and blasts disappear after variable period. No treatment necessary. Some of these children subsequently develop true AML.

Bloom's syndrome – rare, characterised by failure to thrive, telangiectatic facial erythema, molar hypoplasia, short stature and predisposition to leukaemia. Associated with chromosomal instability and structural chromosomal abnormalities including chromatid exchanges and breaks and endoreduplication occur prior to development of frank leukaemia – may be ALL or AML.

Kostmann's syndrome – autosomal recessive, associated with severe neutropenia (<0.2 × 10⁹/l), frequently accompanied by monocytosis and eosinophilia. Severe infection often begins soon after birth. BM seldom shows myeloid maturation beyond the monocyte stage. Leukaemic transformation may occur in those patients who do not succumb to severe infection. BMT and G-CSF may be helpful.

Schwachmann syndrome – constitutional BM disorder (probably autosomal recessive) frequently presents with neutropenia and predisposition to infection. Malabsorption due to exocrine pancreatic insufficiency, growth retardation and metaphyseal dyschondroplasia occur. BM hypoplasia, thrombocytopenia, anaemia and ↑ HbF are features. Some present as aplastic anaemia, others develop MDS, AML or ALL. Most survive to adulthood.

Klinefelter's syndrome – increased incidence of congenital leukaemia and both childhood AML and ALL in individuals with Klinefelter's syndrome.

Indications for BMT in childhood ALL

First CR – high risk patients only

Matched sibling donor BMT

- Ph, t(9;22), +ve.
- Infantile ALL with MLL gene rearrangement.
- Near haploid karyotype.

Matched sibling donor BMT or unrelated donor BMT

- Failure to remit by day 28 of therapy.
- High hazard score.
- True biphenotypic leukaemia defined by morphology, markers, cytogenetics.

Second CR

Bone marrow relapse

- Early relapse (CR1<2.5 years) – unrelated donor BMT or matched sibling donor BMT.
- Intermediate relapse (CR1 2.5–4 yrs) – matched sibling donor BMT, unrelated donor BMT or conventional chemotherapy.
- Late relapse (CR1>4 years) – matched sibling donor BMT or conventional chemotherapy.

Isolated CNS relapse

- Early relapse (CR1<2.5 years) after previous CNS DXT or with a high hazard score – matched sibling donor BMT, unrelated donor BMT or conventional chemotherapy with local DXT.
- Intermediate relapse (CR1 2.5–4 years) after previous CNS DXT – matched sibling donor BMT or conventional chemotherapy with local DXT.

Isolated testicular relapse

- Early relapse (CR1<2.5 years) – matched sibling donor BMT or unrelated donor BMT.

Modified from 1997 recommendations of UKCCSG BMT group

Indications for BMT in childhood

Disease	Status	Matched SIB	Unrelated	Autograft
• Acute myeloid leukaemia	CR1	R[a]	NR	NR
	CR2	R	CRP	R, if CR1>1yr
	Relapse/refractory	D	D	NR
• Acute lymphoblastic leukaemia	High risk CR1	R	R	NR
	CR2	R	R	CRP
• Chronic myeloid leukaemia	Chronic phase	R	R	CRP
	Advanced phase	R	R	CRP
	Blast crisis	D	NR	NR
• Non-Hodgkin's lymphoma	see ALL			
• Hodgkin's disease	CR1	NR	NR	CRP
	1st rel/CR2/CR3	CRP	D	R
	Refractory	NR	NR	D
• Myelodysplasia	JCML/CMML[b]	R	R	NR
	RA[c]/RARS/IMo7	R	CRP	NR
	RAEBt/sAML[d]	R	CRP	NR

Disease	Status	Matched SIB	Unrelated	Autograft
• Immunodeficiency & inborn errors		R	R	–
• Thalassaemia		R	NR	–
• Sickle cell disease		R	NR	–
• Aplastic anaemia & inherited monocytopenia		R	CRP	–
Solid tumours				
• Neuroblastoma	Stage IV	NR	NR	R
• Brain tumour		NR	NR	CRP
• Ewing's sarcoma	High risk	NR	NR	CRP
• Rhabdomyosarcoma		NR	NR	CRP
• Wilm's tumour	Relapsed/refractory	NR	NR	CRP

CR1, CR2 = first and second complete remissions, respectively; 1st rel = first relapse; – = not performed; R = in routine use for selected patients; CRP = to be undertaken in approved Clinical Research Protocols; D = developmental or pilot studies can be approved in specialist units; NR = not generally recommended; a = not t(15;17), t(8;21); inv 16; Down's syndrome; b = if indicated by disease pace; c = if cytogenetics abnormal or blood product dependent; d = RAEBt, AML eligible for AML12 study, except Down's syndrome where BMT unnecessary.

Modified from 1997 recommendations of UKCCSG BMT group

Lymphoma in childhood

Lymphoid neoplasms are the third most common malignancy of childhood. ~60% are NHL and remainder are Hodgkin's disease. In both diseases twice as many boys as girls are affected.

Hodgkin's disease
Uncommon <5 years; incidence increases during the early teenage years.

Stage I
- Radiotherapy.
  Note: TFTs if thyroid irradiated. Muscle wasting may be a problem.

Stage II–IV
- ChlVPP.
  Remember risk of 2° malignancy; male sterility.
- ABVD if unsatisfactory response to ChlVPP.
  Side feffects: cardiotoxicity, lung damage, potentiated by DXT if given in addition.

Non-Hodgkin's lymphoma
- Even age distribution throughout childhood.
- Prognosis of children with NHL has been less good than those with Hodgkin's disease though multiagent chemotherapy has improved results.
- Different spectrum of histological subtypes in childhood NHL compared to adult NHL: 90% of cases are accounted for by Burkitt's lymphoma, T-cell lymphoblastic lymphoma and diffuse large cell lymphoma.

Burkitt's lymphoma
- Characteristic 'starry sky' histological pattern and FAB L3 morphology.
- Associated with chromosomal translocation involving MYC locus on chromosome 8 with Ig heavy chain gene on 14, or less commonly with a κ or λ light chain gene on 2 or 22 with resultant dysregulation of MYC gene transcription; the MYC product functions as a transcription factor.

T-cell lymphoblastic lymphoma
- Related to T-cell acute lymphoblastic leukaemia.
- Associated with non-random chromosomal translocations involving the T-cell receptor β or α/δ loci with dysregulated expression of reciprocal partner gene including the transcription factors HOX11 (t(10;14)) and TAL1 (t(1;14)) and LIM protein RHOMB2 (t(11;14)).

Large cell lymphoma
- May be either B-cell or T-cell tumours.
- 30% are Ki-1⁺ immunoblastic lymphomas, a proportion of which have t(2;5) producing a NPM/ALK fusion transcript which has tyrosine kinase function.

Investigation and staging
- Childhood NHL tends to disseminate early.
- Careful staging important for choosing correct therapy.
- CXR, CT chest, abdomen and pelvis, FBC, serum chemistry, LP and bilateral bone marrow biopsy are standard investigations at diagnosis.

St Jude staging system for Childhood NHL

Stage I	Single tumour (extranodal or single nodal anatomic area), excluding mediastinum or abdomen

Stage II	Single extranodal tumour with regional node involvement
	≥ 2 nodal areas on the same side of the diaphragm
	2 single extranodal tumours $\pm$ regional node involvement on same side of the diaphragm
	Primary GIT tumour, usually ileocaecal, $\pm$ involvement of associated mesenteric nodes
Stage III	≥ 2 extranodal tumours on opposite sides of the diaphragm
	≥ 2 nodal areas above and below the diaphragm
	Presence of 1° intrathoracic tumour (mediastinal, pleural or thymic)
	Presence of extensive primary intra-abdominal disease
	Presence of paraspinal or epidural tumours, regardless of other sites
Stage IV	Any of the above with initial CNS and/or bone marrow involvement

Treatment

Chemotherapy

- Early trials showed that children with stage I or II disease had an excellent outcome with COMP or LSA2L2 regimens irrespective of histology; children with stage III or IV disease and lymphoblastic lymphoma did better with LSA2L2 whilst those with non-lymphoblastic histology did better with COMP.

Burkitt's lymphoma:

- **Localised disease**
  Fully resected – give 2 courses of chemotherapy only (COPAD).

- **All other disease states**
  Chemotherapy consisting of cyclophosphamide, cytarabine, doxorubicin, vincristine, prednisolone, methotrexate $\pm$ etoposide. Duration 4–8 months depending on exact stage and response to treatment.

- **Large B cell lymphoma**
  May increase in size very rapidly. Patients at risk of tumour lysis syndrome.

393

Lymphoblastic lymphoma: intensive ALL type regimens like LSA2L2 including 10 drugs in induction, consolidation and continuation phases over a period of 2–2½ years; 4 year EFS of up to 73% reported with the German BFM 75/81 protocol.

Large cell lymphoma: Treated as per Burkitt's lymphoma.

Surgery

- Indicated for the complete resection of a localised abdominal primary tumour when possible,

Radiotherapy

- Low-dose involved field DXT indicated for airway or spinal cord compression. Mediastinal DXT for persistent local disease.

Principles & Practice of Paediatric Oncology (2nd edition) Pizzo & Poplack 1993

Neuroblastoma

Accounts for ~8% childhood cancers. Most common extracranial solid tumour in childhood. Usually in the under fives, rare >10 years of age.

Pathophysiology

Arises from primitive neural crest cells, therefore found in adrenals or sympathetic chain. 65% tumours found in abdomen. On microscopy tumour consists of small blue cells, often forming rosettes. Some show a degree of differentiation to ganglioneuroma cells. Usually highly malignant, metastasising to lymph nodes, bone and bone marrow. Capable of spontaneous regression, particularly in infants. 90% associated with raised urinary catecholamines. Characteristic changes to chromosomes 1, 2, 17 (1p del, *N-myc* amplification, 17q gain) associated with more advanced disease and poor outcome.

Clinical presentation

- Symptoms of widespread disease usual eg bone pain, abdominal pain, lethargy, periorbital bruising and proptosis.
- Episodic pallor, sweating and diarrhoea due to catecholamine release – rare.
- Symptoms from primary disease, eg palpable mass, respiratory problems, Horner's syndrome.
- BP may be ↑.
- Infants may have hepatomegaly and bluish skin nodules.

Diagnosis

- Abdominal USS, CXR, CT/MRI scan primary site.
- Bone scan for distant metastases. mIBG scan shows uptake at all disease sites (+ve in 90%).
- Bilateral BM aspirates and trephines; immunohistochemical markers useful eg PGP 9.5.
- Random urinary catecholamines (VMA & HVA; creatinine ratio).
- Biopsy of primary tumour (or liver/skin biopsy in infants).
- Serum ferritin, LDH, NSE, are prognostic factors.
- Cytogenetics of primary tumour and BM aspirate.

Treatment

Dependent on stage.

Localised tumours treated by surgery or chemotherapy if symptomatic and surgery not feasible.

Most are stage IV disease and treated by combination chemotherapy or surgery followed by 'megatherapy' – high dose chemotherapy followed by PBSC rescue. Radiotherapy may be targeted to the tumour using ^{131}mIBG treatment. Currently investigating differentiation therapy and immunotherapy as adjuvant treatment.

Outcome

- Related to age, stage and biology of tumour.
- Localised disease and stage IV-S (infants with small primary tumour, liver & bone marrow but not bone disease): 80–90% survival.
- Most children present with stage IV disease (widespread metastases) with dismal outlook: 10–20% survival if >1 year, 50% if <1 year.
- Megatherapy has prolonged remission but little impact on long term survival.

Principles & Practice of Paediatric Oncology (2nd edition) Pizzo & Poplack 1993

Other tumours that spread to bone marrow

Paediatric solid tumours, other than neuroblastoma, which spread to the bone marrow are rare. Mainly soft tissue sarcomas and Ewing's sarcoma. Histologically they have the appearance of small round blue cell tumours.

Soft tissue sarcomas

Mixed group of tumours arising from muscle, connective, adipose, vascular tissue. Account for 6.5% tumours in childhood.

Rhabdomyosarcoma is the commonest type seen in children. Arises from primitive mesenchymal cells committed to developing into striated muscle. Commonest sites of origin: orbit, parameningeal head and neck, GU tract, extremities. Spreads along fascial planes to surrounding tissue. Incidence 4.3/million children <15 years of age. First peak incidence aged 2–5 years, second in adolescence. 20% present with distant metastases: lung, lymph nodes, bone and bone marrow.

Investigations
- CT/MRI of primary lesion with CT scan chest.
- Bone scan.
- Bone marrow aspirates and trephines looking for metastases.
- Biopsy of primary lesion, and where feasible, involved lymph nodes.

Treatment & prognosis
- Multiagent chemotherapy initially.
- Local treatment to residual disease: either DXT or surgery depending on site.
- Survival overall 50–60%.
- Autografting has been performed in the past for children with metastatic disease, but with little impact on survival.
- High dose single agent chemotherapy with stem cell support is being evaluated in this very poor risk group.
- Other types of soft tissue sarcomas show varying degrees of sensitivity to chemotherapy. Some are eminently treatable with surgery alone, others such as peripheral neurectodermal tumour are highly aggressive and should be investigated and treated as for rhabdomyosarcoma.

Ewing's sarcoma accounts for 40% primary bone tumours in childhood. Annual incidence 0.6 per million. Peak incidence 10–15 years. Rare <5 years or >30 years of age. Tumour usually arises in intramedullary cavity. Consists of small blue cells. Immunochemistry may show presence of neural markers. Typically chromosomal translocation t(11;22).

Usually presents with pain and localised swelling. May be associated fever. >60% cases occur in pelvis, femur, tibia and fibula. Differential diagnoses include osteomyelitis, and in young children, neuroblastoma.

Investigations
- X-ray of affected area shows bony destruction, periosteal elevation and soft tissue swelling.
- CT/MRI scan required of affected lesion to determine tumour volume (risk factor for survival).
- CT scan chest looking for pulmonary secondaries.

- Bone scan and bone marrow aspirates/trephines from 2 different sites for metastatic bone disease.
- Serum LDH is a reflection of tumour bulk.
- In young children urinary catecholamines required to exclude neuroblastoma.
- Biopsy of primary lesion should be performed with regard to later definitive treatment.

Overall 15–35% patients present with metastases at diagnosis: 50% pulmonary, 40% diffuse bone marrow or multiple bone metastases.

Treatment & prognosis

- Generally primary chemotherapy to reduce bulk of disease then local treatment followed by further chemotherapy.
- Local treatment consists of surgery or DXT or both depending on site and bulk of disease and response to initial chemotherapy.
- Event free survival ~65% for patients with non-metastatic disease.
- If metastatic disease prognosis <10% survival.
- Myeloablative chemotherapy with stem cell rescue now being given for cases with early relapse or metastatic disease at presentation.

Paediatric Oncology Clinical Practice and Controversies, Plowman & Pinkerton, Chapman & Hall, 1992

Histiocytosis syndromes

A confused and confusing area of haematology – when is a histiocyte reactive and when malignant? The distinction between malignant and non-malignant histiocytic conditions may be arbitrary. Both can kill and kill quickly. Haemophagocytosis is seen in primary histiocytic conditions but is also a reactive phenomenon secondary to infection. Monocytes have a major role in regulating haemopoiesis, immune and inflammatory responses. Formed in the BM they move into the peripheral blood and from there into the tissues where they become tissue specific histiocytes, either in the mononuclear phagocytic system (MPS) or the tissue based dendritic cell system (DCS). The MPS cells are *antigen processing*, are predominantly phagocytic and include many specific organ cells such as the liver Kupffer cells, bone osteoclasts, pulmonary alveolar macrophages. The DCS consists of Langerhans cells (LC) which are *antigen presenting*. Langerhans cell histiocytosis is a disorder of the DCS.

Pathophysiology

In 1991 a new classification of histiocytic syndromes was set out as shown:

Class I	Langerhans cell histiocytosis
	(previously known as Histiocytosis X)
Class II	Histiocytic haemophagocytic syndromes
	Haemophagocytic Lymphohistiocytosis (HLH)
	Infection associated haemophagocytic syndromes
	Associated with pre-existing malignant conditions
Class III	Malignant histiocytic disorders
	Malignant histiocytosis
	Histiocytic lymphoma/monocytic leukaemias

Clinical features

Histiocytic syndromes of all 3 classes are rare. Infection-associated is the most common but the underlying infection is not always clinically obvious. In the differential diagnosis the other histiocytic syndromes will need to be considered and a working knowledge of them is required.

Class I Langerhans cell histiocytosis (LCH)

Characterised by histological evidence of a cellular locally destructive infiltration with the LC. This a well differentiated large cell (15–25µm) with an indented nucleus, inconspicuous nucleolus; it is not phagocytic. Other reactive cells (granulocytes, eosinophils, histiocytes) are often present. Diagnostic criteria of LC include the presence of Burbeck granules on EM and immunochemical staining with S-100 protein and other markers.

Clinical features

1. Eosinophilic granuloma.
2. Letterer-Siwe disease.
3. Hand-Schuller-Christian disease.

Previously considered separate entities have been grouped together under the term LCH, thus a syndrome in which certain patterns of disease are identified. LCH is a disease mainly of infants and young children, ♂ > ♀; occurring in 1 in 2 million population. Lytic bone lesions occur in over ¾ children particularly of the skull and facial bones. Exophthalmos is a common associated finding. Skin and mucous membranes (40%), pulmonary dysfunction (25%), hepatosplenomegaly (25%), lymphadenopathy (30%), BM disease (30%), and pituitary involvement (20%) are seen.

Systemic symptoms eg fever, weight loss, etc. are common. Staging the disease aids in prognosis.

Stage A   Involvement of bones ± local nodes and adjacent soft tissue involvement.

Stage B   Skin ± mucous membranes involvement, ± related nodes.

Stage C   Soft tissue involvement – not Stage A, B or D.

Stage D   Multisystem disease with combinations of A, B, C.

Diagnosis

- Based on biopsy proven material.
- Skeletal survey to define extent of disease; also bone scan, MRI.
- Urine osmolality studies for diabetes insipidus.
- BM aspirate and biopsy.
- Regular review with the foregoing to monitor disease progress.

Treatment

- Relapsing/remitting nature of the disease makes response to treatment difficult to evaluate.
- Many patients survive without any treatment and indeed appear to be cured.
- Options include steroids, chemotherapy and radiotherapy.
- Local curettage of isolated lesion.
- Indications for chemotherapy include multisystem involvement, organ dysfunction, relapse.
- Radiotherapy considered when progressive/threatening bone involvement.

Outcome

Complex; depends on staging; localised bone involvement – good prognosis. Stage C/D – organ involvement/dysfunction indicates poor prognosis. Long term sequelae include pulmonary/liver fibrosis, diabetes insipidus, growth failure.

Class II Histiocytic haemophagocytic syndromes

Primary

Haemophagocytic lymphohistiocytosis (HLH) is disease of infants and young children (⅔ before age 3 months); when familial is known as FHL (also called familial erythrophagocytic lymphohistiocytosis) because predominantly RBCs destroyed.

Clinical

- Fever >7d.
- Splenomegaly.
- Other features eg nodes, rash, jaundice, CNS disease.

Laboratory features

- Peripheral blood cytopenias (≥2 cell lines), hypertrigliceridaemia, hypofibrinogenaemia.
- Histopathology: histiocyte/lymphocyte infiltration, haemophagocytosis in BM, nodes, spleen.

Treatment and prognosis
Seldom effective – steroids/chemotherapy/ALG/cyclosporin A /BMT.
Usually rapidly fatal.

Secondary
- Underlying viral/bacterial infection.
- Clinical picture is similar to HLH.
- Haematology: blood cell cytopenia (≥2 cell lines).
- BM – often hypocellular with striking haemophagocytosis – usually RBCs.
- Outcome: good prognosis if underlying infection treatable. Also seen in immunocompromised/immunodeficient (congenital or acquired) states where prognosis is poor.

Class III Malignant histiocytosis
Also known as histiocytic medullary reticulocytosis.

Clinical features
Rare condition of adults and children presenting with systemic symptoms eg fever, weight loss, lymphadenopathy, hepatosplenomegaly. In children skin rashes and nodules are common.

Laboratory features
- Blood cytopenias.
- Circulating histiocytes.
- ↑ bilirubin.
- ↑ LDH.
- DAT +ve.
- BM may show infiltrating histiocytics which may be erythrophagocytic/ S-100 +ve as are Langerhans cells-confusing.

Diagnosis
Lymph node histology – exclude Hodgkin's and NHL.

Treatment
Aggressive regimes include cyclophosphamide, adriamycin and vincristine. Survival in children and adults is ~ 40%.

Blood 1994 **84** 2840

Systemic disease in childhood

Haematological manifestations of systemic disease and the underlying mechanisms will be similar in children and adults. The incidence of the disorders will differ, marked ↑ acute infection for example, and certain diseases are only seen in children. The following topics are briefly discussed

- Acute infection/inflammation.
- Anaemia of chronic disease.
- Nutritional anaemia.
- AIDS.
- Poisoning.
- Bone marrow infiltration.

Acute infection and inflammatory disorders

Acute viral and bacterial infection is the commonest cause of secondary anaemia in children. Anaemia is mild/moderate (Hb 9–11g/dl) with an incidence of 15–20% in those <4 years, resolves in 3–4 weeks with treatment of the underlying condition. In ¾ children hospitalised for serious infection/inflammation anaemia, usually normochromic normocytic, is present. Mechanism is complex.

Overt haemolytic anaemia May be due to direct RBC destruction (eg malaria, DIC) cold agglutinins, mechanical, oxidative damage. AIHA is rare, transient with a preceding history of infection in ~60%.

Aplastic anaemia parvovirus B19 infection in children with underlying congenital HA. Recovers in 1–2 weeks, but transfusion may be needed. Transient erythroblastopenia of childhood (see p372).

WBC changes – neutrophilia common finding in infection, even leucoerythroblastic in young children. Also neutropenia (see p16)

Platelets ↑ in acute infections; from ~10% in ambulant children to ~45% with HIB meningitis. Thrombocytopenia also noted (see p310).

Kawasaki disease is an acute multisystem disease of young children. Presents with conjunctivitis, rashes, reddening of the mucous membranes, hands and feet with desquamation and lymphadenopathy. Coronary artery aneurysms develop in ~20%; fatal in 3%. Haematological manifestations include anaemia (normochromic normocytic), neutrophilia, ↑ platelets and aggregation (occasionally ↓ platelets), hypergammaglobulinaemia. Treatment is with aspirin and high dose IVIg.

Anaemia of chronic disease (ACD)

Organ specific disorders are covered elsewhere and will not be discussed further. Chronic renal failure (p44), endocrine disease (p46), GIT disease (p50), liver disease (alcohol not a problem here).

Chronic disorders in children include bacterial infections, cystic fibrosis, collagen disorders. The problems of diagnosis are as follows:

Juvenile rheumatoid arthritis (JRA)

Anaemia present in >½ patients with multisystem disease/multiple joint involvement. As well as ACD, iron deficiency with a ↓ ferritin may also be present (normal ferritin does not exclude iron deficiency), ↑ soluble transferrin receptor level indicates IDA as does absent BM iron. A therapeutic trial of iron is useful (3mg/kg/d for 1 month) then check Hb. If Hb ↓, continue ~3 months.

Nutritional anaemia

Iron deficiency occurs in ~⅓ apparently healthy children (*cf.* adults where main cause is blood loss). Linked to marked growth spurts – the first 2 years of life and again at adolescence. Milk, the staple food in the baby and young child, is a poor source of iron and displaces other richer sources of iron. Ferritin stores are normal in term babies and breast feeding prevents IDA for the first 6 months. Premature infants run out of iron by 2 months of age. Children are notoriously finicky about food; do like carbohydrates (impairs Fe absorption), don't like meat/veg. A sick child may eat very little.

Blood loss may be an aggravating factor – ?cow's milk allergy with exudative enteropathy, also intestinal parasites.

Protein deficiency Kwashiorkor is associated with a moderate normocytic normochromic anaemia; occasional aplastic phase follows a high protein diet.

AIDS

Mainly acquired by vertical transmission. HIV/AIDS is not a common problem in children in the UK (<2% of 15,000 UK cases diagnosed by Dec 1997) but world wide is a significant cause of morbidity. AIDS-defining illnesses in children include multiple serious bacterial infections, lymphocytic interstitial pneumonitis, pulmonary lymphoid hyperplasia. Anaemia is present in most children with AIDS. When severe indicates poor prognosis. Leucopenia; ↓ neutrophils, ↓ lymphocytes.

Poisoning

A serious cause of morbidity/mortality in children, particularly in the young (<5 yrs old). Toxic effects of the poison will usually be dominant. Manifestations include *bleeding* – hepatotoxic drugs eg paracetamol, *haemolytic anaemia* – G6PD deficiency, *methaemoglobinaemia* – aniline dyes, oxidant drugs in the neonate.

Lead poisoning – a significant cause of toxicity in children with long-term neurological dysfunction and developmental defects; ↓ since introduction of lead-free paints and petrol. Lead inhibits haem synthesis leading to ↓ RBC survival and in ~10% a hypochromic microcytic anaemia. Iron deficiency frequently co-exists aggravating the lead toxicity and vice versa.

Bone marrow infiltration

Rare cause of anaemia in children. May be neoplastic, non-neoplastic. Excluding the primary blood disorders (leukaemia and NHL) the main cause of malignant infiltration is neuroblastoma (see p394).
Non-neoplastic conditions include storage disorders (Gaucher's, Neimann-Pick, cystine storage disease) and osteopetrosis.

Comment

A working knowledge of how systemic disease affects the haemopoietic system is fundamental for haematological practice. As important, is an awareness of the multiple effects of drugs on the blood and bone marrow.

Lipid storage diseases

These disorders occur as a result of the inherited absence or inactivity of an enzyme which results in the accumulation of abnormal or excessive intermediate metabolites. Most of these conditions follow an autosomal recessive pattern of inheritance (Fabry's disease and Hunter's syndrome are X-linked recessive). Each disorder has characteristic clinical features which are due to the distribution of the accumulated metabolite. Sites may include the reticuloendothelial system (liver, spleen & bone marrow), CNS, skin, bones and cornea. The clinical features of the patient with suspected lipid storage disease will often suggest the most likely diagnosis. The diagnosis is confirmed by enzyme assay of peripheral blood leucocytes, cultured fibroblasts or biopsy tissue. Enzyme replacement offers the prospect of an improved prognosis in some conditions (eg Gaucher's disease) and allogeneic bone marrow transplantation has been effective in some cases. However neither will reverse neurological damage and must be administered early before permanent cellular, skeletal and neurological damage have developed.

Niemann-Pick disease

Due to the inherited deficiency of sphingomyelinase resulting in accumulation of sphingomyelin which produces characteristic foamy cells in the bone marrow, liver, lymph nodes, kidney and CNS. The only effective therapy is early allogeneic bone marrow transplantation. Three types of Niemann-Pick disease have been defined:

Type A   Acute infantile form with cerebral involvement
- Feeding problems, developmental delay & hepatosplenomegaly at 3–6 months.
- Macular cherry red spot in 50%.
- Vacuolation of peripheral blood lymphocytes; large foamy histiocytes in BM.
- Progressive organomegaly, lymphadenopathy, pulmonary infiltrates, hypotonia & CNS deterioration.
- Death in 2–3 years.

Type B   Chronic visceral form
- Failure to thrive, lymphadenopathy, hepatosplenomegaly in infancy or childhood.
- No CNS involvement.
- No lymphocyte vacuolation – sea blue histiocytes and foamy histiocytes in BM.
- Slow progression to death in early adulthood.

Type C   Niemann-Pick-like conditions
- Clinical phenotype of type A or B Niemann-Pick disease without demonstrable deficiency of sphingomyelinase.
- Variable vacuolation of lymphocytes and marrow histiocytes.

405

Gaucher's disease

Inherited (autosomal recessive) disorder resulting in deficiency of the enzyme glucocerebrosidase (β-glucosidase).

Type 1 disease – glycolipid accumulates in cells of spleen, liver and bone marrow; in types 2 and 3 disease lipid accumulation is in brain cells. High incidence in Ashkenazi Jewish populations. Gene has an incidence of 1 in 40,000 in the general population. Not associated with any form of mental handicap or central nervous system manifestation. May be diagnosed at any time during life depending on severity. Some cases are not identified until adult life. There are ~200 cases of Type 1 Gaucher's in the UK.

Type 2 disease – severe progressive neurological deterioration from birth, usually fatal within 1 year.

Clinical signs and symptoms
- Splenomegaly – moderate to massive.
- Hepatomegaly.
- Skeletal problems – failure of bone remodelling, osteopenia, osteonecrosis, osteosclerosis and bone crises with acute episodes of severe bone pain.

Diagnosis
- Anaemia and thrombocytopenia may be present.
- Bleeding abnormalities (thrombocytopenia or inhibition of clotting factors).
- Abnormalities of liver function.
- BM aspirate and/or biopsy will show Gaucher's cells (histiocytes with eccentric nuclei and layered cytoplasm with a 'tissue paper' appearance; cytoplasmic material stains strongly +ve with PAS. Measurement of leucocyte enzymes shows reduction in β-glucosidase activity).
- Molecular analysis will determine the specific type of Gaucher's mutation.
- Radiology may show the 'Erlenmeyer flask' deformity, bony expansion in the distal femora.

Management
- Mild cases – no active therapy but require periodic follow up as gradual progression may still occur.
- Supportive measures eg splenectomy (if massive splenomegaly) and orthopaedic management of specific bony problems.
- Highly specific enzyme therapy with purified β-glucosidase (Ceredase™, prepared from human placenta) or a recombinant preparation is available for progressive/symptomatic cases where tissue infiltration, skeletal problems and organ malfunction are present.
- Therapy is expensive, annual treatment costs for Ceredase™ are ~£75–100,000/year.
- Severe cases have received allogeneic bone marrow transplantation.

Septic shock/neutropenic fever

▶▶ One of the commonest haemato-oncological emergencies.

- May be defined as the presence of symptoms or signs of infection in a patient with an absolute neutrophil count of $<1.0 \times 10^9$/l. In practice, the neutrophil count is often $<0.1 \times 10^9$/l.
- Similar clinical picture also seen in neutrophil function disorders such as MDS despite normal neutrophil numbers.
- **Beware** – can occur without pyrexia, especially patients on steroids.

Immediate action

▶▶ Urgent clinical assessment.

- Follow ALS guidelines if cardiorespiratory arrest (rare).
- More commonly, clinical picture is more like cardiovascular shock ± respiratory embarrassment viz: tachycardia, hypotension, peripheral vasodilatation and tachypnoea. Occurs with both gram +ve (now more common with indwelling central catheters) and gram –ve organisms (less common but more fulminant).
- Immediate rapid infusion of albumin 4.5% or Gelofusin to restore BP.
- Insert central catheter if not *in situ* and monitor CVP.
- Start O_2 by face mask if pulse oximetry shows saturations <95% (common) and consider arterial blood gas measurement – care with platelet counts $<20 \times 10^9$/l – manual pressure over puncture site for 30 mins.
- Perform full septic screen (see p&p guidelines on IV antibiotics).
- Give the first dose of first line antibiotics immediately e.g ureidopenicillin and loading dose aminoglycoside (ceftazidime or ciprofloxacin if pre-existing renal impairment). Follow established protocols.
- If the event occurs while patient on first line antibiotics, vancomycin/ciprofloxacin or vancomycin/meropenem are suitable alternatives.
- Commence full ITU-type monitoring chart.
- Monitor urine output with urinary catheter if necessary – if renal shutdown has already occurred, give single bolus of IV frusemide. If no response, start renal dose dopamine.
- If BP not restored with colloid despite elevated CVP, consider inotropes.
- If O_2 saturations remain low despite 60% O_2 delivered by rebreathing mask, consider ventilation.
- **Alert ITU giving details of current status.**

Subsequent actions

- Discuss with senior colleague.
- Amend antibiotics according to culture results or to suit likely source if cultures negative (see p464, 466).
- Check aminoglycoside trough levels after loading dose and before second dose as renal impairment may determine reducing or withholding next dose. Consider switch to non-nephrotoxic cover e.g ceftazidime/ciprofloxacin.
- Continue antibiotics for 7–10d minimum and usually until neutrophil recovery.
- If cultures show central line to be source of sepsis, remove immediately if patient not responding.

Transfusion reactions

Rapid temperature spike (>40°C) at start of transfusion indicates transfusion should be stopped (suggests acute intravascular haemolysis).

If slow rising temperature (<40°C), providing patient not acutely unwell, slow IVI. Fever often due to antibodies against WBCs (or to cytokines in platelet packs).

▶ Immediate transfusion reaction

Intravascular haemolysis (→ haemoglobinaemia & haemoglobinuria). Usually due to anti-A or anti-B antibodies (in ABO mismatched transfusion). Symptoms occur in minutes/hours.

Immediate transfusion reaction or bacterial contamination of blood

Symptoms	Signs
Patient restless/agitated	Fever
Flushing	Hypotension
Anxiety	Oozing from wounds or venepuncture sites
Chills	Haemoglobinaemia
Nausea & vomiting	Haemoglobinuria
Pain at venepuncture site	
Abdominal, flank or chest pain	
Diarrhoea	

If predominantly extravascular may only suffer chills/fever 1h after starting transfusion – commonly due to anti-D. Acute renal failure is *not* a feature.

Mechanism

Complement (C3a, C4a, C5a) release into recipient plasma → smooth muscle contraction. May develop DIC (see p422); oliguria (10% cases) due to profound hypotension.

Initial steps in management of acute transfusion reaction

- Stop blood transfusion immediately.
- Replace giving set, keep IV open with 0.9% saline.
- Check patient identity against donor unit.
- Insert urinary catheter and monitor urine output.
- Give fluids (IV colloids) to maintain urine output >1.5ml/kg/h.
- If urine output <1.5ml/kg/h insert CVP line and give fluid challenge.
- If urine output <1.5ml/kg/h and CVP adequate give frusemide 80–120 mg.
- If urine output still <1.5 ml/kg/h consult senior medical staff for advice.
- Contact Blood Transfusion Lab before sending back blood pack and for advice on blood samples required for further investigation.

Complications

Overall mortality ~10%.

413

Immediate-type hypersensitivity reactions

May occur soon (30–90 min) after transfusion of blood/component. Antibody often unknown but in some cases is due to antibody directed against IgA (in recipients who have become sensitised).
- Mild reaction: urticaria, erythema, maculopapular rash, periorbital oedema.
- Severe reaction: bronchospasm.
- Hypotension.

Management
- Stop transfusion immediately.
- Change giving set.
- IV colloids to maintain BP/circulatory volume.
- Give
  - **adrenaline 1:1000 1ml IM stat**
  - **hydrocortisone 100 mg IV stat**
  - **chlorpheniramine 10 mg IV stat**

Febrile transfusion reactions

Seen in 0.5–1.0% blood transfusions. Mainly due to anti-HLA antibodies in recipient serum or granulocyte-specific antibodies (eg sensitisation during pregnancy or previous blood transfusion).

Treatment
- Slow down rate of transfusion.
- Antipyretic.
- Leucocyte (WBC) depleted blood.

Delayed transfusion reaction

Occurs in patients immunised through previous pregnancies or transfusions. Antibody weak (so not detected at pretransfusion stage). 2° immune response occurs – antibody titre ↑.

Symptoms/signs
- Occur 7–10d after blood transfusion.
- Fever, anaemia and jaundice.
- ± haemoglobinuria.

Management
- Check DAT and repeat compatibility tests.
- Transfuse patient with freshly cross-matched blood.

Bacterial contamination of blood products

Uncommon but potentially fatal adverse effect of blood transfusion (affects red cells and blood products eg platelet concentrates). Implicated organisms include gram –ve bacteria, including *Pseudomonas*, *Yersinia*, and *Flavobacterium*.

Features
- Fever.
- Skin flushing.
- Rigors.
- Abdominal pain.
- DIC.
- ARF.
- Shock.
- Cardiac arrest.

Management – as per *Immediate transfusion reaction*
- Stop transfusion
- Urgent resuscitation.
- IV broad-spectrum antibiotics if bacterial contamination suspected.

Post-transfusion purpura

Profound thrombocytopenia occurring 5–10d after blood or platelet transfusion. Usually due to high titre of anti-HPA-1a antibody in HPA-1a –ve patient.

Features
- Rare.
- Multiparous ♀ most commonly (previous pregnancies or transfusions).
- Caused by platelet-specific alloantibodies (usually anti-HPA-1a).
- Platelets ↓↓ with associated bleeding/bruising – may be severe and even life-threatening.

Management
- Random donor platelets are of little value. Request HPA-1a –ve platelet donations.
- Corticosteroids 1mg/kg/d.
- High dose IVIg.
- If other treatments fail consider plasmapheresis (physical removal of anti-platelet antibody).

Hypercalcaemia

Clinical symptoms
- General – weakness, lassitude, weight loss.
- Mental changes – impaired concentration, drowsiness, personality change, and coma.
- GIT – anorexia, nausea, vomiting, abdominal pain (peptic ulceration and pancreatitis are rare complications).
- Genitourinary – polyuria, polydipsia.

Clinical effects
- Cardiovascular – reduced QT interval on ECG, cardiac arrhythmias and hypertension.
- Renal – dehydration, renal failure and renal calculi.

Haematological causes
1. Myeloma.
2. High grade lymphoma.
3. Adult T-cell leukaemia/lymphoma (ATLL).
4. Acute lymphoblastic leukaemia.

Hypercalcaemia occurs in other clinical situations including metastatic carcinoma of breast, prostate and lung. Theories for occurrence in haematological malignancy include increased bone resorption mediated by osteoclasts under the influence of locally or systemically released cytokines such as PTH-related peptide, TGF, TNF, M-CSF, interleukins and prostaglandins. Increased intestinal absorption of calcium secondary to increased 1,25-hydroxycholecalciferol.

Normal range for plasma Ca^{2+} 2.12–2.65mmol/l. 40% of plasma Ca^{2+} is bound to albumin. Most laboratories measure the total plasma Ca^{2+} although only unbound Ca^{2+} is physiologically active. For accurate measurement of plasma or serum Ca^{2+} blood sampling should be taken from an uncuffed arm, ie without the use of a tourniquet.

Correct for albumin
Albumin <40g/l   corrected calcium = (Ca^{2+}) + 0.02 [40–(Albumin)]
Albumin >45g/l   corrected calcium = (Ca^{2+}) – 0.02 [(Albumin)–45]

Management
▶ An emergency if Ca^{2+} >3.0mmol/l.
1. Rehydrate with normal saline 4–6L/24h.
2. Beware fluid overload – use loop diuretics and CVP monitoring if necessary.
3. Stop thiazide diuretics and consider regular loop diuretics.
4. Give bisphosphonates eg disodium pamidronate 60–90mg IV stat (table).
5. Treat underlying malignancy.
6. Consider dialysis if complicating factors (CCF, advanced renal failure).
7. Other therapeutic options:
   - calcitonin 200IU 8-hourly
   - corticosteroids (eg prednisolone 60mg/d PO)
   - mithromycin 25µg/kg IV × 3 weekly
   - plicamycin.

Treatment of hypercalcaemia with disodium pamidronate

Serum Ca^{2+} (mmol/l)	Pamidronate (mg)
Up to 3.0	15-30
3–3.5	30-60
3.5–4.0	60-90
>4.0	90

- Infuse slowly (*see BNF*).
- Response often takes 3–5d.

Hyperviscosity

Common haematological emergency. Defined as increase in whole blood viscosity as a result of an increase in either red cells, white cells or plasma components, usually Ig.

Commonest situations arise as a result of
- ↑ in red cell volume in polycythaemia rubra vera.
- High blast cell numbers in peripheral blood eg AML or ALL at presentation.
- Presence of monoclonal Ig eg Waldenström's macroglobulinaemia.

Clinical features – polycythaemia (eg PRV)
- Lethargy, itching, headaches, hypertension, plethora, arterial thromboses viz: MI, CVA and visual loss (central retinal artery occlusion).

▶ Emergency treatment
Isovolaemic venesection. Remove 500ml blood volume from large bore vein (antecubital usually) with simultaneous replacement into another vein of 500ml 0.9% saline. Repeat daily until microhaematocrit PCV (spun PCV) <0.45.

Clinical features – high WBC (eg AML)
- Dyspnoea and cough (pulmonary leucostasis); confusion, ↓ conscious level, isolated cranial nerve palsies (cerebral leucostasis), visual loss (retinal haemorrhage or CRVT).

▶ Emergency treatment
- Unless machine leucapheresis can be obtained immediately, venesect 500ml blood from large bore vein and replace isovolaemically with packed red cells if Hb <7.0g/dl – otherwise replace with 0.9% saline to avoid increasing whole blood viscosity.
- Arrange leucapheresis on cell separator machine. Use white cell interface programme to apherese with replacement fluids depending on Hb as above. 2h is usually maximum tolerated.
- Initiate tumour lysis prophylactic protocol (see p470) in preparation for chemotherapy.
- Start chemotherapy as soon as criteria allow (high urine volume of pH>8 and allopurinol commenced). This is crucial as leucapheresis in this situation is only a holding manoeuvre while the patient is prepared for chemotherapy.
- Continue leucapheresis daily until leucostasis symptoms resolved or until WBC <50 × 10^9/l.

Hypergammaglobulinaemia (eg Waldenström's)
Lethargy, headaches, memory loss, confusion, vertigo, visual disturbances from cerebral vessel sludging – rarely MI, CVA.

▶ Emergency treatment
- Unless immediate access to plasma exchange machine available, venesect 500 ml blood from large bore vein with isovolaemic replacement with 0.9% saline unless Hb <7.0g/dl when use packed red cells.
- Arrange plasmapheresis on a cell separator machine using plasma exchange programme (see p496). Replacement fluids on criteria as above. Aim for 1–1.5 × blood volume exchange (usually 2.5–4.0L) starting at lower end of range initially. Repeat daily until symptoms resolved.
- Maintenance plasma exchanges at 3–6 weekly intervals may be sufficient treatment for some forms of Waldenström's macroglobulinaemia. However,

if hyperviscosity due to IgA myeloma or occasionally IgG myeloma, chemotherapy will need to be initiated.

Note

Diseases in which the abnormal Ig shows activity at lower temperature eg cold antibodies associated with CHAD (see p114) require maintenance of plasma-pheresis inlet and outlet venous lines and all infusional fluids at 37°C. Polyclonal ↑ in Ig (eg some forms of cryoglobulinaemia) can also rarely cause hyperviscosity symptoms. Management is as above for monoclonal immunoglobulins.

Disseminated intravascular coagulation

Pathological process characterised by generalised intravascular activation of the haemostatic mechanism producing widespread fibrin formation, resultant activation of fibrinolysis, and consumption of platelets/coagulation factors (esp I, II, V). Usually the result of serious underlying disease but may itself become life-threatening (through haemorrhage or thrombosis). Mortality in severe DIC may exceed >80%. Haemorrhage usually the dominant feature and is the result of excessive fibrinolysis, depletion of coagulation factors and platelets and inhibition of fibrin polymerisation by FDPs. Wide range of disorders may precipitate DIC.

Pathophysiology – DIC may be initiated by

- Exposure of blood to tissue factor (eg after trauma).
- Endothelial cell damage (eg by endotoxin or cytokines).
- Release of proteolytic enzymes into the blood (eg pancreas, snake venom).
- Infusion or release of activated clotting factors (factor IX concentrate).
- Massive thrombosis.
- Severe hypoxia and acidosis.

Causes of DIC

Tissue damage (release of tissue factor) eg trauma (esp brain or crush injury), thermal injury (burns, hyperthermia, hypothermia), surgery, shock, asphyxia/hypoxia, ischaemia/infarction, rhabdomyolysis, fat embolism.

Complications of pregnancy (release of tissue factor) eg amniotic fluid embolism, abruptio placentae, eclampsia & pre-eclampsia, retained dead fetus, uterine rupture, septic abortion, hydatidiform mole.

Neoplasia (release of tissue factor, TNF, proteases) eg solid tumours, leukaemias (esp acute promyelocytic).

Infection (endotoxin release, endothelial cell damage) eg gram –ve bacteria (eg meningococcus), gram +ve bacteria (eg pneumococcus), anaerobes, *M tuberculosis*, toxic shock syndrome, viruses (eg Lassa fever), protozoa (eg malaria), fungi (eg candidiasis), Rocky Mountain spotted fever.

Vascular disorders (abnormal endothelium, platelet activation) eg giant haemangioma (Kasabach Merritt syndrome), vascular tumours, aortic aneurysm, vascular surgery, cardiac bypass surgery, malignant hypertension, pulmonary embolism, acute MI, stroke, subarachnoid haemorrhage.

Immunological (complement activation, release of tissue factor) anaphylaxis, acute haemolytic transfusion reaction, heparin-associated thrombocytopenia, renal allograft rejection, acute vasculitis, drug reactions (quinine).

Proteolytic activation of coagulation factors eg pancreatitis, snake venom, insect bites.

Neonatal disorders eg infection, aspiration syndromes, small-for-dates infant, respiratory distress syndrome, purpura fulminans.

Other disorders eg fulminant hepatic failure, cirrhosis, Reye's syndrome, acute fatty liver of pregnancy, ARDS, therapy with fibrinolytic agents, therapy with factor IX concentrates, massive transfusion, acute intravascular haemolysis familial ATIII deficiency, homozygous protein C or S deficiency.

Clinical features

Acute (uncompensated) DIC	Rapid and extensive activation of coagulation, fibrinolysis or both, with depletion of procoagulant factors and inhibitors and significant haemorrhage.
Chronic (compensated) DIC	Slow consumption of factors with normal or increased levels; often asymptomatic or associated with thrombosis.

Clinical features may be masked by those of the disorder which precipitated it and rarely is the cause of DIC obscure. DIC should be considered in the management of any seriously ill patient. The specific features of DIC are:

- Ecchymoses, petechiae, oozing from venepuncture sites and post-op bleeding.
- Renal dysfunction, ARDS, cerebral dysfunction and skin necrosis due to microthrombi.
- MAHA.

Laboratory features

The following investigations are useful in establishing the diagnosis of DIC though the extent to which any single test may be abnormal reflects the underlying cause of DIC.

- **D-dimers** – more specific and convenient than FDP titre (performed on plasma sample). Significant ↑ of D-dimers plus depletion of coagulation factors ± platelets is necessary for diagnosis of DIC.
- **PT** – less sensitive, usually ↑ in moderately severe DIC but may be normal in chronic DIC.
- **APTR** – less useful. May be normal or even <normal, particularly in chronic DIC.
- **Fibrinogen** – ↓ or falling fibrinogen levels are characteristic of many causes of DIC in the presence of D-dimers. Greatest falls are seen with tissue factor release.
- **Platelet count** – ↓ or falling platelet counts are characteristic of acute DIC, most notably in association with infective causes.
- **Blood film** may show evidence of fragmentation (schistocytes) though the absence of this finding does not exclude the diagnosis of DIC.
- **ATIII levels** are frequently ↓ in DIC and degree of reduction in plasma ATIII and plasminogen may reflect severity.
- **Factor assays** rarely necessary or helpful. In severe DIC levels of most factors are reduced with the exception of FVIIIc and von Willebrand factor which may be increased due to release from endothelial cell storage sites.

423

Management of DIC

1. Identify and, if possible, remove the precipitating cause.
2. Supportive therapy as required (eg volume replacement for shock).
3. Replacement therapy if bleeding: platelet transfusion if platelets $<50 \times 10^9/l$, cryoprecipitate to replace fibrinogen, and FFP to replace other factors (10 units cryoprecipitate for every 3 units FFP).
4. Prophylactic platelet transfusion may be helpful if platelets $<20 \times 10^9/l$.
5. Monitor response with platelet count, PT, fibrinogen and D-dimers.
6. Heparin (IVI 5–10iu/kg/h) for DIC associated with APML, carcinoma, skin necrosis, purpura fulminans, microthrombosis affecting skin, kidney, bowel and large vessel thrombosis.
7. ATIII concentrate in intractable shock or fulminant hepatic necrosis.
8. Protein C concentrate in acquired purpura fulminans or severe neonatal DIC.

Overdosage of thrombolytic therapy

- Large doses of any thrombolytic agent (streptokinase, urokinase, t-PA) will cause primary fibrinolysis by proteolytic destruction of circulating fibrinogen and consumption of plasminogen and its major inhibitor α2-antiplasmin.
- Overdosage is associated with high risk of severe haemorrhage particularly at recent venepuncture sites or surgical wounds; intracranial haemorrhage occurs in 0.5–1% of patients treated with thrombolytic therapy.
- Superficial bleeding at venepuncture site may be managed with local pressure and the infusion continued.
- Bleeding at other sites or where pressure cannot be applied necessitates cessation of thrombolytic therapy (t½ <30mins) and determination of the thrombin time (if used to monitor thrombolytic therapy) or fibrinogen level. If strongly indicated and bleeding minimal or stopped the infusion may be restarted at 50% the initial dose when the thrombin time has returned to the lower end of the therapeutic range (1.5 × baseline).

Treatment of serious bleeding after thrombolytic therapy
- Stop thrombolytic infusion immediately.
- Discontinue any simultaneous heparin infusion and any antiplatelet agents.
- Apply pressure to bleeding sites, ensure good venous access and commence volume expansion.
- Check fibrinogen and APTR.
- Transfuse 10 units cryoprecipitate.
- Monitor fibrinogen, repeat cryoprecipitate to maintain fibrinogen >1.0g/l.
- If still bleeding, transfuse 2–4 units FFP.
- If bleeding time >9 mins, transfuse 10 units platelets.
- If bleeding time <9 mins, commence tranexamic acid.

Haematological emergencies

Heparin overdosage

The most serious complication of heparin overdosage is haemorrhage. The therapeutic range using the APTT is 1.5–2.5 × average normal control. The plasma t½ following IV administration is 1–2h. The t½ after SC administration is considerably longer.

Management guidelines – APTT > therapeutic range

Without haemorrhage

Continuous IV infusion
stop infusion, if markedly elevated, recheck after 0.5–1h; restart at lower dose when APTT in therapeutic range

Intermittent SC heparin
reduce dose recheck 6h after administration

With haemorrhage

Continuous IV infusion
stop infusion; if bleeding continues, administer protamine sulphate by slow IV injection (1mg neutralises 100iu heparin, max dose 40mg/injection)

Intermittent SC heparin
if protamine is required, administer 50% of calculated neutralisation dose 1h after heparin administration and 25% after 2h

Warfarin overdosage

Haemorrhage is a potentially serious complication of anticoagulant therapy and may occur with an INR in the therapeutic range if there are local predisposing factors eg peptic ulceration or recent surgery, or if NSAIDs are given concurrently.

Management guidelines

INR	Action
>7.0	Without haemorrhage: stop warfarin & consider a single 5–10 mg oral dose of vitamin K if high bleeding risk; review INR daily
4.5–7.0	Without haemorrhage: stop warfarin & review INR in 2d
>4.5	With severe life-threatening haemorrhage: give Factor IX concentrate (50U/kg) or FFP (1L for an adult), consider a single 2–5 mg IV dose of vitamin K
>4.5	With less severe haemorrhage: eg haematuria or epistaxis, withhold warfarin for ≥1d and consider a single 0.5–2 mg IV dose of vitamin K
2.0–4.5	With haemorrhage: investigate the possibility of an underlying local cause; reduce warfarin dose if necessary; give FFP/Factor IX concentrate only if haemorrhage is serious or life-threatening

Vitamin K administration to patients on warfarin therapy

Effect of vitamin K is delayed several hours even with IV administration. Doses >2 mg cause unpredictable and prolonged resistance to oral anticoagulants and should be avoided in most circumstances where prolonged warfarin therapy is necessary. Particular care must be taken in patients with prosthetic cardiac valves who may require heparin therapy for several weeks to achieve adequate anti-coagulation if a large dose of vitamin K has been administered.

Massive blood transfusion

Massive transfusion defined as replacement of >1 blood volume (5l) in less than 24h. Haemostatic failure may result from dilution or consumption of coagulation factors and platelets, DIC, systemic fibrinolysis or acquired platelet dysfunction.

Pathophysiology

- **Dilution/consumption** eg replacement of intravascular volume with fluids lacking coagulation factors or platelets eg packed red cells and crystalloids.
- **DIC** may follow tissue damage, hypoxia, acidosis, sepsis or haemolytic transfusion reaction. Causes coagulopathy due to consumption of platelets and coagulation factors, fibrinolysis and circulating fibrin degradation products (see p422).
- **Systemic fibrinolysis** particularly associated with liver disease; causes rapid lysis of thrombi at surgical sites and plasmin-induced fibrinogenolysis; may be assessed by the euglobulin lysis time.
- **Platelet dysfunction** may be due to circulating FDPs, exhausted platelets activated by intravascular trauma or effects of transfusion of stored platelets.

Investigations

- Baseline tests
  - haematocrit
  - platelet count
  - fibrinogen
  - PT
  - APTT ratio
  - D-dimers
- Frequent reassessment of tests to monitor effect of, and need for, further replacement therapy.

Management

Haematocrit <0.30	transfuse red cells
Platelet count <75 × 10^9/l	transfuse platelets
Fibrinogen <1.0g/l	transfuse cryoprecipitate
PT ± APTT ratio >1.5 × control	transfuse fresh frozen plasma

Red cell transfusion

- Full crossmatch takes 30–40 minutes.
- Uncrossmatched group-specific blood can be available in 10 minutes.
- Uncrossmatched group O Rh (D) –ve blood may be transfused in the emergency situation until group-specific blood can be made available; group O Rh (D) +ve red cells may be given to males and older women if necessary.

Platelet transfusion

- Usually available within 10–15 minutes.
- Standard adult dose (6 units equivalent) will raise platelet count by ~60×10^9/l in absence of dilution or consumption.
- As platelets do not carry Rh antigens, type incompatible platelets may be administered when necessary; Rh immune globulin should be administered when a Rh –ve patient has received Rh +ve platelets.
- 6 units of platelets contain ~300ml plasma.

Haematological emergencies

Fresh frozen plasma
- Takes up to 30 minutes to thaw; dose required ~10ml/kg.
- Use immediately for optimum replacement of coagulation factors.
- Each unit contains ~200–280ml plasma and 0.7–1.0iu/ml activity of each coagulation factor
- ABO group compatible FFP should be administered – no crossmatch is required.
- If large volumes infused, serum [Ca^{2+}] should be monitored to exclude hypocalcaemia due to citrate toxicity.

Cryoprecipitate
- Precipitate formed when FFP is thawed at 4°C; resuspended in 10–15ml plasma and refrozen at –18°C; takes up to 15 minutes to thaw and pool.
- No grouping required.
- Contains 80–100 IU FVIIIC, 100–250mg fibrinogen, 50–60mg fibronectin and 40–70% of the original von Willebrand factor.
- Should be used immediately for optimum replacement of fibrinogen and factor VIIIC.
- Infusion of 8–10 bags raises fibrinogen concentration by 0.6–1.0g/l in a 70 kg patient.

Paraparesis/spinal collapse

May be due to tumour in the cord, spinal dura or meninges or by extension of a vertebral tumour into the spinal canal with compression of the cord or as a result of vertebral collapse.

Spinal cord compression from vertebral collapse in a haematological patient is most commonly due to myeloma (in up to 20% of patients) but may occur in a patient with Hodgkin's disease (3–8%) or occasionally non-Hodgkin's lymphoma. Spinal cord involvement by leukaemia is most common in AML, less so in ALL and CGL and least common in CLL.

Onset of paraplegia may be preceded for days or weeks by paraesthesia but in some patients the onset of paraplegia may follow initial symptoms by only a few hours.

Symptoms suggestive of spinal cord compression require urgent assessment by CT or MRI and referral to a neurosurgical unit for assessment for surgical decompression. Where this is not possible early radiotherapy may provide symptomatic improvement. However if treatment is delayed until paraparesis has developed, this often proves to be irreversible despite surgery and/or radiotherapy.

Leucostasis

Term is applied both to organ damage due to 'sludging' of leucocytes in the capillaries of a patient with high circulating blast count and to the lodging and growth of leukaemic blasts, usually in AML, in the vascular tree eroding the vessel wall and producing tumours and haemorrhage.

Features

- More common in AML and blast crisis of CML.
- Leucostatic tumours are associated with an exponential increase in blasts in the peripheral blood and, prior to the development of effective chemotherapy, haemorrhage from intracerebral tumours was not an uncommon cause of death.
- Pulmonary or cerebral leucostasis are serious complications which may occur in patients who present with a blast count >50 × 10^9/l.
- Leucocyte thrombi may cause plugging of pulmonary or cerebral capillaries. Vascular rupture and tissue infiltration may occur.
- Less common manifestations are priapism and vascular insufficiency.
- Pulmonary leucostasis causes progressive dyspnoea of sudden onset associated with fever, tachypnoea, hypoxaemia, diffuse crepitations and a diffuse interstitial infiltrate on CXR.
- Pulmonary haemorrhage and haemoptysis may occur. More common with monocytic leukaemias and the microgranular variant of acute promyelocytic leukaemia. Differentiation from bacterial or fungal pneumonia may be difficult.
- Cerebral leucostasis may cause a variety of neurological abnormalities.
- Anaemia may protect a patient with marked leucocytosis from the effects of increased whole blood viscosity. Transfusion of RBCs to correct anaemia prior to chemotherapy may initiate leucostasis.

Management

Urgent leucapheresis is required for a patient with marked leucostasis (>200×10^9/l) or in any patient in whom leucostasis is suspected. Chemotherapy may be commenced concomitantly to further reduce the leucocyte count but may be associated with a high incidence of pulmonary and CNS haemorrhage.

Haematological emergencies

Thrombotic thrombocytopenic purpura

Definition
Fulminant disease of unknown aetiology characterised by increased platelet aggregation and occlusion of arterioles and capillaries of the microcirculation. Considerable overlap in pathophysiology and clinical features with HUS – fundamental abnormality may be identical.

Incidence:
Rare, ~1 in 500,000 per year. ♀:♂ = 2:1. HUS much commoner in children, TTP commoner in adults – peak age incidence is 40 years, and 90% of cases <60 years old. There is some case clustering.

Clinical features
- Classical description is of a *pentad* of features:
  1. microangiopathic haemolytic anaemia
  2. severe thrombocytopenia
  3. neurological involvement
  4. renal impairment
  5. fever.
  In practice, few patients have the full monty. 50–70% have renal abnormalities (*cf.* nearly all with HUS) and they are less severe. Neurological involvement is more prevalent in TTP than HUS. 40% of TTP patients have fever.
- *Haemolysis* – severe and intravascular causing jaundice.
- *Thrombocytopenia* – severe, mucosal haemorrhage likely and intracranial haemorrhage may be fatal.
- *Neurological* – from mild depression and confusion → visual defects, coma and status epilepticus.
- *Renal* – haematuria, proteinuria, oliguria and ↑ urea and creatinine. HUS > TTP.
- *Fever* – very variable, weakness and nausea common.
- *Other disease features*: serious venous thromboses at unusual sites (eg sagittal sinus – microthrombi in the brain seen on MRI scan). Abdominal pain severe enough to mimic an acute abdomen is sometimes seen due to mesenteric ischaemia. Diarrhoea is common particularly bloody in HUS.

Diagnosis and investigations
- Made on the clinical features above – exclude other diseases eg cerebral lupus, sepsis with DIC.
- FBC shows severe anaemia and thrombocytopenia.
- Blood film shows gross fragmentation of red cells, spherocytes and nucleated red cells with polychromasia.
- Reticulocytes ↑↑ (>15%).
- LDH ↑↑ (>1000 iu/l).
- Clotting screen including fibrinogen and FDPs usually normal (*cf.* DIC).
- Serum haptoglobin low or absent.
- Urinary haemosiderin +ve.
- Unconjugated bilirubin ↑.
- DAT –ve.
- BM hypercellular.
- U & E show increases (HUS > TTP).

- Proteinuria and haematuria.
- Renal biopsy shows microthrombi.
- Stool culture for *E.coli* 0157 +ve in most cases of HUS in children, less often in adult TTP.
- MRI brain scan shows microthrombi and occasional intracranial haemorrhage.
- **Lumbar puncture – do not proceed with LP unless scans clear and there is suspicion of infective meningitis.**
- Look for evidence of viral infection. Association of syndrome with HIV, SLE, cyclosporin usage and the 3rd trimester of pregnancy.

Treatment is a haematological emergency – seek expert help immediately

1. Unless antecubital venous access is excellent, insert a large bore central apheresis catheter (may need blood product support).
2. May need ITU level of care and ventilation.
3. *Initiate plasmapheresis as soon as possible.*
   Exchange 1–1.5 × plasma volume daily until clinical improvement.
   May need 3–4l exchanges. Replacement fluid should be solely FFP.
   In the event of delayed access to cell separator facilities, start IV infusions of FFP making intravascular space with diuretics if necessary.
   Once response achieved, ↓ frequency of exchanges gradually.
   If no response obtained within one week, change FFP replacement to *cryosupernatant* (rationale: it lacks high molecular weight multimers of von Willebrand factor postulated in endothelial damage disease triggers).
4. Give RBC as necessary but reserve platelet transfusions for severe mucosal or intracranial bleeding as reports suggest they may worsen the disease.
5. Cover for infection with IV broad spectrum antibiotics including teicoplanin if necessary to preserve the apheresis catheter.
6. Start anticonvulsants if fitting.
7. Most would start high dose steroids (prednisolone 2mg/kg/d PO) with gastric protection although evidence is equivocal.
8. Aspirin/dipyridamole/heparin may be considered for non-responders.
9. Refractory patients (~10%) should be considered for IV vincristine.
10. Still refractory patients may achieve remission with splenectomy.
11. Response to treatment may be dramatic eg ventilated, comatose patient watching TV in the afternoon after plasma exchange in the morning!

Prognosis

- 90% respond to plasma exchange with FFP replacement.
- ~30% will relapse. Most respond again to further plasma exchange but leaves 15% who become chronic relapsers.
- Role of prophylaxis for chronic relapsers unclear. Intermittent FFP infusions or continuous low dose aspirin may help individual cases.

Sickle crisis

Management

▶ Early and effective treatment of crises essential (hospital).

▶ Rest patient and start IV fluids and O_2 (patients often dehydrated through poor oral intake of fluid + excessive loss if fever).

▶ Start empirical antibiotic therapy (eg ampicillin) if infection is suspected whilst culture results (blood, urine or sputum) are awaited.

▶ Analgesia usually required – eg intravenous opiates (diamorphine/morphine) especially when patients are first admitted to hospital. Switch later to oral medication after the initial crisis abates.

▶ Consider exchange blood transfusion (if neurological symptoms, stroke or visceral damage). Aim to ↓ Hb S to <30%.

▶ Exchange transfusion if PaO$_2$ <60mm on air.

▶ α-adrenergic stimulators for priapism.

▶ Seek advice of senior haematology staff.

▶ Consider regular blood transfusion if crises frequent or anaemia is severe.

▶ Top-up transfusion if Hb <4.5 g/dl (hunt for cause).

Transfusion and splenectomy may be lifesaving in children with splenic sequestration.

Supportive care 13

Quality of life

In managing any disease problem a key objective is to improve the quality of a patient's survival as well as its duration. Part of the clinical decision-making process takes into account quality of life (QOL) in judging the most appropriate treatment.

Defining quality of life precisely is not easy; it has been described as a measure of the difference at a particular time point between the hopes and expectations of the individual and that individual's present experiences. QOL is multifaceted and can only be assessed by the individual since it takes into account many aspects of that individual's life and their current perception of what, for them, is good QOL in their specific circumstances.

A clear distinction exists between performance scores (eg Karnofsky or WHO) which record functional status and assess independence; these are assessed by the physician according to pre-set criteria. They have erroneously been considered to be surrogate markers of QOL.

Patient QOL as assessed by the treating physician has been shown to be unreliable in an oncological setting.

There is no single determinant of good QOL. A number of qualities which go to make up QOL are capable of assessment; these include *ability to carry on normal physical activities, ability to work, to engage in normal social activities, a sense of general well-being* and a *perception of health*.

Several validated instruments now exist to measure QOL; these mainly involve questionnaires completed by the patient. They are simple to complete and involve 'yes' or 'no' answers to specific questions, answers on a linear analogue scale or the use of four or seven point Likert scales.

Available QOL instruments include
- Functional Living Index – Cancer (FLIC)[1]
- Functional Assessment of Cancer Therapy (FACT)[2]
- European Organisation for Research and Treatment in Cancer (EORTC) Quality of Life Questionnaire C-30 (QLQ C30)[3]

Data from validated QOL questionnaires is now accepted as a requirement and a clinical end point in many major clinical trials, especially in malignancies, particularly those where survival differences are minimal between contrasting therapy approaches. Where survivals are minimally affected it is then essential to focus on treatments which will offer the best QOL.

1 H Schipper 1984 J Clin Oncol **2** 472
2 DF Cella 1993 J Clin Oncol **11** 570
3 NK Aaronson 1993 J Natl Cancer Inst **85** 365

Pain management

Pain is a clinical problem in diverse haematological disorders, notably in sickle cell disease, haemophilia & myeloma. Acknowledgement of the need to manage pain effectively is an essential part of successful patient care and management in clinical haematology.

Pain may be local or generalised. More than one type of pain may be present and causes may be multifactorial. It is most important to listen to the patient and give him/her the chance to talk about their pain(s). Not only will this help determine an appropriate therapeutic strategy, the act of listening and allowing the patient to talk about their pains and associated anxieties is part of the pain management process.

Engaging the patient in 'measuring' their pain is often helpful; it enables specific goals to be set and provides a means to assess the effectiveness of the analgesic strategy.

Basic to the control of pain is to manage and remove the pathological process causing pain, wherever this is possible. Analgesia must be part of an integrated care plan which takes this into account.

Analgesic requirements should be recorded regularly as these form a valuable 'semi-quantitative' end point of pain measurement. Reduction in requirements, for example, is an indicator that attempts to remove or control the underlying cause are succeeding.

Managing pain successfully involves patient and family/carer participation, a collaborative multidisciplinary approach in most categories of haematological disorder related pain; medication should aim to provide continuous pain relief wherever possible with a minimum of drug related side effects

Analgesics

Simple non opioid analgesics	Paracetamol: 1g 4–6 hourly, oral as tablets or liquid; suppositories available. No contraindication in liver disease; useful in mild to moderate pain.
Antiinflammatory drugs	Ibuprofen 800mg or diclofenac 75–100mg bd as slow release formulations can be synergistic with other analgesics; combined formulations of diclofenac with misoprostol may reduce risks of gastric irritation bleeding; useful in combination with paracetamol or weak opioids
Weak opioids	Dextropropoxyphene 100mg usually combined with paracetamol 1g as coproxamol tablets; usual dosage is 2 tablets 6 hourly or codeine 30–60mg or dihydrocodeine 30–60mg up to 4 hourly provide effective analgesia for moderate pain. Confusion, drowsiness may be associated with initial usage in some. Weak (and strong) opioids cause constipation; usually requires simple laxatives
Strong opioids	Morphine available as liquid or tablets commencing at 5–10mg and given 4 hourly is treatment of choice in

severe pain. Once daily requirements are established patients can be 'converted' to 12 hourly slow release morphine preparations. Breakthrough pain can be treated with additional doses of 5–10mg morphine. Diamorphine preferred for parenteral usage. Highly soluble and suitable for use in a syringe driver for continuous administration or as a 4 hourly injection.

Alternatives to opioids Tramadol may be given orally. Fentanyl given as slow release transdermal patches may be a valuable alternative to slow release morphine for moderate to severe chronic pain.

For chronic pain give analgesia PO regularly, wherever possible.

- Pain control is very specific to the individual patient, there is no 'correct' formula other than the combination of measures which alleviate the pain.
- The clinician should work 'upwards' or 'downwards' through the levels of available analgesics to achieve control.
- Constipation due to analgesics should be managed with aperients.
- Nausea or vomiting may occur in up to 50% patients with strong opiates; cyclizine 50mg 8 hourly, metoclopramide 10mg 6 hourly or haloperidol 1.5mg 12 hourly are available options to limit nausea or vomiting.
- Additional general measures include
  - radiotherapy for localised cancer pain
  - physical methods eg TENS or consideration of nerve root block
  - surgery, especially in myeloma where stabilising fractures and pinning will relieve pain and allow mobility
  - encouraging/allowing patients to utilise 'alternative' approaches including relaxation techniques, aromatherapy, hypnosis, etc.
- Additional drug therapy
  - antidepressants eg amitriptyline may help in neuropathic pain
  - anticonvulsants eg carbamazepine may be helpful in neuropathic pains especially in post-herpetic neuralgia
  - corticosteroids, particularly dexamethasone, to relieve leukaemic bone pain in late stage disease.

447

Many hospitals also run specific pain clinics. The support and expertise available should be enlisted particularly for difficult problems with persistent localised pain, eg post-herpetic neuralgia. For long term painful conditions it is essential to work with medical & nursing colleagues in Primary Care and in Palliative Care so that the patient receives appropriate support in the community setting.

Psychological support

Many haematological disorders are long term conditions; the specific diagnosis can be seen to 'label' the patient as different or ill and therefore will exert a profound influence on their life and that of their immediate family or carers. Patients (and their families) experience and demonstrate a number of reactions to their diagnosis, the clinical haematologist needs to have an awareness of this and respond accordingly.

Reactions to serious diagnosis include
- Numbness.
- Denial.
- Anger.
- Guilt.
- Depression.
- Loneliness.

Ultimately most patients come to acceptance of their condition; carers /partners will also go through a similar range of reactions. The clinician needs to be aware of the way in which news of a diagnosis is likely to affect a patient and his/her family/carers and respond appropriately. In the first instance this will often involve the need to impart the diagnosis, what it means and what needs to be done clinically. There is no 'right way' to impart bad or difficult news. It is very important to make and take time to tell the patient of the diagnosis. Wherever possible this should be done in a quiet, private setting. Numbness at learning of a serious diagnosis often means that very little is taken in initially other than the diagnostic label. The various reactions listed above may subsequently emerge during the time the patient comes to accept the diagnosis, what it means and what is to be done clinically.

Within the haematological team there should be support available to the patient and family/carers which can provide them with practical information about the disease and its management. Simply knowing there is a sympathetic ear may be all that is required in the way of support, however for some patients and families/carers more specialised support may be needed eg availability of formal counselling or access to psychological or psychiatric support.

Use can be made of local or national patient support groups; knowledge of others in similar predicaments can help diffuse anger and loneliness. Support groups can also be a valuable resource in providing information and experience which patients and families/carers find helpful.

The most effective psychological support for haematological patients is to see them as individuals and not 'diseases'.

Protocols and procedures

14

Note
Please check local protocols since these may differ to those outlined in this handbook.

Acute leukaemia – investigation

Haematology
- FBC, blood film, reticulocytes, ESR.
- Serum B_{12}, red cell folate, and ferritin.
- Blood group, antibody screen and DAT.
- Coagulation screen, INR, APTT, fibrinogen (and XDPs if bleeding).
- BM aspirate for morphology, cytogenetics, immunophenotype (and peripheral blood if relevant) plus samples required by the MRC trials.
- BM trephine biopsy.

Biochemistry
- U & E, LFTs.
- Ca^{2+}, phosphate, random glucose.
- LDH.
- Serum and urine lysozyme (if AML M4 or M5 AML suspected).

Virology
- Hepatitis BsAg.
- Hepatitis A antibody.
- Hepatitis C antibody.
- HIV I and II antibody (counselling and consent required).
- CMV IgG and IgM.

Immunology
- Serum immunoglobulins.
- Autoantibody screen profile.
- HLA type – Class 1 always in case HLA matched platelets are required, Class 1 and 2 if allogeneic transplant indicated.

Bacteriology
- Baseline blood cultures.
- Throat swab.
- MSU.
- Stool for fungal culture.
- Nose swab for MRSA if transferred from another hospital/unit.

Cardiology
- ECG.
- Echocardiogram, only if in cardiac failure or IE suspected or significant cardiac history.

Radiology
- CXR.
- Sinus radiographs.

Other
- If any evidence of severe dental caries or gum disease refer patient for dental assessment *before* chemotherapy.
- Consider semen storage.

Protocols and procedures

Platelet transfusion support

See p456 and p552.

Platelet storage and administration

Storage

Platelets should be stored at room temperature (20–22°C) in a platelet agitator until infused. Helps to retain function. Use before expiry date on pack.

- Platelet packs should be inspected before infusion – platelet packs that look visibly pink due to RBC contamination should not be used. Occasionally fine fibrinoid strands may be seen in concentrates (give a slightly stringy or cloudy appearance). Such strands disperse with gentle massage and are safe to use. Occasionally larger aggregates of platelets and/or white cell clumps are seen in the bags which do not disperse with gentle massage. Such bags are dangerous and should *never* be infused.

Dosage and timing

- A single dose of platelets is generally supplied as a single bag.
- Represents a standard transfusion dose although twice this amount may be required to cover insertions of central lines or minor surgery.
- Occasionally double doses may be required for patients becoming refractory.
- The frequency of platelet transfusion will be determined by clinical circumstances. In general, a patient who is well, afebrile and with no evidence of new bruising or bleeding need only have a platelet count maintained above 10×10^9/l. May be achieved with platelets given as infrequently as every 2–4 days with this estimate being guided on daily platelet counts.
- Patients who are infected or bleeding have much greater platelet requirements – aim to keep the platelet count >20×10^9/l. This will usually mean daily platelet infusions for the duration of this clinical episode.
- Platelet counts of <10×10^9/l should always be avoided but within these constraints the less platelets transfused the better since this reduces the risk of alloimmunisation to HLA and platelet antigens.
- Anyone with a *persistent* platelet count <10×10^9/l should be started on tranexamic acid 1g qds PO or IV unless specific contraindications exist such as genitourinary tract bleeding.

Choice of blood group for platelet support

At diagnosis, all patients should have a blood group and CMV antibody status determined. Patients should receive platelets of their own blood group as far as possible. Due to fluctuations in supply, this is not always possible and the choice is less critical than for red cell transfusions as platelet ABO blood group antigen expression is weak and the recipient is exposed only to donor plasma.

Patient's blood group	first choice	second choice
O	O	A
A	A	O
B	B (if available)	A preferably or O
AB	A	O

- Rh (D) +ve patients may receive Rh (D) +ve or Rh (D) –ve products.
- Rh (D) –ve patients should receive Rh (D) –ve platelets.
- Occasionally necessary to give Rh (D) +ve platelets to Rh (D) –ve patients. The Blood Bank should be informed as all future red cell transfusions must be Rh (D) –ve. Anti-D administration may be given to such patients routinely or may be reserved for women of child-bearing age (dose: 250iu (50μg). Anti-D SC immediately after the transfusion.

Platelet reactions and refractoriness

Reactions to platelet transfusion are common and range from mild temperatures to rigors. The development of an urticarial rash is also frequently seen. When a transfusion reaction develops, the following steps should be taken:

▶ Stop the transfusion.
▶ Give 10mg chlorpheniramine IV and 1g of paracetamol PO.
▶ Cover future transfusions with chlorpheniramine and paracetamol 30 mins pre-transfusion.

Occasionally, troublesome reactions remain despite giving platelets with cover. Try the addition of an in-line white cell filter (eg Pall PL100). If effective, may be used for all future transfusions, or use products leucodepleted at source which should be used for all subsequent transfusions together with chlorpheniramine and paracetamol.

- Hydrocortisone 100mg IV stat may be (sparingly) used for refractory reactions
- Pethidine is a suitable alternative for severe reactions and is almost invariably effective. Give 25mg IV stat with repeat dose if necessary or set up an IVI of 25–50mg IV over 8 h.
- The possibility of generation of HLA and platelet-specific antibodies should also be considered (see below).

Platelet refractoriness

Occasionally patients show little/no increment in the platelet count after platelet transfusions. This is called platelet refractoriness. May be due to physical or immunological mechanisms in the patient. The commonest physical mechanism is of platelet circulatory half-life reduction caused by concurrent sepsis or coagulopathy eg DIC. Immunological causes include induction of anti-HLA antibodies due to allosensitisation from previous transfusions or generation of anti-platelet antibodies such as in ITP. Investigation should be considered if platelet transfusions fail to maintain a platelet count $>10 \times 10^9/l$ at all times.

Proceed as follows

1. Check FBC pre-platelet infusion, 1 and 12h post-infusion to assess the rate of platelet count decay. Failure to show a rise of platelet count by at least $10 \times 10^9/l$ at 1h or any rise after 12h post-infusion merits further testing.
2. Samples should be sent to a blood transfusion centre for HLA and platelet antibody screening (10ml EDTA samples and 20ml serum).
3. The patient's own HLA type should be checked.
4. If HLA or platelet antibodies are identified, the provision of HLA or platelet antigen matched platelet products may improve the platelet transfusion responsiveness.

Platelet refractoriness >⅔ patients receiving multiple transfusion with random platelets develop anti-HLA antibodies. Refractoriness defined as failure of 2 consecutive transfusions to give corrected increment of $>7.5 \times 10^9/l$ 1h after platelet transfusion in absence of fever, infection, severe bleeding, splenomegaly, or DIC.

GvHD Rare complication where there is engraftment of donor lymphocytes in platelet concentrate in severely immunocompromised patients.

Protocols and procedures

Calculating platelet increment $[(P_1 - P_0) \times SA]/n$

P_0 = platelet count pre-transfusion ($\times 10^9$/l)
P_1 = platelet count post-transfusion ($\times 10^9$/l)
SA = surface area
n = number of units of platelets transfused

Corrected increment 60 min after transfusion $>7.5 \times 10^9$/l indicates successful platelet transfusion $(P_1 - P_0)$.

459

JM Hows & R Brozovic 1992 in *ABC of Transfusion* 2nd edn BMJ Publications

Prophylactic regimen for neutropenic patients

Infective risk is related to the severity and duration of neutropenia. Higher risk is associated with concurrent immunological defects eg hypogammaglobulin-aemia in myeloma, T cell defects eg HIV disease, additional immunosuppressive agents eg Cyclosporin post-transplant, and older patients. Principal risk is from bacterial organisms but fungi and viruses, especially Herpes (HSV, HZV) and CMV are also seen in prolonged neutropenia.

Typical protocols include

- **Isolation procedures** – strict handwashing by all patient contacts is the only isolation measure of universally proven benefit. Others include visitor restriction, gloves, aprons, gowns, masks and full reverse barrier nursing. Isolation rooms with positive pressure filtered air will prevent fungal infection.
- **Drinks** – avoid mains tap water/still mineral water (use boiled water or sparkling mineral water). Avoid unpasteurised milk and freshly squeezed fruit juice.
- **Food** – avoid cream, ice-cream, soft, blue or ripened cheeses, live yoghurt, raw eggs or derived foods eg mayonnaise and soufflés, cold chicken, meat paté, raw fish/shellfish, unpeeled fresh vegetables/salads, unpeeled fruit, uncooked herbs and spices, ground pepper (contains *Aspergillus* spores).
- **General mouthcare** – antiseptic mouthwash eg Corsadyl 10ml 4 hourly swish and spit. If soreness develops, substitute Difflam mouthwash. For discrete oral ulcers, use topical Adcortyl in Orobase; for generalised ulceration use 0.9% saline mouthwash hourly, swish and spit. Corsodyl toothpaste should replace standard preparations. Oral antifungal prophylaxis should be Nystatin susp. 1ml 4 hourly swish and spit or swallow, or amphotericin lozenges one to suck slowly 4 hourly.
- **Antibacterial prophylaxis** – aim to alter gut flora (decontamination) and prevent exogenous colonisation. Principal agents: ciprofloxacin 250mg bd or cotrimoxazole 480mg bd or Colistin 1.5 megaunits tds and Neomycin 500mg qds. All given PO starting 48h after antifungal prophylaxis.
- **Antifungal prophylaxis** – a systemic imidazole compound is most routinely used eg fluconazole 100mg PO od. Itraconazole liquid 2.5mg/kg bd PO may offer additional protection against *Aspergillus*.
- **Antiviral prophylaxis** – Acyclovir is the most useful drug at preventing Herpes reactivation. Dose is dependent on degree of immunosuppression and thus the likely organism to be encountered. 400mg bd will prevent HSV reactivation eg post-standard chemotherapy; 400mg qds may prevent HZV reactivation eg post-SCT; 800mg tds or more may prevent CMV reactivation post-allogeneic SCT.
- **Additional prophylaxis for specials situations** – history of, or radiological evidence of, tuberculosis (TB). Consideration should be given to standard anti-TB prophylaxis eg rimactazid/pyridoxine particularly if prolonged neutropenia expected. Splenectomised patient – at extra risk from encapsulated organisms particularly *Streptococcus pneumoniae*, *Haemophilus influenzae* and *Neisseria meningitidis*. Use penicillin V 500mg od PO or Erythromycin 250 mg od PO if penicillin allergic as prophylaxis switching to high dose amoxycillin/cefotaxime if febrile. Post-SCT (see p218).

Protocols and procedures

461

Guidelines for use of IV antibiotics in neutropenic patients

▶▶ When neutropenic patient develops any of the following, action should be taken urgently:

- Single fever spike >38°C.
- 2 fever spikes >37.5°C within 24h.
- Symptoms and signs of sepsis even in the absence of fever.

Assessment should include

1. Search for any localising symptoms or signs of infection.
2. Full examination including pulse and BP.
3. O_2 saturation (pulse oximetry).
4. Perform a 'Septic Screen' consisting of the following investigations
   - peripheral blood cultures
   - blood cultures taken from each lumen of the indwelling central venous catheter and labelled clearly with colour code.
   - throat swab (for both microbiology and virology)
   - swab of central venous catheter exit site
   - sputum culture
   - MSU plus urinalysis
   - stool culture including *Cl. difficile*
   - CXR
   - other investigations as clinically indicated, eg sinus x-rays.

Start patient on appropriate first line IV antibiotics which aim to give a broad spectrum cover. Prophylactic oral ciprofloxacin should be stopped on commencing IV antibiotics. Follow local protocol if available.

Suggested algorithm is as follows

If patient is NOT penicillin allergic–

- Azlocillin 5g tds IV + gentamicin.
- Use loading dose if creatinine normal, and subsequent doses according to renal function and gentamicin levels. (Consult local gentamicin policy for adjustments in impaired renal function and for subsequent doses.)

If patient IS penicillin allergic–

- Ceftazidime 2g tds IV + gentamicin (as above).
- If patient has not responded to these antibiotics after 24h, and in absence of definitive microbiological diagnosis, patient should be changed to second line antibiotics as follows:

If patient is NOT penicillin allergic–

- Ceftazidime 2g tds IV + teicoplanin 400mg 12-hrly × 2 doses, daily thereafter (split teicoplanin dose if double lumen line *in situ*).

If patient IS penicillin allergic–

- Ciprofloxacin 400mg bd IV + teicoplanin 400mg 12-hrly × 2 doses, daily thereafter. (Ciprofloxacin dosage may be changed to 750mg bd PO after 48h if no problem with systemic absorption and fever resolved.)

If patient remains unresponsive to second line antibiotics after 48h, or there are signs of fungal infection, amphotericin should be added (see p252). If prophylactic fluconazole is used, it should be stopped at this point.

At all times, close cooperation with Microbiology Department should be maintained for advice and further information. If any +ve isolate identified with sensitivities, preferred antibiotic combination to be used should be discussed with expert advice.

Additional notes

- Where there is strong evidence of line infection at onset of fever, it may be reasonable to start with a combination of teicoplanin + gentamicin. In a proven line infection, leave teicoplanin within the line lumen for 1h prior to flushing.
- Metronidazole may be added to any stage of the protocol where anaerobic sepsis is suspected, eg periodontal or perianal disease.

Treatment of neutropenic sepsis when source unknown

▶▶ One of the commonest haemato-oncological emergencies.

- May be defined as the presence of symptoms or signs of infection in a patient with an absolute neutrophil count of $<1.0 \times 10^9/l$. In practice, the neutrophil count is often $<0.1 \times 10^9/l$.
- Similar clinical picture also seen in neutrophil function disorders such as MDS despite normal neutrophil numbers.
- **Beware** – can occur without pyrexia, especially patients on steroids.

Immediate action

▶▶ Urgent clinical assessment.

- Follow ALS guidelines if cardiorespiratory arrest (rare).
- More commonly, clinical picture is more like cardiovascular shock ± respiratory embarrassment viz: tachycardia, hypotension, peripheral vasodilatation and tachypnoea. Occurs with both gram +ve (now more common with indwelling central catheters) and gram –ve organisms (less common but more fulminant).
- Immediate rapid infusion of albumin 4.5% or Gelofusin to restore BP.
- Insert central catheter if not *in situ* and monitor CVP.
- Start O_2 by face mask if pulse oximetry shows saturations <95% (common) and consider arterial blood gas measurement – care with platelet counts $<20 \times 10^9/l$ – manual pressure over puncture site for 30 mins.
- Perform full septic screen (see p462).
- Give the first dose of first line antibiotics immediately e.g ureidopenicillin and loading dose aminoglycoside (ceftazidime or ciprofloxacin if pre-existing renal impairment). Follow established protocols.
- If the event occurs while patient on first line antibiotics, vancomycin/ciprofloxacin or vancomycin/meropenem are suitable alternatives.
- Commence full ITU-type monitoring chart.
- Monitor urine output with urinary catheter if necessary – if renal shutdown has already occurred, give single bolus of IV frusemide. If no response, start renal dose dopamine.
- If BP not restored with colloid despite elevated CVP, consider inotropes.
- If O_2 saturations remain low despite 60% O_2 delivered by rebreathing mask, consider ventilation.
- **Alert ITU giving details of current status.**

Subsequent actions

- Discuss with senior colleague.
- Amend antibiotics according to culture results or to suit likely source if cultures negative.
- Check aminoglycoside trough levels after loading dose and before second dose as renal impairment may determine reducing or withholding next dose. Consider switch to non-nephrotoxic cover e.g ceftazidime/ciprofloxacin.
- Continue antibiotics for 7–10d minimum and usually until neutrophil recovery.
- If cultures show central line to be source of sepsis, remove immediately if patient not responding.

Protocols and procedures

Treatment of neutropenic sepsis when source known/suspected

Central indwelling catheters

Very common. Organisms usually *Staph. epidermidis* but can be other *Staph* spp. and even gram –ve organisms. Signs may be erythema/exudate around entry or exit sites of line, tenderness/erythema over subcutaneous tunnel or discomfort over line tract. Blood cultures must be taken from each lumen and peripherally and labelled individually.

Add Teicoplanin 400mg bd IV if not in standard protocol. Split dose between all lumens unless cultures known to be +ve in one lumen only. Lock and leave in line for 1h, then flush through. If no response within 3 doses or if teicoplanin resistant *Staph. epidermidis* is cultured, switch to vancomycin with loading dose then levels. If still no response or clinical deterioration, ***remove line immediately.***

Perianal or periodontal

Both are common sites of infection in neutropenic patients. Perianal lesions may become secondarily infected if skin abraded. Add metronidazole 500mg IV tds to standard therapy. Painful SC abscesses may form and may require surgical incision. Gum disease and localized tooth infections/abscesses are frequently seen. Add metronidazole to therapy as above, arrange OPG and dental review as surgical intervention may be required in non-responders. If possible, best delayed until neutrophil recovery in most cases – then do electively before next course of chemotherapy.

Lung

Atypical organisms

Risk group

HIV infection, HCL, post-SCT.
Mycoplasma and other atypicals are commonly found and usually community acquired (except *Legionella*) – typically occur shortly after return to hospital and in patients with chronic lung disease.

Treatment

Azithromycin (or clarithromycin if IV preparation needed) is now treatment of choice – well absorbed and fewer SEs than erythromycin. 5d rather than 3d course may be needed.

Pneumocystis carinii pneumonia

Risk group

Lymphoid malignancy long-term treatment esp. ALL, steroid usage, purine analogues eg fludarabine and 2-CDA.

Treatment

High dose cotrimoxazole IV initially – watch renal function and adjust dose to creatinine. Give short pulse of steroid 0.5mg/kg at start of treatment. At risk patients should remain on long-term prophylaxis until chemo finished and absolute CD4 lymphocyte count >500 × 10^6/l. Use cotrimoxazole 480mg bd on Mon, Wed and Fri only, provided neutrophil count maintained >1.0 × 10^9/l. Otherwise use nebulised pentamidine 300mg every 3weeks with preceding nebulised salbutamol 2.5mg.

Protocols and procedures

Fungal

Risk group

Prolonged, severe neutropenia, chronic steroid and antibiotic usage, GvHD. *Aspergillus* and other moulds increasingly common with intensive chemotherapy protocols and post-stem cell transplant esp. MUDs.

Treatment

- Amphotericin IV (see p252–253).
- Once neutrophil recovery has occurred, maintenance treatment may be with oral itraconazole liquid 2.5mg/kg bd – may also be used for prophylaxis.

Viral – CMV

Risk group

Allogeneic SCT especially MUDs where either donor or recipient is CMV seropositive. Disease usually due to reactivation rather than *de novo* infection. Apart from pneumonitis, may cause graft suppression, gastritis and oesophagitis, weight loss, hepatitis, retinitis, haemorrhagic cystitis and vertigo.

Treatment

Ganciclovir or foscarnet (see CMV p254) + IV immunoglobulin. Lack of response, switch to the other drug.

Viral – HSV/HZV

Risk group

Rare causes of lung disease. SCT recipients at greatest risk esp. MUDs and intensively treated lymphoid malignancy.

Treatment

High dose IV acyclovir 5–10mg/kg tds IV for minimum 10d.

Viral – RSV

Risk group

Post-SCT recipients esp. MUDs.

Treatment

Consider Ribovarin therapy.

TB and atypical Mycobacteria

Risk group

Prolonged T cell immunosuppression eg chronic steroid or cyclosporin therapy, chronic GvHD, previous history and/or treatment for TB, HIV related disease.

Treatment

Often difficult to diagnose – empirical treatment required with standard triple therapy.

Prophylaxis for patients treated with purine analogues

The purine analogues fludarabine and 2-CDA used in standard lympho-proliferative protocols induce neutropenia in all cases. Nadir ~14d post-treatment initiation and neutrophil counts may fall to zero for several days or even weeks. They are therefore associated with the usual neutropenic infections. In addition, purine analogues have a particular property of inhibition of T4 helper lymphocyte subsets within weeks of initiation of therapy (nadir at 3 months) and may last for >1 year following cessation of therapy. This profound T4 function inhibition predisposes to fungal infection, as well as a higher incidence of herpes zoster infection and PCP. ↓ lymphocyte function also predisposes to transfusion associated GvHD in passenger lymphocytes of donor blood transfusions.

The following preventive measures are recommended

Recommended

1. Irradiation of cellular blood products (2500 cGy) from day 1 of initiation of therapy and continue until 2 years post-treatment.
2. PCP prophylaxis from start of therapy – usually cotrimoxazole 1 tablet bd Mondays, Wednesdays and Fridays. In patients who are already severely neutropenic, cotrimoxazole may be substituted by pentamidine nebulisers 300mg 3-weekly with 2.5 mg of salbutamol nebuliser pre-treatment. PCP prophylaxis should continue until a year after the end of treatment.
3. HZV prophylaxis – acyclovir 400mg qds is the minimum continuous dose required to prevent HZV reactivation. Most physicians will not wish to have patients continuously on this dosage throughout the treatment cycle and for a year post-treatment so suggest: counsel patients about the risk of shingles and advised to contact the hospital immediately if shingles suspected. Patients who have already had a zoster reactivation should be maintained continuously on acyclovir 400 mg qds and continuation of the purine analogue reviewed.

Optional

1. Anti-bacterial prophylaxis – consider use of ciprofloxacin 250mg bd PO from day 7 → 21 of each course.
2. Anti-fungal prophylaxis: Patients with no history of fungal reactivation should perform nystatin suspension 1ml qds mouthcare from day 7 → 21 of each course, taught symptoms of oral and genital thrush and supplied with fluconazole 200mg to be taken daily for 7d in the event of thrush.
3. Patients with previous history of suspected fungal infection with a mould-type organism eg *Aspergillus* – give itraconazole capsules 400mg daily or oral liquid 2.5mg/kg bd throughout treatment.

Protocols and procedures

Acute tumour lysis syndrome

Initiation of chemotherapy in patients with high tumour load may result in rapid cellular breakdown and release of intracellular contents into the circulation. This may be severe in patients with high count leukaemias and high grade lymphomas. Profound metabolic disturbances can occur within a few hours of commencing chemotherapy, may persist for several days and may result in permanent renal damage and fatality.

- *Hyperkalaemia* – especially if very large tumour burdens and with preexisting renal impairment.
- ↑ *urea and creatinine* – usually commencing within 24h of chemotherapy as result of tumour lysis and direct effect of breakdown products on the kidneys.
- *Hyperphosphataemia and hypocalcaemia* – rising phosphate levels frequently the earliest sign of tumour lysis syndrome.
- *Hyperuricaemia.*

Tumour lysis syndrome should be anticipated – and best treatment is *avoidance of its occurrence.*

Identify 'at risk' patients
- High count ALL (WCC >50 × 10^9/l).
- High count AML (WCC>100 × 10^9/l).
- High count CML (WCC>100 × 10^9/l).
- High count CLL (WCC>200 × 10^9/l and extensive disease).
- High grade NHL.

Establish adequate hydration should be commenced at least 24h prior to the commencement of chemotherapy. A diuresis of more than 100ml/h should be achieved for at least 6h prior to chemotherapy. Aim for total fluid intake of at least 4l/d. Strict fluid balance should be maintained at all times and the patient should be weighed bd. Small amounts of IV frusemide (20mg) may be given if evidence of fluid retention.

Allopurinol ideally, this should be started 24h prior to chemotherapy. If renal function is normal give 300mg bd PO. However, if creatinine >100μmol/l, give 100mg alternate days.

Alkalinisation may be achieved PO or IV depending on venous access. IV regimen reserved for patients with central venous access. *Oral regimen:* 3g sodium bicarbonate PO 2 hourly. *Intravenous regimen:* cycles are repeated every 6h.

250ml	2.74% NaHCO$_3$ over 1h
1000ml	5% dextrose over 4h
500ml	0.9% NaCl over 1h

▶ *Never use full strength IV bicarbonate.*

All urine passed should be pH tested and the chemotherapy should not be started until two urines of pH 8 have been passed at least 1h apart. Tumour lysis regime must be continued until WCC <10 × 10^9/l.

Patient monitoring
Monitor at least bd during the first 24h of treatment: serum K^+, urea and creatinine, Ca^{2+}, phosphate, and uric acid. Perform ECG pre-treatment, subsequently if indicated by the K^+/Ca^{2+}. If hyperkalaemia develops, the following measures should be undertaken:

Protocols and procedures

1 Measure arterial blood gases (severe acidosis will make the hyperkalaemia more difficult to correct).
2 If K⁺ >5mmol/l, start calcium resonium 15g PO qds and increase hydration. Repeat K⁺ 2h later.
3 If K⁺ >6mmol/l, ECG stat and if obvious hyperkalaemic changes give 10ml 10% calcium chloride IV. Commence insulin/dextrose infusion (50ml 50% dextrose with 20u actrapid insulin over 1h).

Indications for haemodialysis
- K⁺ not controlled by above measures.
- Rising urea, creatinine or phosphate despite the above.
- Fluid overload unresponsive to diuretics.

Management of chronic bone marrow failure

Introduction
Common haematological problem. Occurs as result of marrow infiltrated with disease eg MDS, or following chemotherapy or other causes of marrow aplasia. Extent of RBC, WBC and platelet production failure varies greatly in individual clinical situations. Production failure may not affect all three cell lines equally.

Management
- Mainstay is supportive treatment with blood products and antibiotics.
- Underlying disease should be treated where possible.

Red cell production failure
- Where anaemia is due solely to absence of RBC production, transfusion requirement should be ~1 unit packed red cells/week. Suitable protocol is 3 unit transfusion every 3 weeks as day case.
- If requirement is greater, investigate for bleeding and haemolysis.
- If requirement is chronic eg a young patient with MDS, consider giving red cells leucodepleted by filtration to prevent HLA sensitisation and give desferrioxamine as long-term iron chelation (see p85).
- Erythropoietin may be tried where some red cell production capacity remains and transfusion needs to be avoided or minimised eg Jehovah's Witnesses.

White cell production failure
- Mainstay of treatment is with antibiotics.
- Prompt treatment of fever in neutropenic patient with combination IV antibiotics is lifesaving.
- Simple mouthcare with Corsadyl or similar mouthwash, plus nystatin suspension orally reduces risk of bacterial and fungal colonisation in oropharynx. Dietary modifications may also be helpful.
- Role of prophylactic antibiotics remains controversial as resistance generation is an increasing problem.
- Ciprofloxacin 250 mg bd PO is probably the best single agent.
- Patients with recurring foci of infection may have prophylaxis targeted to their usual or most likely organisms.
- Patients with neutropenia and low Igs who have developed bronchiectasis may benefit from regular infusions of IVIg 200mg/kg every 4 weeks ± rotating antibiotic courses.
- WBC infusions are not generally useful except in rare situations – they are toxic and cause HLA sensitisation.
- Haemopoietic growth factors should not be used routinely.
- Life-threatening infections despite IV antibiotics and anti-fungals can be considered for trial of G-CSF or GM-CSF at 5µg/kg/d SC.

Platelet production failure
Where low platelets are due solely to absence of platelet production, transfusion requirement should be ~1–2 adult dose packs/week. If requirement is chronic eg young MDS patient, consider giving platelets leucodepleted by filtration to prevent HLA sensitisation and platelet refractoriness (see p458). Tranexamic acid 1g qds PO may reduce clinical bleeding episodes and transfusion requirement. Thrombopoietin (TPO) is a potent *in vitro* platelet growth and maturation factor but its clinical role remains to be defined.

Venepuncture

Blood samples are best taken from an antecubital vein using a 21G needle and a Vacutainer™ system or syringe. If a large volume of blood is required a 21G butterfly may be inserted to facilitate changing the vacutainer sample bottle or the syringe.

A tourniquet should be gently applied to the upper arm and the antecubital fossa inspected and palpated for veins. In an obese individual antecubital veins may be more easily palpated than seen. The skin over the vein should be 'sterilised' (alcohol swab or Mediswab™) and allowed to dry. The needle should then be gently introduced along the line of the chosen vein at an angle of 45° to the skin surface. It may be helpful to attempt to penetrate the skin with the initial intro-duction of the needle and then slowly penetrate the vessel wall by continuing the forward movement of the needle. The tourniquet on the upper arm should be loosened once the needle has been inserted into the vein to reduce haemocon-centration. If a syringe is used the piston should be withdrawn slowly to prevent collapse of the vein. Once an adequate sample has been obtained, the tourniquet should be completely removed, a dry cotton wool ball applied gently above the site of venepuncture and gentle pressure increased as the needle is removed. Firm pressure should be directly applied to the venepuncture site for 3–5 minutes to ensure haemostasis and prevent extravasation and bruising. A small elastoplast or if allergic, suitable light dressing, should be applied to the venepuncture site.

In patients in whom it is difficult to obtain a sample, the arm should be kept warm, a sphygmomanometer cuff inflated on the upper arm to the diastolic pressure and the vein may be dilated by smacking the overlying skin. With patience it is rarely impossible to obtain a venous sample. In very obese individuals or those in whom iatrogenic thrombosis or sclerosis has occurred in the antecubital veins, the dorsal veins of the hand may be used for sampling though a smaller gauge needle (23G) or butterfly is often necessary.

Protocols and procedures

Venesection

Aim of venesection or phlebotomy is the removal of blood for donation to the Blood Transfusion Service or as a therapeutic manoeuvre for a patient with haemochromatosis or polycythaemia rubra vera or for a patient who requires an exchange transfusion. In patients with haemochromatosis or PRV the therapeutic effect of the venesection programme to date should be assessed on a full blood count sample taken prior to venesection.

Procedure

- Patient or donor is best placed lying on a couch with the chosen arm placed comfortably on a supporting pillow.
- A large gauge needle attached to a collection pack containing anticoagulant is inserted in an antecubital vein or forearm vein after application of a sphygmomanometer cuff to the upper arm (inflated to diastolic pressure) and sterilisation of the skin. It is widespread practice to infiltrate the skin over the chosen vein with local anaesthetic (1% lignocaine) prior to insertion of the large bore needle.
- Inflation of the sphygmomanometer cuff is maintained until the desired volume of blood is collected.
- The patient may assist the flow of blood by squeezing a soft ball or similar object in the hand of the arm from which the blood is drawn.
- Blood is allowed to drain into the collection pack until the desired volume has been obtained (usually 500ml).
- The volume collected may be monitored by suspension of the pack from a simple spring measuring device.
- The positioning of the collection pack below the patient's (or donor's) level facilitates blood flow into the bag.
- Once the desired volume has been collected the cuff is deflated, the line should be clamped and the needle removed and a dry cotton wool ball used to apply pressure to the venesection site.
- Direct firm pressure should be applied for five minutes and the site inspected for haemostasis prior to application of a firm bandage.
- The patient should slowly adopt the erect posture and should remain seated for several minutes if symptoms of lightheadedness occur.
- Patients should not be permitted to drive after venesection.
- The collected blood from a therapeutic venesection should be disposed of by incineration.

Note: for patients with PPP/PRV isovolaemic venesection is recommended to minimise volume depletion whilst still reducing Hct. See p188.

Protocols and procedures

477

Bleeding time

A useful global test of *platelet function*, the BT is defined as the time taken for an incision to stop bleeding. The initial BT involved stabbing an earlobe (Duke's BT); next came the Ivy BT with 2–3 small stabs with a lancet on the forearm.

Recommended method

Use a template device (eg Simplate™, General Diagnostics), a small spring loaded sterile disposable blade(s) to deliver a 5mm × 1mm deep cut(s) on the forearm, with a constant cuff pressure of 40mm Hg. Serially blot (every 30 sec) with filter paper the blood flowing from the wound till bleeding stops – *do not touch the wound edge.*

Adult normal range 2.5–9.5 min (a paediatric Simplate™ and range is available).

Advantage a simple bedside test of overall platelet function. Used as a pre-surgical screening test eg before renal or liver biopsy.

Disadvantage not sensitive to minor platelet dysfunction.

Aspirin and other NSAIDs can prolong the BT and should not be taken within 10 days of testing. The effect may not be marked; the BT could ↑ from 4 to 8 min ie still within the normal range.

Time consuming if grossly prolonged (stop test if BT >15 min). Leaves small scar.

Practical application

- BT is ↑ in thrombocytopenia, platelet function disorders and some congenital and acquired bleeding disorders. Prolonged with severe anaemia.
- In a patient with otherwise unexplained bleeding, an ↑ BT is a clue and points to the need for further platelet function tests.
- In vWD, it helps quantify the vWD defect but with limitations – not always closely related to Factor VIII activities and clinical bleeding.
- Can be used to monitor the therapeutic response to eg platelet transfusion.
- Increased in certain vascular abnormalities eg Ehlers-Danlos syndrome.
- Note drug induced prolongation (*see above*).

Tunnelled central venous catheters

A tunnelled central venous catheter is required in all patients undergoing intensive cytotoxic chemotherapy and those undergoing bone marrow or peripheral blood stem cell transplantation. Also indicated for some patients on long-term regular transfusion programmes.

Catheter type

A double or triple lumen catheter preferred, and essential for patients undergoing transplantation procedures. Hickman catheters are available from Vygon UK and the Groshong lines (Bard) are available for use in all patients except those needing stem cell collections who will require apheresis catheters (Kimal).

Requirements

An X-ray screening room with facility for aseptic procedures or an operating theatre is required. A trained radiographer must be available for X-ray screening throughout the procedure. In addition a minimum of two staff are required for the safe execution of this procedure. One should be a member of medical staff (Radiologist/Surgeon/Anaesthetist/Haemato-oncologist) to insert the catheter and administer sedation and antibiotics and the other to generally assist. The second person can be an IV trained nurse.

Patient assessment

Assess for fitness for sedation and the ability to lie flat. Plan position of central venous catheter in advance. The first choice is the right subclavian vein, followed by the left subclavian vein. Check FBC and clotting screen. Platelets should be available if platelet count is less than 50×10^9/l.

Patient preparation

The patient should be well hydrated ($\downarrow$ CVP makes procedure difficult), and fasting for 6 hours prior to the procedure as sedative drugs will be administered. Good peripheral venous access must be established (with Venflon™) before commencing central venous cannulation, for the administration of sedative drugs and prophylactic antibiotics as well as for emergency venous access.

Technique

Follow manufacturer's instructions. Sequence of stages during insertion is as follows:

1. Cannulation of the central vein, placement of guide wire and creation of the upper central wound.
2. Creation of lower peripheral wound, formation of subcutaneous tunnel and threading of the catheter through subcutaneous tunnel with cuff buried.
3. Placement of the vessel dilator/sheath in the central vein over the guide wire.
4. Placement of the catheter into the sheath.
5. Careful removal of the sheath whilst retaining position of catheter.
6. Suturing of the upper and lower wounds with suture around the body of the catheter close to the exit site to hold the catheter in position.
7. Manipulate catheter so tip lies in SVC above right atrium. Patency must be confirmed by easy aspiration of blood, and the catheter flushed with heparinised saline. Check position with standard PA chest radiograph.

Sedation and analgesia

IV sedation is used if the patient is particularly anxious before or during the procedure.

Prophylactic antibiotics

- Teicoplanin 400mg is administered by peripheral vein immediately prior to central venous cannulation.
- 400mg teicoplanin is also administered into the central venous catheter immediately after the insertion procedure (200mg is locked into each lumen for 1h and then the catheter is flushed with heparinised saline.

Catheter aftercare

- Catheter may be used immediately after above procedures. All patients should be educated in the care of their indwelling tunnelled intravenous catheter. This may include self-flushing of the catheter. Catheter should be flushed after each use with saline and locked with heparinised saline. Flush twice weekly when not in use.
- Urokinase may be used if line blockage occurs, insert urokinase and leave for 4–12h and remove.
- Clindamycin roll-on lotion may be applied to the exit site to minimise local infections.
- Upper wound suture is removed 7d post-insertion.
- Lower exit site suture can be removed at 2 weeks post-insertion for most lines and 3 weeks for apheresis lines to ensure SC embedding of the cuff.

Bone marrow examination

Bone marrow is the key investigation in haematology. It may prove *diagnostic* in the follow-up of abnormal peripheral blood findings. It is an important *staging* procedure in defining the extent of disease, especially lymphoprolifera-tive disorders. It is a helpful *investigative* procedure in unexplained anaemia, splenomegaly or selected cases of pyrexia of unknown origin (PUO). Preferred site for sampling → posterior iliac crest; aspirate and biopsy material can easily be obtained from this location. The anterior iliac crest is an alternative. The sternum is suitable only for marrow aspiration (see below for contraindications).

Marrow aspirate material provides information on
- Cytology of nucleated cells.
- Qualitative and semi-qualitative analysis of haematopoiesis.
- Assessment of iron stores.
- Smears for cytochemistry of atypical cells.

Suspensions of marrow cells in medium are suitable for
- Chromosomal (cytogenetic) analysis.
- Immunophenotype studies using monoclonal antibodies directed against cell surface antigens.
- Aliquots of marrow can be cryopreserved for future molecular analysis.

Marrow trephine biopsy yields information on
- Marrow cellularity.
- Identification/classification of abnormal cellular infiltrates.
- Immunohistochemistry on infiltrates.

Note: Cytology of trephine imprints can be helpful, especially when aspirate yields a 'drytap'. Trephine biopsy information complements that obtained at aspiration.

Contraindications
None, other than physical limitations eg pain or restricted mobility. Avoid sites of previous radiotherapy (inevitably grossly hypocellular and not representative).

Procedure
Bone marrow aspiration may be performed under local anaesthesia alone, but short acting intravenous benzodiazepines (eg midazolam) preferred when trephine biopsy is performed. General anaesthesia rarely used (except in children). Best position is with patient in L or R lateral position. Skin and periosteum over the posterior iliac spine are infiltrated with local anaesthetic. A small cutaneous incision is made, the aspirating needle is introduced through this and should penetrate the marrow cortex 3–10mm before removal of the trocar. No more than 0.5–1ml marrow should be aspirated initially, and smear made promptly. Further material can be aspirated and placed in EDTA or other anti-coagulant media for other studies. An Islam or Jamshidi needle is preferred for trephine biopsy. The needle is advanced through the same puncture site to penetrate the cortex. The trocar is removed and using firm hand pressure the needle is rotated clockwise and should be advanced as far as possible. The needle is removed by gentle anti-clockwise rotation. In this manner an experienced operator should regularly obtain biopsy samples of 25–35mm in length. Simple pressure dressings are sufficient aftercare and minor discomfort at the location may be dealt with by simple analgesia such as paracetamol.

Administration of chemotherapy

Cytotoxic chemotherapeutic drugs may cause serious harm if not prescribed, dispensed and administered with great care. Drugs should be prescribed, dispensed and administered by an experienced multidisciplinary team with shared clear information on:

- The fitness of the patient to receive chemotherapy (eg recent FBC for myelosuppressive agents, renal function studies for cisplatinum).
- Appropriate protocol and chemotherapeutic regimen for the patient.
- Prescribed drugs and individualised dosage for the patient's surface area (see p484), taking note of cumulative maximum doses (eg anthracyclines).
- Appropriate supportive treatment required eg allopurinol, antiemetic prophylaxis, anti-infective prophylaxis, and hydration.

Chemotherapy for IV administration should be reformulated carefully in accordance with the manufacturer's instructions by an experienced pharmacist using a class B laminar airflow hood. Care should be taken to ensure that the drug is administered within the expiry time after it has been reformulated in the form chosen.

Many cytotoxic drugs are best administered as a slow IVI in dextrose or 0.9% saline over 30 minutes to 2h. *Vesicants* eg vincristine, daunorubicin, adriamycin and mitozantrone should be administered as a slow IV 'push'. However this should only be administered through the side access port of a freely flowing infusion of 0.9% saline or dextrose and should *never be injected directly into a peripheral vein*.

If the patient does not have an indwelling intravenous catheter (Hickman line), a teflon or silicone intravenous cannula of adequate bore (≤21G) should be inserted into a vein of sufficient diameter to permit a freely flowing 0.9% saline infusion to be commenced. Site chosen should be one where cannula can be easily inserted and observed, can be fastened securely and will not be subject to movement during drug administration. The veins of the forearm are the most suitable for this purpose followed by those on the dorsum of the hand. Antecubital fossae and other sites close to joints are best avoided. The risk of extravasation (see p484) is increased by the use of a cannula which has not been inserted recently and by the use of steel (butterfly) cannulae.

A slow 'push' injection should be administered carefully into the side access port on the IV line with continuous observation of the drip chamber ensure that the infusion is continuing to run during injection of the cytotoxic drug. The patient should be asked whether any untoward sensations are being experienced at the site of the infusion and the site should be carefully observed to ensure that no extravasation is occurring. Patency of the IV site should be verified regularly throughout the procedure. The saline or dextrose infusion should be continued for 30 minutes after the chemotherapy administration has been completed before the cannula is removed.

The administration of potentially extravasable chemotherapy, site of cannulation, condition of the site and any symptoms associated with administration should be clearly documented in the patient's notes.

485

Antiemetics for chemotherapy

Classification of drugs

Dopamine antagonists – block D_2 receptors in the chemoreceptor trigger zone (CTZ). Examples are metoclopramide and domperidone – both have additional effect on enhancing gastric emptying. SEs include extrapyramidal reactions and occasionally oculogyric crisis.

Phenothiazines – examples are prochlorperazine and cyclizine – particular benefit in opioid-induced nausea. SEs include anticholinergic effects and drowsiness.

Benzodiazepines – lorazepam commonest used. Advantages are long $t\frac{1}{2}$ and additional anxiolytic effect. SEs include drowsiness.

5HT₃ antagonists – block $5HT_3$ receptors in the CTZ. Examples include ondansetron, granisetron and tropesitron. SEs include headaches, bowel disturbance and rashes.

Cannabinoids – nabilone is the major drug. SEs include depersonalisation experiences.

Steroids – examples are dexamethasone and prednisolone. SEs include fungal infection predisposition, hypertension, irritability and sleeplessness, gastric erosions and, with chronic use, diabetes and osteoporosis.

Emesis with chemotherapy

Categorised as: anticipatory, early or late.

Anticipatory occurs in advance of chemotherapy. Psychogenic in origin, it occurs in patients with previous bad experiences of nausea and vomiting and almost unknown prior to first dose. May be largely prevented by ensuring a positive experience with first dose by use of prophylactic antiemetics.

Early occurs within minutes of IV chemotherapy administration or within hours of oral chemotherapy. The easiest to respond to antiemetics generally.

Late occurs after the end of a chemotherapy course – up to 7d. The most difficult form to treat – requires continuation of antiemetics throughout post chemo period and even the newer agents such as the $5HT_3$ receptor antagonists are relatively ineffective.

Antiemetics may be used singly or in combination. Choices determined largely by patient preferences and degree of emetic potential of the chemo regimen to be used. These may be divided into high, medium and low.

Highly emetogenic regimens
Examples include CisPlatinum, high dose cyclophosphamide and TBI. Suitable cocktail might be domperidone, $5HT_3$ antagonist and dexamethasone ± lorazepam.

Medium emetogenic regimens
Examples include anthracyclines, cytosine arabinoside. Suitable cocktail might be domperidone, cyclizine ± $5HT_3$ antagonist ± lorazepam.

Low emetogenic regimens
Examples include chlorambucil, vinca alkaloids, 6MP, fludarabine and most steroid-containing protocols. Suitable choice would be metoclopramide or domperidone as single agent.

Protocols and procedures

Intrathecal chemotherapy

Usage
- Given for both prophylaxis and treatment of CNS disease.
- May be used in addition to other CNS disease strategies such as high dose IV methotrexate or cranial irradiation.
- CNS involvement is detected by presence of blasts on CSF cytospin.
- The ONLY cytotoxic drugs used intrathecally are:
    methotrexate
    cytosine arabinoside
    hydrocortisone.
- All have strict upper dosage limits – *follow the protocol.*

▶▶ *Never use any other cytotoxic drugs for intrathecal injection – fatal consequences may ensue.*

Common protocols
1. CNS prophylaxis for ALL and high grade NHL:
  – methotrexate $10mg/m^2$ (max 12.5mg) × 6 injections at weekly intervals.
2. CNS prophylaxis for AML:
  – Ara-C $30mg/m^2$ (max 50mg), dosage schedule varies.
3. CNS treatment for ALL:
  Triple IT regimen viz:
    methotrexate $15mg/m^2$ (max 12.5–15mg)
    ara-C $30mg/m^2$ (max 50mg)
    hydrocortisone $15mg/m^2$.
Usually given twice weekly until CSF clear of blasts then weekly to a maximum of 6 total courses. Consider using folinic acid rescue.

Technique
- Standard contraindications to lumbar puncture apply – alternatives will be needed in these situations. Cytotoxics should be made up freshly in smallest possible volume in a sterile pharmacy.
- Consider GA for children and IV sedation for adults.
- Use special LP 'blunt' needle or small gauge bevelled LP needle.
- Aim to remove the same volume of CSF as you are injecting intrathecally (may be several ml if giving triple chemotherapy).
- Take samples for CSF cytospin to determine blast cell concentration, microbiology for M/C/S, biochemistry for protein and glucose.
- Check syringe cytotoxic dose carefully with another person before connecting.
- Connect syringe and aspirate gently to confirm position in CSF. Inject slowly, drawing back at intervals to reconfirm position. Disconnect syringe and connect other syringes in turn if giving 'triple'.
- Follow standard post-LP precautions. Document procedure in notes.
- Repeated IT chemotherapy carries risk of CSF leakage and post-LP headache. Manometry pre-injection may help assess whether less CSF should be withdrawn pre-injection.
- A syndrome of methotrexate-induced neurotoxicity occurs in a few patients presenting with features of meningo-encephalitis. Aetiology is unknown. Treat with short pulse of high dose steroids.
  ▶ *Do not give further IT methotrexate to these patients.*

Protocols and procedures

Management of extravasation

Inappropriate or accidental administration of chemotherapy into subcutaneous tissue rather than into the intravenous compartment causes pain, erythema and inflammation which may lead to sloughing of the skin and severe tissue necrosis. Appropriate early treatment can prevent the most serious consequences of extravasation. All chemotherapy units should have a protocol with which all staff administering chemotherapy are familiar and a regularly updated extravasation kit for the management of extravasation giving first aid instructions and further directions.

The risk of tissue damage relates to the drug's ability to bind to DNA, to kill replicating cells, to cause tissue or vascular dilatation and its pH, osmolarity, concentration, volume and formulation components eg alcohol, polyethylene glycol.

Drugs may be divided into three risk groups:

Group 1:   Vesicants
Aclarubicin; amsacrine; carmustine; cisplatinum; dacarbazine; dactinomycin; daunorubicin; docetaxel; doxorubicin; epirubicin; idarubicin; mitomycin; mustine; paclitaxel; plicamycin; treosulfan; vinblastine; vincristine; vindesine.

Group 2:   Irritants (may cause local inflammation, pain and necrosis)
Carboplatin; etoposide; liposomal daunorubicin; methotrexate; mitozantrone.

Group 3:   Non-vesicants
Asparaginase; bleomycin; cladribine; cyclophosphamide; cytarabine; fludarabine; fluorouracil; gemcitabine; ifosfamide; melphalan; pentostatin; raltitrexed; thiotepa; aldesleukin (IL-2).

Symptoms and signs
- Burning, stinging or pain at the injection site.
- Induration, swelling, venous discolouration or erythema at the injection site.
- No blood return.
- Reduced flow rate.
- Increased resistance to administration.

Pre-extravasation syndrome
- Severe phlebitis and/or local hypersensitivity.
- Local risk factors eg difficult cannulation and one patient symptom.
- Withdraw IV therapy immediately to prevent progression to extravasation.

Type I extravasation
- Bleb or blister with defined area of induration around site of extravasation.
- Often due to rapid iv bolus injection with excessive pressure.

Type II extravasation
- Diffuse boggy tissue injury with dispersal into the intracellular space.
- Associated with IV infusion or IV bolus into side arm port of infusion with dislodged cannula.

Protocols and procedures

General treatment guidelines

- Stop the infusion, disconnect the IV line but do not remove the cannula.
- Mark the area of injury around the cannula tip.
- Seek the help of a more experienced individual if available.
- Aspirate the site of extravasation to remove as much of the offending drug as possible through cannula with a fresh 10ml syringe; this may be facilitated with SC injection of 0.9% saline.
- Remove the cannula.
- Administer 100mg hydrocortisone intravenously at another site.
- Administer a further 100mg hydrocortisone locally by 6–8 SC injections around the area of injury.
- Administer SC injections of specific antidote where available.
- Apply 1% hydrocortisone cream to the area and repeat bd whilst erythema persists.
- Cover with gauze and apply heat to disperse the drug or cool to localise the extravasation.
- Administer oral antihistamine (terfenadine 60mg/chlorpheniramine 4mg).
- Administer analgesia if required (indomethacin 25mg tds).
- Document site and extent of extravasation and treatment in the case notes.
- Photograph site if possible.
- Complete a 'Green Card' to report the extravasation episode.
- Monitor injured site twice daily for erythema, induration, blistering or necrosis.
- Photograph injured site weekly until healed.

Specific procedures

Group 1: vesicant drugs

All vesicants except vinca alkaloids & cisplatinum	Apply cold pack instantly. SC dexamethasone 4mg around margins. Elevate limb but encourage movement. Reapply cold pack for 24h.
Actinomycin D	Infiltrate area with 1–3ml 3% sodium thiosulphate.
Aclarubicin Daunorubicin Doxorubicin Epirubicin Idarubicin Mitomycin	Topical DMSO painted every 2h followed by hydrocortisone cream and 30 mins cold compression. Repeated for 24h thereafter DMSO and hydrocortisone should be alternated every 3h; if blistering occurs stop DMSO.
Cisplatinum	Infiltrate area with 1-3ml 3% sodium thiosulphate, aspirate off then administer 1500 units hyaluronidase and apply heat and compression.
Carmustine	Infiltrate area with 1-3ml sodium bicarbonate diluted to plicamycin 2.1%, avoid normal tissue at the margins, leave 2 mins then aspirate off.
Docetaxel Paclitaxel	Infiltrate area with 1–3ml of a mixture of 100mg hydrocortisone and 4mg chlorpheniramine as 0.2ml pincushion injections, followed by 1500U of hyaluronidase then warm compression alternated with topical antihistamine cream; hydrocortisone and antihistamine creams should be applied alternately for 3d. In severe cases administer 1g sodium cromoglycate po as soon as possible.
Mustine	Infiltrate area with 1-3ml 3% sodium thiosulphate then infiltrate with 100mg hydrocortisone, apply cold compression intermittently for 12h.
Vincristine, vinblastine, vindesine	Infiltrate area with 1500 units of hyaluronidase as 0.2ml sc over and around the affected area; apply heat and compression for 24h then apply topical non-steroidal anti-inflammatory cream to the area qds.

Group 2: irritant drugs
- Aspirate as much as possible.
- Administer 100mg hydrocortisone IV.
- Administer 100mg hydrocortisone SC at multiple sites around the margins of the extravasation.
- Apply topical hydrocortisone.
- Cover area with an ice pack.
- Manage symptoms.

Group 3: non-vesicant drugs
- Aspirate as much as possible.
- Disperse extravasated drug with SC hyaluronidase injection around the area.
- Apply heat and compression to aid dispersal.
- Manage symptoms.

Splenectomy

Splenectomy is an established procedure in management of selected haematological disorders. Its removal is usually required for one or more of the following reasons:

- Extreme enlargement.
- Hyperfunction.
- Autoimmune activity.
- Diagnostic and therapeutic purposes.

Indications include:

- **Lymphoproliferative disorders**, eg CLL, mantle zone lymphoma, hairy cell leukaemia. Reasons include massive organomegaly, occurrence of autoimmune complications and for diagnostic and/or therapeutic purposes.
- **Myeloproliferative disorders** – commonly used in myelofibrosis to reduce transfusion requirements, abdominal discomfort from massive splenic enlargement and may reduce constitutional symptoms eg weight loss and night sweats. Occasionally used in the management of chronic myeloid leukaemia.
- **Autoimmune conditions** – an accepted treatment in autoimmune thrombocytopenic purpura and autoimmune haemolytic anaemia following the failure of immunosuppression with corticosteroids and immunoglobulin (in the case of thrombocytopenic purpura). The procedure is not curative but may result in prolonged remissions and certainly will have steroid-sparing effect.
- **Hereditary disorders** – reduces red cell sequestration and transfusion requirements in homozygous β-thalassaemia. Recurrent, severe hereditary spherocytosis. Rare indications include pyruvate kinase deficiency and type 1 Gaucher's disease. Other circumstances where splenectomy may help include Felty's syndrome.
- **Staging splenectomy** is no longer a routine procedure for non-Hodgkin's lymphoma or Hodgkin's disease.

The clinician has to balance the risks and benefits of the procedure in an individual patient bearing in mind the *long-term risk of post-splenectomy sepsis* as well as immediate surgical factors. There are now established consensus guidelines for carrying out splenectomy.

Pre-operatively the need for the procedure is agreed with the patient and surgical team. At least 2 weeks pre-operatively immunisation with Pneumococcal and Haemophilus vaccine should be given. Meningococcal vaccine may be offered but this covers sub-types A and C only and does not give long-lasting immunity. Peri-operative thromboembolic risks should be considered (eg standard surgical risks and those posed by the rebound thrombocytosis after splenectomy). Low dose heparin may be appropriate peri-operatively followed by low dose aspirin (may require modification in thrombocytopenia or if platelet dysfunction). Before discharge, patients must be given a leaflet/card which they carry. Lifelong prophylaxis with penicillin V 250mg bd recommended or Erythromycin 250mg bd if the patient is allergic to penicillin. The patient and his/her family must be advised to report urgently profound systemic symptoms, most promptly to their nearest local A & E Department.

Re-vaccination with Pneumococcal vaccine every 5 years recommended. Asplenic patients travelling to malarial areas must be meticulous in taking anti-malarial prophylaxis (greater risk of severe illness from *Plasmodium falciparum*).

Plasma exchange (plasmapheresis)

Plasmapheresis is the therapeutic removal of plasma from the peripheral blood usually carried out by a cell separator machine. The removed plasma is replaced isovolaemically usually by albumin/saline combinations depending on indication, plasma albumin level and frequency of exchange. Blood products may also be given as part of replacement which is useful in patients with fluid intolerance eg on renal dialysis. The exception to this is TTP where the replacement fluid is always FFP or cryosupernatant. ~1–1.5 × plasma volume is exchanged in each procedure ie 2.5–4l for average adult. Procedure takes 2–4h depending on volume to be exchanged and the line flow rates. Procedure may need to be repeated daily until response eg TTP, or until a total volume exchange has been achieved eg 10–15l over 2 weeks as for Guillain-Barré syndrome, or monthly to control hyperviscosity eg Waldenström's macroglobulinaemia.

Indications – generally accepted in:
- Hyperviscosity syndromes.
- Guillain-Barré syndrome resistant to IVIg.
- Myasthenia gravis: peri-operatively for thymectomy, and refractory disease.
- Paraproteinaemic neuropathy.
- Goodpasture's syndrome.
- Thrombotic thrombocytopenia purpura.
- Post-transfusion purpura.
- Cold haemagglutinin disease.

Efficacy contentious but may be indicated in:
- Severe warm type AIHA.
- Lupus, Wegeners and other vasculitides.
- Rheumatoid arthritis.
- Peripheral neuropathies other than paraproteinaemic neuropathy.
- Multiple sclerosis.
- Chronic inflammatory demyelinating polyradiculopathy.
- Eaton Lambert syndrome.
- Renal transplant rejection.

Venous access

If exchange is to be performed via peripheral veins, one large antecubital vein is required sufficient to tolerate cannulation by a 16 gauge butterfly needle as the drawing line (return line need only be 18 gauge). If not possible, make arrangements for insertion of a central line prior to the planned exchanges inserting a double lumen renal dialysis type catheter of 16 gauge or larger.

Regular medication due immediately prior to exchange may be best deferred until immediately post-exchange particularly for drugs which are predominantly protein bound (see p498).

Problems with apheresis

General Patient anxiety, discomfort and boredom.

Citrate toxicity Parasthesiae, tremors, tetany.

Vascular and cardiac poor venous access giving poor flow rates. Extravasation, with haematoma at puncture sites, local vein thrombosis – during and after procedure, sepsis at puncture sites, hypo/hypervolaemia, vasovagal attacks, arrhythmias.

Metabolic and pharmacological Hypoalbuminaemia, hypoglycaemia, removal of drugs (plasma bound).

Allergic reactions Including anaphylaxis.

Drugs >75% bound

If drugs on the list below are due immediately prior to exchange delay administration until after procedure.

Beta blockers
Propranolol
Timolol
Penbutolol

Ca channel blockers
Diltiazem
Nifedipine
Verapamil

Anti-arrhythmics
Amiodarone
Propofenone
Quinidine
Digitoxin (Digoxin is OK)

Diuretics
Frusemide
Metolazone
Bendrofluazide
Diazoxide
Acetazolamide

Hypolipidaemics
Clofibrate

Gout drugs
Probenecid
Sulphinpyrazone

Analgesics
NSAIDs (all)
Aspirin
Coproxamol

Benzodiazepines
All

Antidepressants
All

Antiepileptics
Carbamazepine
Phenytoin
Sodium Valproate

Antipsychotics
Chlorpromazine
Haloperidol
Thioridazine

Antifungal agents
Amphotericin B
Ketoconazole

Antihistamines
Chlorpheniramine

Antimalarials
Mepacrine
Pyrimethamine

Antibiotics
Cloxacillin
Flucloxacillin
Penicillin V
Sulphonamide
Doxycycline

Anti-TB
Rifampicin

Anticoagulants
Heparin
Warfarin

Thyroid Drugs
Thyroxine
Tri-iodothyronine
Propylthiouracil

Oestrogens and progestogens
All

Hypoglycaemics
Tolbutamide
Glipizide
Gliclazide
Glibenclamide
Chlorpropamide

Leucapheresis

Leucapheresis is the removal from the peripheral blood of white blood cells, usually leukaemic blasts, via a cell separation machine.

Procedure

Usually now a standard computer controlled programme on modern machines eg Cobe Spectra™ or Fenwall CS™. May be performed manually in an emergency (see p420).

Indications

In patients with high WBC eg AML, CML and with symptoms or signs of leucostasis, leucapheresis should be performed urgently. Leucostatic features are less common in lymphoid than in myeloid malignancies.

Leucostatic features

- Confusion.
- Decreased conscious level.
- Fits.
- Retinal haemorrhages.
- Papilloedema.
- Hypoxia and miliary shadowing on CXR.
- Bleeding and coronary ischaemia.

Should not be performed routinely just because of a high WBC. Leucostatic clinical features are the indication. Conversely, leucostasis may occur in some patients with AML without a very high blast count but these patients should be considered for leucapheresis.

Chemotherapy should be started as soon as possible after leucapheresis as WBC will 'rebound' quickly due to outpouring of cells from marrow. Leucapheresis may need to be repeated daily until chemotherapy has suppressed marrow.

Other indications

- Leucapheresis should be performed routinely at diagnosis of CML in patients <60 for stem cell cryopreservation which can be used in the future as a stem cell rescue procedure.
- Leucapheresis may be used as an alternative to chemotherapy in low grade haematological malignancies in pregnancy.

Protocols and procedures

Anticoagulation therapy – heparin

For acute thrombosis DVT/PE start with heparin and warfarin simultaneously. Essential to confirm diagnosis – but start treatment whilst awaiting results of investigations. When warfarin stable – stop heparin.

Heparin

Main advantage over oral anticoagulation is immediate anticoagulant effect and short t½. Two main products: **standard unfractionated heparin (UFH)**, a mixture of polysaccharide chains, mean MW 15,000, t½ 1.0–1.5h, and **low molecular weight heparin (LMWH)**, fragments of UFH (mean MW 5000) with longer t½ (3–6h) and greater bioavailability. Heparins act by potentiating coagulation inhibitor antithrombin (AT) resulting in anti-AT and anti Xa activity. These are equal in UFH; in LMWH anti-Xa > AT activity. Both UFH and LMWH depend on renal clearance.

Administration

Standard IV UFH – initial IV bolus 5000iu in 0.9% saline given over 30 mins (lower loading dose for small adult/child). Follow with 15–25iu/kg/h using a solution of 25,000iu heparin in 50ml 0.9% saline (= 500iu/ml) and a motorised pump, eg for 80 kg adult dose is $80 \times 25 = 2000$iu/h. Monitor IVI with APTT ratio, aim for ratio 1.5–2.5, check 6h after starting treatment. Adjust dose as shown opposite.[1]

Check APTT ratio 10h after dose change; daily thereafter. Use fresh venous sample – do not take from line. Continue heparin until INR in therapeutic range for warfarin – takes ~5 days; massive ileo-femoral thrombosis and severe PE may require 7–10 days' heparin.

Subcutaneous route – eg venous access difficult or outpatient treatment. Use either UFH with concentration 25,000iu/ml, initial dose 250iu/kg 12-hrly, check APTT ratio mid-point, ie 6h after injection or LMWH given SC is effective alternative for VTE allowing OP treatment for selected patients. In ischaemic stroke, LMWH for 10d ↓ mortality/severe dependency from ~65% to 50% in placebo group. Main advantage is fixed dose, longer half-life,[2] ↓ bleeding and interaction with platelets, thrombocytopenia and osteoporosis. No lab control required (usually); in high risk patients can use anti-Xa assay to monitor.

Contraindications Caution if renal, hepatic impairment, recent surgery, known bleeding diathesis, severe hypertension.

Immediate complications of therapy

Bleeding – Occurs even when APTT ratio within the therapeutic range but risk ↑ with ↑APTT ratio. Treatment: Stop heparin until APTT ratio <2.5. In life threatening bleeding use protamine sulphate: 1mg/100iu of heparin given in preceding hour. *Thrombocytopenia* – Mild ↓ platelets common early in heparin therapy; not significant. Severe thrombocytopenia rare; occurs 6–10d after therapy begun; may be associated thrombosis. Stop heparin. Give platelets if patient bleeding. LMWH can be substituted but can cross react. Patient usually warfarinised by day 5–7 so is rarely a problem.

Prophylactic treatment

General surgery – In low/moderate risk patients: UFH SC 5000iu 2h before surgery and bd until patient is mobile, ↓ risk of VTE 2–3 fold. LMWH given

2h pre-op and once daily (*see BNF for dosage*) is an effective alternative. In high risk patient ↑ dose – usually × 2 (see BNF).

Orthopaedic surgery – A high risk situation in which LMWH is more effective; several regimens available using fixed dose eg dalteparin, or weight based dose eg tinzaparin (*see BNF*). No lab control required.

Medical conditions – Ischaemic stroke (42% incidence of DVT in paralysed leg), low dose od LMWH ↓ DVT risk.

Pregnancy – UFH is the treatment of choice in high risk women with prosthetic heart valves. LMWH usage is growing but is not yet licensed for use.

Conclusions

The increased convenience and proven efficacy means that for most clinical situations LMWH will now be preferred to UFH. High cost remains a significant factor.

503

Heparin infusion adjustment[1]						
APTR	>5.0	4.1–5.0	3.1–4.0	2.5–3.0	**TARGET** (1.5–2.5)	<1.2	1.5–2.5
DOSE	Stop* ↓500U/h	↓300U/h	↓100U/h	↓50U/h	No change	↑200U/h	↑400U/h

* Nil for 0.5–1.0h; check APTT ratio

1 Drugs & Therapeutics Bulletin 1992 **30** 77
2 NEJM 1997 **337** 688

Oral anticoagulation

▶ **Doctors do this badly: computers not much better. USE these guidelines.**

Warfarin is the drug of choice; few side effects, well tolerated. A vitamin K antagonist, it takes ~72h to be effective; stable state takes 5–7d. t½ ~35h. Circulates mainly bound to albumin; free warfarin is active. Many drugs ↑ warfarin effect by displacing it from albumin. Monitored by PT using the international normalised ration (INR).

Administration

Given daily around ~6 pm. Usually given with heparin on Day 1. If massive thrombosis, delay warfarin for 2–3d. Standard adult regimen = 10mg/d for 2d. Load with caution using reduced dose if liver disease, interacting drugs, patient >80 years. Check INR <1.4 before loading. Check INR on Day 3, ~16h after 2nd dose, and adjust as follows:[1]

INR	<1.4	1.4	1.5–1.7	1.8–1.9	2.0–2.3	2.4–2.7	2.8–3.1	3.2–3.5	3.6–4.0	4.1–4.5	>4.5
DAY 3	10*	10	10	10	5	4	3	1.5	0	0	0
DAY 4	10	8	7	6	5	4	4	3.5	3	Miss 1d 2 mg	Miss 2d Test

*Warfarin (mg)

Check again Day 4 and dose as shown; Day 4 dose near maintenance daily dose. Think in *weekly* dose eg day 4 dose = 5mg, weekly dose = 35mg. When 2 consecutive doses in therapeutic range, move to weekly check. Concomitant heparin does not affect INR as long as APTT ratio in therapeutic range.

Therapeutic range: set target INR

INR 2.0–3.0: Prophylaxis of DVT – target 2.2. Treatment DVT/PE/TIA; prophylaxis post MI; atrial fibrillation (AF) – target 2.5.
INR 3.0–4.5: Recurrent thrombosis; mechanical prosthetic valves; arterial disease – MI 2° prevention, antiphospholipid syndrome – target 3.5.

Duration

No underlying cause – treat ~3 months; ≥6 months if life threatening episode. Post-op thrombosis, warfarin for 6 weeks; stop when patient fully active. *No need to tail off.* Anticoagulate indefinitely for recurrent thrombosis, heart valves, arterial disease.

Contraindications

First trimester pregnancy (warfarin induced embryopathy), cerebral thrombosis, severe hypertension.

Complications

Haemorrhage. Easy bruising common within therapeutic range – is patient on aspirin? Rate of major bleeds ~2.7/100 treatment years, ↑ age ↑ INR. Rare side effects – alopecia, warfarin-induced skin necrosis (check for congenital thrombophilia defect), hypersensitivity, purple toe syndrome.

Management of over-anticoagulation: See p430 for details

Asymptomatic patient

INR >5.0, withhold warfarin 1–2d, alert GP if outpatient, check INR before restarting.

Protocols and procedures

Symptomatic patient

Moderate bleeding, INR 5.0–8.0, give vitamin K 1mg slowly IV. INR >8.0: give vitamin K 1mg and FFP 12–15ml/kg, ~2 units. Severe bleeding: vitamin K 5mg IV, and prothrombin concentrate if available (factor IX 50U/kg) or FFP. Observe in hospital. Vitamin K reverses over-anticoagulation in 24h. Look for causes of over-anticoagulation eg heart failure, alcohol, drugs.

Special considerations

Dental and minor surgery[2]: stop warfarin 36h before operation/dental extraction. Proceed if INR <2.5. Can give FFP to ↓ INR if necessary. Use tranexamic acid mouthwash.

Major surgery

Omit 3 doses of warfarin pre-op. Day before surgery check INR. If >2.0 consider giving vitamin K 1mg SC. If <2.0 in high risk patients (eg acute VTE <1 month history, prosthetic heart valve) give IV heparin full dose until 6h before surgery. Other patients give SC heparin as for high risk prophylaxis (*see BNF for details*). *Day of operation* most surgeons will proceed if INR 2.0. *Post-op* restart warfarin on evening of surgery. Cover high risk patients with IV heparin starting 12h post-op; risk of bleeding is significant so keep period of full heparinisation to a minimum. Other groups continue as for pre-op regimen. Continue heparin until warfarin back in therapeutic range.

Pregnancy: warfarin contraindicated in first trimester. Best avoided throughout pregnancy. Use heparin SC until delivery. Warfarin safe in puerperium and for breast feeding.

Drug interactions: Always check INR if major interacting agent added or removed. *See BNF for details of drugs interacting with warfarin.*

AF: Rheumatic and non-valvular (cardiovascular and other systemic disease) AF carry a major risk of stroke which ↑ with age to >5% over 80 years. Warfarin prevents ⅔ strokes and is indicated unless risk of haemorrhage outweighs benefits. Target INR 2.5 effective in stroke prevention. Lone AF (no cause found) in <60 years has low risk of stroke – does not benefit from anticoagulation.

505

1 Drugs & Therapeutics Bulletin 1992 **30** 77
2 NEJM 1997 **336** 1506

Management of needlestick injuries

Every doctor dealing with high risk patients is concerned to prevent exposure to blood and body fluids, particularly a needlestick injury. The UK DoH published guidance on post-exposure prophylaxis (PEP) for HIV in 1997 (tel 0171-9724385 for copy). Your hospital/GP surgery should have a policy for the prevention and management of contamination incidents – check this out.

Risk to health care workers

2 types of injury – **sharps injury** where intact skin is breached by sharp object contaminated with blood/blood-stained body fluids or unfixed tissue, and **contamination injury** where blood/blood-stained body fluid comes into contact with mucous membranes or non-intact skin. HBV and HIV are the 2 major concerns. All health care workers should be vaccinated against HBV. Risk of contracting HIV from percutaneous exposure to HIV-infected blood is ~0.3%. The amount of blood injected and a high viral load in the patient's blood increase the risk.

General guidelines

Prevention

All health care workers must adopt universal precautions when handling blood/blood stained fluids – wear gloves, avoid blood spillage, use decontamination procedures if spillage occurs, label high risk specimens, care with needles (**do not resheath**), disposal in burn bins, etc.

Immediate action in event of exposure

- Encourage bleeding and/or wash under running water.
- Contact Occupational Health/A & E departments for help.
- Establish patient status re blood-borne viruses.
- Take blood from patient/test for viruses (with consent).
- Take blood from needlestick victim and store. Check HBV immunity/later tests if necessary.

Treatment

Decision to treat will be made by an experienced medical staff member. Treatment recommended for '*all health care workers exposed to high risk body fluids or tissues known to be, or strongly suspected to be, infected with HIV through percutaneous exposure, mucous membrane exposure or through exposure of broken skin.*' Zidovudine alone given as soon as possible ↓ risk of seroconversion by 80% but failures are well described. Prophylaxis with triple therapy now recommended. Treat for 4 wks as soon as possible with:

- Zidovudine 200mg tds/250mg bd + Lamivudine 150mg bd + Indinavir 800mg tds. A 'starter pack' should be available in an accessible place at all times.
- Known exposure to Hepatitis B
  – no immunity – give HepB Ig 500mg IM; vaccinate immediately
  – known immunity with HepB Ab >100 IU/l in past 2 yr – no action
  – immunity – HepB Ab status not known – give booster dose.

Follow up

Occupational Health Department appointment for advice re further management and tests. Counselling as required. Six months after the incident a –ve test indicates infection has not occurred. Report incident to PHLS CDSC tel 0181-200-6868. In Scotland to SCIEH tel 0141-946-7120.
NEJM 1997 337 1485

507

Chemotherapy protocols
ABVD

Adriamycin (doxorubicin), bleomycin, vinblastine, dacarbazine

Indication
Hodgkin's disease

Schedule

28 day cycle		Day 1 (A)	Day 15 (B)
Doxorubicin	$25mg/m^2$ IV	x	x
Bleomycin	10 units/m^2 IV	x	x
Vinblastine	$6mg/m^2$ IV (max l0mg)	x	x
Dacarbazine	$375mg/m^2$ IVI in normal saline	x	x

Administration
- Out-patient regimen.
- Consider sperm banking in males.
- Add allopurinol 300mg/day throughout first treatment cycle.
- Anti-emetic therapy for moderate emetogenic regimens.
- Consider doxorubicin dose reduction if significant liver impairment.
- Repeat treatment if WCC $>3.5 \times 10^9/l$ and platelet count $>100 \times 10^9/l$.
- 25% dose reduction if WCC $2.5–3.5 \times 10^9/l$ or platelet count $75–100 \times 10^9/l$.
- Delay treatment one week if WCC $<2.5 \times 10^9/l$ or platelet count $<75 \times 10^9/l$.
- Treat to complete remission + 2 cycles.

Protocols and procedures

ChlVPP

Chlorambucil, vinblastine, procarbazine, prednisolone

Indication

Hodgkin's disease

Schedule

28 day cycle

Chlorambucil	6mg/m^2 PO	days 1–14
Vinblastine	6mg/m^2 IV (max l0mg)	days 1 & 8
Procarbazine	100mg/m^2 PO (max 150mg)	days 1–14
Prednisolone	40mg PO	

Administration

- Out-patient regimen.
- Consider sperm banking in males.
- Add allopurinol 300mg/d throughout first treatment cycle.
- Antiemetic therapy for moderate emetogenic regimens.
- Alcohol prohibited with procarbazine; avoid monoamine oxidase inhibitors.
- Repeat treatment when WCC >3.0 × 10^9/l and platelet count >100 × 10^9/l.
- Treat to complete remission + 2 cycles.

MOPP

Mustine, vincristine, procarbazine, prednisolone.

Indication
Hodgkin's disease

Schedule

28 day cycle

Mustine	6mg/m^2 IV	days 1 & 8
Vincristine	1.4mg/m^2 IV (max 2mg*)	days 1 & 8
Procarbazine	100mg/m^2 PO (max 150mg)	days 1–14
Prednisolone	100mg/m^2 PO	days 1–14

*Original protocol put no maximum limit on vincristine dosage; higher doses are associated with severe neuropathy.

Administration
- Out-patient regimen.
- Consider sperm banking in males.
- Add allopurinol 300mg/d throughout first treatment cycle.
- Antiemetic therapy for highly emetogenic regimens.
- Alcohol prohibited with procarbazine; avoid monoamine oxidase inhibitors.
- Repeat treatment if WCC >3.5 × 10^9/l and platelet count >100 × 10^9/l.
- 25% dose reduction if WCC 2.5–3.5 × 10^9/l or platelet count 75–100×10^9/l.
- Delay treatment one week if WCC <2.5 × 10^9/l or platelet count <75×10^9/l.
- Treat to complete remission + 2 cycles.

Protocols and procedures

513

MOPP/ABVD

Mustine, vincristine, procarbazine, prednisolone, adriamycin (doxorubicin), bleomycin, vinblastine, dacarbazine.

Indication
Hodgkin's disease

Schedule

8 week cycle

Mustine	$6mg/m^2$ IV	days 1 & 8		
Vincristine	$1.4mg/m^2$ IV (max 2mg*)	days 1 & 8		
Procarbazine	$100mg/m^2$ PO (max 150mg)	days 1–14		
Prednisolone	$100mg/m^2$ PO	days 1–14		

		Day 29	**Day 43**
Doxorubicin	$25mg/m^2$ IV	x	x
Bleomycin	10 units/m^2 IV	x	x
Vinblastine	$6mg/m^2$ IV (max 10mg)	x	x
Dacarbazine	$375mg/m^2$ IVI in normal saline	x	x

*Original protocol put no maximum limit on vincristine dosage; higher doses are associated with severe neuropathy.

Administration
- Out-patient regimen.
- Consider sperm banking in males.
- Add allopurinol 300mg/d throughout first treatment cycle.
- Antiemetic therapy for highly emetogenic regimens.
- Alcohol prohibited with procarbazine; avoid monoamine oxidase inhibitors.
- Consider doxorubicin dose reduction if significant liver impairment.
- Repeat treatment if WCC >35 × 10^9/l and platelet count >100 × 10^9/l.
- 25% dose reduction if WCC 2.5–3.5 × 10^9/l or platelet count 75–100×10^9/l.
- Delay treatment one week if WCC <2.5 × 10^9/l or platelet count <75×10^9/l.
- Treat for 12 months (6 cycles).

CHOP

Cyclophosphamide, vincristine, doxorubicin, prednisolone.
Indications
- Intermediate and high grade non-Hodgkin's lymphoma.
- Low grade non-Hodgkin's lymphoma resistant to first-line therapy.

Schedule

21 day cycle		day 1	2	3	4	5
Cyclophosphamide	750mg/m^2 IV	x				
Vincristine	1.4mg/m^2 IV (max 2mg)	x				
Doxorubicin	50 mg/m2 IV	x				
Prednisolone	100mg PO	x	x	x	x	x

Administration
- Out-patient regimen.
- Consider sperm banking in males.
- Add allopurinol 300mg/d throughout first treatment cycle.
- Antiemetic therapy for moderately emetogenic regimens.
- Consider doxorubicin dose reduction if significant liver impairment.
- Repeat treatment when WCC >3.0 × 10^9/l and platelet count >100× 10^9/l.
- Treat to complete remission + 2 cycles.

Protocols and procedures

CVP

Cyclophosphamide, vincristine, prednisolone.

Indications
- Low grade non-Hodgkin's lymphoma.
- Advanced chronic lymphocytic leukaemia.

Schedule

21 day cycle		day 1	2	3	4	5
Cyclophosphamide	750mg/m^2 IV	x				
Vincristine	1.4mg/m^2 IV (max 2mg)	x				
Prednisolone	100mg PO	x	x	x	x	x

Administration
- Out-patient regimen.
- Consider sperm banking in males.
- Add allopurinol 300mg/d throughout first treatment cycle.
- Antiemetic therapy for moderately emetogenic regimens.
- Consider doxorubicin dose reduction if significant liver impairment.
- Repeat treatment when WCC >3.0×10^9/l and platelet count >100×10^9/l.
- Treat to complete remission + 2 cycles.

Protocols and procedures

ABCM

Adriamycin (doxorubicin), BCNU (carmustine), cyclophosphamide, melphalan

Indication
Multiple myeloma.

Schedule

6 week cycle	day	1	2	3	4
Doxorubicin	30mg/m^2 IV	x			
Carmustine	30mg/m^2 IV	x			
Cyclophosphamide	100mg/m^2 PO	x	x	x	x
Melphalan	6mg/m^2 PO	x	x	x	x

Administration
- Out-patient regimen.
- Consider sperm banking in males.
- Add allopurinol 300mg/day throughout first treatment cycle.
- Add infection prophylaxis with cotrimoxazole 2 tabs triweekly and nystatin mouthwash/fluconazole 100mg/day.
- Antiemetic therapy for moderately emetogenic regimens.
- Repeat treatment when WCC >3.0 × 10^9/l and platelet count >100 × 10^9/l.
- Treat to plateau phase (normally 4–8 courses).

Protocols and procedures

C-VAMP

Cyclophosphamide, vincristine, adriamycin (doxorubicin), methylprednisolone

Indications
Multiple myeloma

Schedule

21 day cycle		1	2	3	4	5	8	15
Vincristine	0.4mg/day continuous IVI	x	x	x	x			
Doxorubicin	9mg/m^2/day continuous IVI	x	x	x	x			
Methylprednisolone	1.5g IV/PO	x	x	x	x	x		
Cyclophosphamide	500mg/m2 IV		x				x	x

(column header group: DAY)

Administration
- Out-patient regimen.
- Indwelling central venous catheter required with ambulatory infusion pump.
- Consider sperm banking in males.
- Add allopurinol 300mg/day throughout first treatment cycle.
- Add infection prophylaxis with cotrimoxazole 2 tabs triweekly and nystatin mouthwash/fluconazole 100mg/day.
- Antiemetic therapy for mildly emetogenic regimens.
- Repeat treatment when WCC >2.0 $\times$ 10^9/l and platelet count >100 $\times$ 10^9/l.
- Treat until maximum paraprotein and bone marrow response (normally 4–8 courses).

523

VAD

Vincristine, adriamycin (doxorubicin).

Indication
Multiple myeloma.

Schedule

21 day cycle		day 1	2	3	4
Vincristine continuous IVI	0.4mg/d	x	x	x	x
Doxorubicin continuous IVI	9mg/m^2/d	x	x	x	x
Dexamethasone	40mg PO	x	x	x	x

(repeated days 9–12 and days 17–20 on first cycle only)

Administration
- Out-patient regimen.
- Indwelling central venous catheter required with ambulatory infusion pump.
- Consider sperm banking in males.
- Add allopurinol 300mg/day throughout first treatment cycle.
- Add infection prophylaxis with cotrimoxazole 2 tabs triweekly and nystatin mouthwash/fluconazole 100mg/day.
- Antiemetic therapy for mildly emetogenic regimens.
- Repeat treatment when WCC >2.0 × 10^9/l and platelet count >100×10^9/l.
- Treat until maximum paraprotein and bone marrow response (normally 4–8 courses).

Protocols and procedures

Full blood count

Rapid analysis by the latest generation automated blood counters using either forward angle light scatter or impedance analysis provides enumeration of leucocytes, erythrocytes and platelets and quantification of haemoglobin, MCV plus derived values for haematocrit, MCH and MCHC, red cell distribution width (a measure of cell size scatter), mean platelet volume and platelet distribution width and a 5 parameter differential leucocyte count. The counter also flags samples which require direct morphological assessment by examination of a blood film.

Sample: peripheral blood EDTA; the sample should be analysed in the laboratory within 4h.

Blood film

Morphological assessment of red cells, leucocytes and platelets should be performed by an experienced individual of all samples in which the FBC has revealed any result significantly outside the normal range, samples in which a flag has been indicated by the automated counter and if clinically indicated. A manual differential leucocyte count may be performed and may differ from that produced by the automated counter most notably in patients with haematological disease affecting the leucocytes.

Sample: peripheral blood EDTA; the sample should be analysed in the laboratory within 4h. May be made directly from drop of blood or EDTA sample, air-dried and fixed.

Plasma viscosity

This test is a sensitive but non-specific index of plasma protein changes which result from inflammation or tissue damage. The PV is unchanged by haematocrit variations and delay in analysis up to 24h and is therefore more reliable than the ESR. It is not affected by sex but is affected by age, exercise and pregnancy.

Sample: peripheral blood EDTA; the sample should be analysed in the laboratory within 24h.

ESR

This test is a sensitive but non-specific index of plasma protein changes which result from inflammation or tissue damage. The ESR is affected by haematocrit variations, red cell abnormalities (eg poikilocytosis, sickle cells) and delay in analysis and is therefore less reliable than measurement of the plasma viscosity. The ESR is affected by age, sex, menstrual cycle, pregnancy and drugs (eg OCP, steroids).

Sample: peripheral blood EDTA; the sample should be analysed in the laboratory within 4h.

Haematinic assays

Measurement of the serum B_{12} and red cell folate are necessary in the investigation of macrocytic anaemia, and serum ferritin in the investigation of microcytic anaemia in order to assess body stores of the relevant haematinic(s). *Serum* folate levels are an unreliable measurement of body stores of folate. The serum ferritin may be elevated as an acute phase protein in patients with underlying neoplasia or inflammatory disease (eg rheumatoid arthritis) and may give an erroneously normal level in an iron deficient patient.

Sample: clotted blood sample and peripheral blood EDTA.

Haemoglobin electrophoresis

This test is performed in the diagnosis of abnormal haemoglobin production (haemoglobinopathies or thalassaemia). It is usually performed on cellulose acetate at alkaline pH (8.9) but may be performed on citrate agar gel at acid pH (6.0) to detect certain haemoglobins more clearly. Haemoglobin electrophoresis has been largely replaced by HPLC analysis.

Sample: peripheral blood EDTA.

Haptoglobin

The serum haptoglobin should be measured in patients with suspected intravascular haemolysis and is frequently reduced in patients with extravascular haemolysis. It should generally be accompanied by estimation of the serum methaemalbumin, free plasma haemoglobin and urinary haemosiderin.

Sample: clotted blood.

Schumm's test

This spectrophotometric test for methaemalbumin (which has a distinctive absorption band at 558nm) should be measured in patients with suspected intravascular haemolysis and may be abnormal in patients with significant extravascular (generally splenic) haemolysis. It should generally be accompanied by estimation of the serum haptoglobin level, free plasma haemoglobin and urinary haemosiderin.

Sample: heparinised blood or clotted blood.

Kleihauer test

The Kleihauer test which exploits the resistance of fetal red cells to acid elution should be performed on all Rh(D) negative women who deliver a Rh(D) positive infant. Fetal cells appear as darkly staining cells against a background of ghosts. An estimate of the required dose of anti-D can be made from the number of fetal cells in a low power field.

Sample: maternal peripheral blood EDTA.

Reticulocytes

Definition
- Immature RBCs formed in marrow and found in normal peripheral blood.
- Represent an intermediate maturation stage in marrow between the nucleated red cell and the mature red cell.
- No nucleus but retain some nucleic acid.

Detection and measurement
- Demonstrated by staining with supravital dye for the nucleic acid.
- Appear on blood film as larger than mature RBCs with fine lacy blue staining strands or dots.
- Some modern automated blood counters using laser technology can measure levels of retics directly.
- Usually expressed as a % of total red cells eg 5%, though absolute numbers can be derived from this and total red cell count.

Causes of ↑ retic counts

Marrow stimulation due to
- Bleeding.
- Haemolysis.
- Response to oral Fe therapy.
- Infection.
- Inflammation.
- Polycythaemia (any cause).
- Myeloproliferative disorders.
- Marrow recovery following chemotherapy or radiotherapy.
- Erythropoietin administration.

Causes of ↓ retic counts

Marrow infiltration due to
- Leukaemia.
- Myeloma.
- Lymphoma.
- Other malignancy.

Marrow underactivity (hypoplasia) due to
- Fe, folate or B_{12} deficiency
  note: return of retics is earliest sign of response to replacement therapy.
- Immediately post-chemotherapy or radiotherapy.
- Autoimmune disease especially RA.
- Malnutrition.
- Uraemia.
- Drugs.
- Aplastic anaemia (see p118).
- Red cell aplasia (see p368).

Haematological investigations

Urinary haemosiderin

Usage
The most widely used and reliable test for detection of chronic intravascular haemolysis.

Principle
Free Hb is released into the plasma during intravascular haemolysis. The haemoglobin binding proteins become saturated resulting in passage of haem-containing compounds into the urinary tract of which haemosiderin is the most readily detectable.

Method
1. A clean catch sample of urine is obtained from the patient.
2. Sample is spun down in a cytocentrifuge to obtain a cytospin preparation of urothelial cells.
3. Staining and rinsing with Perl's reagent (Prussian Blue) is performed on the glass slides.
4. Examine under oil-immersion lens of microscope.
5. Haemosiderin stains as blue dots within urothelial cells.
6. Ignore all excess stain, staining outside cells or in debris all of which are common.
7. True positive is only when clear detection within urothelial squames is seen.

Cautions
An iron-staining +ve control sample should be run alongside test case to ensure stain has worked satisfactorily. Haemosiderinuria may not be detected for up to 72 hours after the initial onset of intravascular haemolysis so the test may miss haemolysis of very recent onset – repeat test in 3–7 days if –ve. Conversely, haemosiderinuria may persist for some time after a haemolytic process has stopped. Repeat in 7 days should confirm.

Causes of haemosiderinuria

Common causes	Red cell enzymopathies e.g. G6PD and PK deficiency but only during haemolytic episodes
	Mycoplasma pneumonia with anti-I cold haemagglutinin
	Sepsis
	Malaria
	Cold haemagglutinin disease
	TTP/HUS
	Severe extravascular haemolysis (may cause intravascular haemolysis)
Rarer causes	PNH
	Prosthetic heart valves
	Red cell incompatible transfusion reactions
	Unstable haemoglobins
	March haemoglobinuria

Haematological investigations

Ham's test

Usage

The principal diagnostic test for paroxysmal nocturnal haemoglobinuria (PNH).

Principle

- Abnormal sensitivity of RBCs from patients with PNH to the haemolytic action of complement.
- Complement is activated by acidification of patient's serum to pH of 6.2 which induces lysis of PNH red cells but not normal controls.

Specificity High – similar reaction is produced only in the rare syndrome HEMPAS (a form of congenital dyserythropoietic anaemia type II) which should be easily distinguished morphologically.

Sensitivity Low – as the reaction is crucially dependent on the concentration of magnesium in the serum.

It appears to be a technically difficult test in most laboratories. Patients with only a low % of PNH cells may be missed ie at an early stage of the disease. Markedly abnormal PNH cells are usually picked up in ~75% of patients. Less abnormal cells are detected in only ~25% of patients.

Alternative tests

- Sucrose lysis – an alternative method of complement activation is by mixing serum with a low ionic strength solution such as sucrose. **Sensitivity** of this test is high but **specificity** is low – ie the opposite of the Ham's test.
- Immunophenotypic detection of the deficiency of the PIG transmembrane protein anchors in PNH cells is becoming a more widely used alternative cf PNH section. Monoclonal antibodies to CD59 or CD55 (DAF) are used in flow cytometric analysis. Major advantage is that test can be performed on neutrophils and platelets in PB which are more numerous than the PNH red cells.

Immunophenotyping

Definition
Identification of cell surface proteins by reactivity with monoclonal antibodies of known specificity.

Uses
- Aids diagnosis and classification of haematological malignancy.
- Assess cellular clonality.
- Identify prognostic groups.
- Monitor minimal residual disease (MRD).

Terminology and methodology
Cell surface proteins are denoted according to their Cluster Differentiation (CD) number. These are allocated after international workshops define individual cell surface proteins by reactivity to monoclonal antibodies. Most cells will express many such proteins and pattern of expression allows cellular characterisation.

Monoclonal antibodies (MoAbs) are derived from single B lymphocyte cell lines and have identical antigen binding domains known as ***idiotypes***. It is easy to generate large quantities of MoAbs for diagnostic use.

- Cell populations from eg PB or BM samples are incubated with a panel of MoAbs eg anti-CD4, anti-CD34 which are directly or indirectly bound to a fluorescent marker antibody eg FITC.
- Sample is passed through a fluorescence activated cell sorter (FACS) machine.
- FACS instruments assign cells to a graphical plot by virtue of cell size and granularity detected as forward and side light scatter by the laser.
- Allows subpopulations of cells eg mononuclear cells in blood sample to be selected.
- The reactivity of this cell subpopulation to the MoAb panel can then be determined by fluorescence for each MoAb.
- A typical result for a CD4 T lymphocyte population is shown:
  CD3, CD4 +ve; CD8, CD13, CD34, CD19 –ve.

Common diagnostic profiles

AML	CD13+, CD33+, ± CD 34, ± CD14 +ve.
cALL	CD10 and TdT +ve.
T-ALL	cCD3, CD7, TdT +ve.
B-ALL	CD10, CD19, surface Ig +ve.
CLL	CD5, CD19, CD23, weak surface Ig +ve.

Clonality assessment
Particularly useful in determining whether there is a monoclonal B cell or plasma cell population.

▶ Monoclonal B cells from eg NHL will have surface expression of κ or λ light chains *but not both*.

▶ Polyclonal B cells from eg patient with infectious mononucleosis will have both κ *and* λ expression.

Cytogenetics

Acquired somatic chromosomal abnormalities are common in haematological malignancies. Determination of patterns of cytogenetic abnormalities is known as *karyotyping*.

Uses
- Aid diagnosis and classification of haematological malignancy.
- Assess clonality.
- Identify prognostic groups.
- Monitor minimal residual disease (MRD).
- Determine engraftment and chimerism post-allogeneic transplant.

Terminology
- Normal somatic cell has 46 chromosomes; 22 pairs and XX or XY.
- Numbered 1–22 in decreasing size order.
- 2 arms meet at centromere – short arm denoted *p*, long arm denoted *q*.
- Usually only visible during condensation at metaphase.
- Stimulants and cell culture used – colchicine to arrest cells in metaphase.
- Stained to identify regions and bands eg p1, q3.

Common abnormalities
- Whole chromosome gain eg trisomy 8 (+8).
- Whole chromosome loss eg monosomy 7 (–7).
- Partial gain eg 9q+ or partial loss eg 5q– .
- Translocation – material repositioned to another chromosome; usually reciprocal eg t(9;22) – the Philadelphia translocation.
- Inversion – part of chromosome runs in opposite direction eg inv(16) in M4Eo.
- Many translocations involve point mutations known as oncogenes, eg bcr, ras, myc, bcl-2.

Molecular cytogenetics
- Molecular revolution is further refining the specific abnormalities in the genesis of haematological malignancies.
- Techniques such as FISH (fluorescence *in situ* hybridisation) and PCR (polymerase chain reaction) can detect tiny amounts of abnormal genes.
- Bcr-abl probes are now used in diagnosis and monitoring of treatment response in CML.
- IgH and T cell receptor (TCR) genes are useful in determining clonality of suspected B and T cell tumours respectively.
- Specific probes may be used in diagnosis and monitoring of subtypes of AML e.g. PML-RARA in AML M3.

Common karyotypic abnormalities

CML
t(9;22)   Philadelphia chromosome translocation creates bcr-abl chimeric gene.

AML
t(8;21)   AML M2, involves AML-ETO genes – has better prognosis.
t(15;17)   AML M3 involves PML-RARA genes – has better prognosis.
inv(16)   AML M4Eo – has better prognosis.
−5, −7   Complex abnormalities have poor prognosis.

MDS
−7, +8, +11   Poor prognosis.
5q– syndrome   Associated with refractory anaemia and better prognosis.

MPD
20q– and +8   Common associations.

ALL
t(9;22)   Philadelphia translocation, poor prognosis.
t(4;11)   Poor prognosis.
Hyperdiploidy   Increase in total chromosome number – good prognosis.
Hypodiploidy   Decrease in total chromosome number – bad prognosis.

T-ALL
t(1;14)   Involves tal-1 oncogene.

B-ALL and Burkitt's lymphoma
t(8;14)   Involves myc and IgH genes, poor prognosis.

CLL
+12, t(11;14)

ATLL
14q11

NHL
t(14;18)   Follicular lymphoma, involves bcl-2 oncogene.
t(11;14)   Small cell lymphocytic lymphoma, involves bcl-1 oncogene.
t(8;14)   Burkitt's lymphoma, involves myc and IgH genes.

543

HLA typing

HLA (human leucocyte antigen) system or MHC (major histocompatibility Complex) is name given to highly polymorphic gene cluster region on chromosome 6 which codes for cell surface proteins involved in immune recognition.

The gene complex is subdivided into 2 regions

Class 1   The A, B and C loci.
            These proteins are found on most nucleated cells and interact with CD8 positive T lymphocytes.

Class 2   Comprised of DR, DP, DQ loci present only on B lymphocytes, monocytes, macrophages and activated T lymphocytes. Interact with CD4+positive T lymphocytes.

- Class 1 and 2 genes are closely linked so one set of gene loci is usually inherited from each parent though there is a small amount of cross-over.
- There is ~1:4 chance of 2 siblings being HLA identical.
- There are other histocompatibility loci apart from the HLA system but these appear less important generally except during HLA matched stem cell transplantation when even differences in these minor systems may cause GvHD.

Typing methods

Class 1 and 2 antigens were originally defined by serological reactivity with maternal antisera containing pregnancy-induced HLA antibodies. Many problems with technique and too insensitive to detect many polymorphisms. Molecular techniques are increasingly employed such as SSP. Molecular characterisation is detecting vast Class 2 polymorphism.

Importance of HLA typing

- Matching donor/recipient pairs for renal, cardiac and marrow stem cell transplantation.
- Degree of matching more critical for stem cell than solid organ transplants.
- Sibling HLA matched stem cell transplantation is now treatment of choice for many malignancies.
- Unrelated donor stem cell transplants are increasingly performed but outcome is poorer due to HLA disparity. As molecular matching advances, improved accuracy will enable closer matches to be found and results should improve.

Functional tests of donor/recipient compatibility

- MLC (mixed lymphocyte culture) – now rarely used.
- CTLp (cytotoxic T lymphocyte precursor assays) – determine the frequency of cytotoxic T lymphocytes in the donor directed against the recipient – provides an assessment of GvHD occurring.

HLA related transfusion issues

- HLA on WBC and platelets may cause immunisation in recipients of blood and platelet transfusions.
- May cause refractoriness and/or febrile reactions to platelet transfusions.
- WBC depletion of products by filtration prevents this.
- Diagnosis of refractoriness confirmed by detection of HLA or platelet specific antibodies in patient's serum.
- Platelet transfusions matched to recipient HLA type may improve increments.

Blood transfusion 16

Using the blood transfusion laboratory

Requests for compatibility testing or blood grouping

Transfusion samples and forms must be clearly identified and clerical details match exactly. The form and sample should be signed by the person taking the sample as vouching for the identity of the potential recipient.

- 3 points of identification are required: patient's full name, date of birth, hospital number.
- Requests must be legible and clearly labelled with the name of the responsible clinician.
- Indication for transfusion should be specified.
- Indicate time for planned surgery.
- For major elective surgery where transfusion is usual with the procedure the laboratory should receive a G & S sample in advance (7 days) – allows identification of alloantibodies – the lab will arrange for appropriate blood units to be available.
- In genuine haemorrhagic emergencies ABO ± Rh (D) group compatible blood can be given *without* matching as the slight risk of this action far outweighs the immediate risk of death from exsanguination.
- Unmatched O Rh (D) Neg blood should *only* be used in extreme emergency when the patient's blood group is unknown or, if known, blood of the same ABO and Rh type is unavailable. Emergency grouping can be conducted in ~15 min; full laboratory compatibility testing can be completed in ≤1h. Can be ~20 min in emergencies (sending G & S sample to laboratory may save valuable time).

Hazards

- Most serious is ABO mismatch – almost invariably arises through clerical errors (at time of sampling) or when blood given to patient.
- The blood transfusion laboratory groups the blood sample received and assumes the sample has been correctly identified at the time of collection.

Issue & administration of blood & blood products

1. Units of blood are labelled as being matched for an individual patient.
2. Before administering the patient/recipient identity must be checked (see 3 point identity above).
3. Label details are rechecked by trained nursing staff at the bedside immediately prior to the transfusion *any discrepancies identified must be referred urgently to the blood bank and the clinician responsible for the patient – transfusion of that unit cannot proceed until any ambiguity about identity has been resolved.*
4. Unit of blood must be given within its expiry date.
5. Check for damage to the pack, discolouration of the contained red cells, or evidence of haemolysis.
6. Administration of the unit must commence <30 mins after leaving the blood bank and be completed within 4 hours of commencing infusion.
7. Administration of blood products must be recorded in the case notes.
8. The unique number of given RBCs or blood products should be entered in the notes.
9. If given warm, ensure a safe approved warming procedure is used.

Blood transfusion

Maximum surgical blood ordering schedule (MSBOS)

A system of tailoring blood requirements to particular elective surgical procedures, including – importantly – procedures which do not usually require blood cover.

- The ABO group and Rh (D) type of the patient is determined on duplicate samples, and the serum screened for significant RBC ('atypical') antibodies. If there are no antibodies, the serum is kept available ('saved') for a determined period (usually a week) – this is the 'Group, Screen and Save' (G & S) procedure.
- If there are no atypical antibodies, and the planned surgery is likely to need peri-operative transfusion, the required number of red cell units are matched by routine tests, labelled and set aside in an accessible refrigerator. Storage conditions must meet certain standards (continuous recording of appropriate temperature, alarms, etc).
- If more blood is required than anticipated, extra units must be readily available. If the need is urgent, suitable arrangements – such as rapid matching (using the 'saved' serum) and despatch procedures – must enable the timely supply of blood.
- If there *are* atypical antibodies, which may occur in up to 10% patients, their specificity must be determined and, if clinically significant, sufficient (extra) red cell units *lacking* the relevant antigen provided and matched by detailed techniques. (These are often referred to as 'phenotyped red cells'.)
- If there is no 'MSBOS' more units must be matched than are usually required for transfusion, in order to give rapid access if extra blood is needed. Matched 'bespoke' blood is therefore unavailable for other patients for the 2–3 days set aside.
- A good MSBOS gives better access to blood stocks and enables more efficient use, in particular of O Rh(D) –ve blood. There is no good reason for regarding O Rh(D) –ve blood as a 'Universal' donation type. It can be antigenic; and it is a precious resource, being available from <8% population.
- The surgical team must be confident in the system, and the blood bank staff committed to 'minimal barriers'. The cross-match : transfusion ratio of a blood bank may well become lower than 2 (ie, overall <2 units matched for every unit transfused) which is an indication of efficient practices. It could even be nearer to 1 than to 2.
- MSBOS schedules will vary between hospitals – depending on demographic factors, general layout, access to the blood bank refrigerators, types of surgery etc.

Transfusion of red blood cells

Used acutely in the management of 'significant' blood loss following trauma or surgery electively to manage anaemia *which is not correctable by other means*, eg correction of iron deficiency is by giving iron supplements, not by blood transfusion.

Indications for red cell transfusion

Blood loss	Massive/Acute
Bone marrow failure	Post-chemotherapy, leukaemias, etc.
	Supportive therapy with concentrated cells
Inherited RBC disorders	Homozygous β-thalassaemia
	Red cell aplasia, etc
	Hb SS (some circumstances)
Acquired RBC disorders	Myelofibrosis
	Myelodysplasia
	Some chronic disorder anaemias
	Selected use in renal failure
Neonatal &	Haemolytic disease of the newborn
exchange transfusions	Meningococcal septicaemia
	Falciparum malaria

RBC transfusion is contraindicated in chronic iron deficiency anaemia; iron supplements will raise the haemoglobin in a safer and less costly manner. If patients are suffering marked anaemic symptoms then use of 2 units of concentrated cells will deal with this problem pending a response to iron. In severe megaloblastic anaemias RBCs should not be used; a rapid response to haematinics is expected. Transfusion can precipitate severe cardiac failure.

- Red cells have a shelf life of 35 days at 4°C and are supplied as concentrated red cells with PCV between 0.55 and 0.75. Most units in the UK are supplied in 'optimal additive solution', SAG-M* which allows removal of all the plasma for preparation of other blood components and results in a less viscous product. The volume of a unit of concentrated cells is 280 ± 20ml. With adequate venous access it will flow easily through a standard blood giving set.
- In acute blood loss concentrated RBCs are adequate (whole blood not currently available in practice). Concentrated RBCs allow maintenance of oxygen delivery, and are often infused at same time as other colloids.
- Leucodepletion is needed clinically for individuals who experience febrile transfusion reactions usually due to leucocyte derived cytokines. Standard RBCs have $<1.2 \times 10^9$ leucocytes present. Leucocyte depleted RBCs through filtration at source have lower numbers of contaminating WBCs, $<5 \times 10^6$. Their use will reduce the development of leucocyte alloantibodies, also an alternative to CMV negative RBCs.
- Irradiated RBCs are indicated to stop transfusion transmitted graft versus host disease, eg following total body irradiation, bone marrow allografting or therapy with purine analogues (Fludarabine, 2-CDA).

Blood transfusion

- Frozen RBCs similarly have plasma and some other constituents removed. They are expensive to process, store and handle; they must be used within 24h after thawing. Clinical usage is restricted to patients with extremely rare blood groups or with highly problematic blood group alloantibodies.

In autoimmune haemolytic disorders transfusion can be lifesaving as a short term support pending a response to immunosuppression. As a general rule, most otherwise fit adult patients with chronic anaemia will tolerate Hb levels around 9.0–10.0g/dl without major problems. Transfusion therapy is more likely to be needed below this level

Transfusion procedure

Although fussy, strictly laid down hospital protocols must be followed for administration of blood and blood products. *Errors carry the potential for major morbidity or fatality.*

1. Identity of label on each matched unit must match EXACTLY with the patient's identity.
2. The ABO & Rh groups on the blood pack and the compatibility report must correspond as must the donor number on the pack and compatibility form.
3. Units must show no sign of leakage or damage and be used within their expiry period.
4. The prescription of blood must be made by a registered medical practitioner and details of the product's administration must be recorded in the case record.
5. An IV line should be established and flushed with 0.9% saline solution *before the pack is opened.*
6. No drug or other infusion solution should be added to any blood component.
7. Monitoring of the patient involves recording temperature, pulse and blood pressure before transfusion, every 15 minutes for the first hour and hourly until transfusion is finished.
8. Adverse events should be recorded meticulously.
9. Major reactions require immediate cessation of the transfusion and instigation of a full investigative protocol (see *Emergencies: Transfusion reactions, p 412–414*).
10. Minor febrile reactions are not uncommon, their occurrence should be recorded, simple measures such as slowing the rate of infusion or administration of an antihistamine may deal with the problem; if not transfusion of the specific unit should be stopped.
11. An RBC pack should be given within 30 minutes of removal from the blood bank; the target infusion time for an individual unit should be ≤4hours.

Platelet transfusion

May be given as prophylaxis against bleeding eg in patients undergoing intensive chemotherapy or to arrest overt haemorrhage eg in DIC. Platelets may be required to cover surgery and dentistry.

Required in following pathophysiological situations

↓ **production due to BM failure/infiltration**	Acute and chronic leukaemias
	Myelodysplasia
	Myeloproliferative disorders and myelofibrosis
	Marrow infiltration with other malignant tumours
	Post-chemotherapy or TBI
	Aplastic anaemia
↑ **platelet destruction in peripheral circulation**	Hypersplenism 2° splenic infiltration or portal hypertension
	Consumptive coagulopathies eg DIC
	Avoid in TTP (p438)
	Acute and chronic ITP (in emergencies only)
	Alloimmune thrombocytopenias e.g. PTP and perinatal thrombocytopenia (need to be HPA typed)
	Sepsis
	Drug induced
Platelet function abnormalities	Aspirin and NSAIDs
	Myelodysplasia
	Rare congenital disorders e.g. Bernard Soulier (*p298*)
Dilutional	Massive blood transfusion – in practice not usually required unless some other haemostatic abnormality (eg consumption)
Cardiac bypass	Dilution and damage to platelets in extracorporeal circulation.

Indications for irradiated platelets

Recommended in immunosuppressed patients and haemopoietic stem cell transplant recipients to prevent transfusion-associated GvHD.

Indications for leucodepleted platelets

Platelet transfusions contain white cells – may result in febrile transfusion reactions, generation of alloimmunisation to HLA and platelet antigens and transmission of CMV infection. Leucodepleted platelets can be obtained by filtration of the product at source (usually by Blood Transfusion Centres) or may be achieved by bedside filters used in-line on the platelet infusions eg Pall. The value of leucodepletion has only been established in a few key situations: patients undergoing long-term RBC eg young patients with β thalassaemia major, myelodysplasia, aplastic anaemia, in utero and neonatal transfusions, in lieu of CMV negative platelet products to prevent CMV transmission.

Indications for CMV negative platelets

1. Where CMV transmission may cause disease.
2. BM and PBSCT recipients who are CMV –ve.
3. Solid organ transplant recipients who are CMV –ve.
4. *In utero* and neonatal transfusion.
5. Aplastic anaemia.
6. GvHD.
7. Primary immunodeficiency syndromes.

Fresh frozen plasma (FFP)

FFP is prepared by removing plasma from a single donor unit by centrifugation within 8h of donation, snap frozen at −80°C and maintained deep frozen until use. Serological testing excludes HBV, HCV, HIV and the product is ABO and Rh (D) grouped. Group AB Rh (D) −ve FFP is suitable for all groups since it lacks anti-A and B, and will not sensitise Rh(D) −ve patients to Rh(D). New products will be virally inactivated but the current National Blood Service (NBS) product is not.

Range and median concentrations of vitamin K dependent coagulation factors in FFP

Factor	II	VII	IX	X
range u/dl	53–121	41–140	32–102	61–150
median	82.5	92.0	61.0	90.5

Indications for use
- Warfarin overdose – *see p430.*
- DIC (common causes include obstetric haemorrhage, postoperative complications, following trauma, severe infection, septicaemic shock, acute blood loss–*see p422–424*).
- Liver disease and biopsy.
- Massive blood transfusion–use of prophylactic FFP (1–2 units FFP/10 units of blood) and platelets is *not supported by documented clinical benefit*. Give as dictated by coagulation tests.
- Isolated coagulation deficiencies where no specific concentrate is readily available.
- Treatment of thrombotic thrombocytopenia purpura/haemolytic uraemic syndrome (*see p374, 438*).
- Non-specific haemostatic failure in a bleeding patient eg following surgery, in intensive care with disturbed coagulation tests where no definite diagnosis is made.

Instructions for use
The average volume of 1 unit is 220–250 ml.

Half life of infused coagulation factors in FFP
<12h	Factors V, VII, VIII, and Protein C
>12 <24h	Factor IX and Protein S
>24 <48h	Factor X
>48h	Fibrinogen, Factors XI, XII, XIII, ATIII

- Defrost the bag in a waterbath (5 min) or at room temperature (20 min).
- Give as soon as possible and at least within the hour through a filter needle.
- Must be group compatible; if blood group not known, give 'all groups'.
- If recipient Rh (D) −ve ♀ of child bearing age given Rh (D) +ve plasma give anti-D (250u-check).
- Dose 10–15 ml/kg body wt (usual starting dose in an adult = 2–4 units depending on the PT).
- Check PT & APTT before and 5 min after infusion to assess response.
- Note clinical response in bleeding patients; repeat as necessary, *remember short half life*.

Thrombosis Haemostasis 1997 77 477–80

Cryoprecipitate

- Prepared by slow thawing of FFP at 4–6°C. Fresh plasma taken from a single donor is snap frozen then thawed at 4°C and a cryoprecipitate forms.
- Precipitate formed is cryoprecipitate which is then stored at –30°C.
- Rich in factors VIII, XIII, fibrinogen and von Willebrand factor.
  Per unit (bag):
  Factor VIII and vWF ~80–100 iu
  Fibrinogen ~250mg
  Factor XIII and Fibronectin
  Does not contain other coagulation factors
  May contain anti-A and anti-B blood group antibodies.
- Formerly (but no longer) used for management of bleeding in factor VIII deficiency and von Willebrand's disease.
- Main clinical use for cryoprecipitate is as additional support for the clotting defects induced by massive transfusion and DIC.
- Not virally inactivated by heat or solvent detergents at present.
- All donations are screened for HIV, HBV and HCV.

Indications for use

- Haemophilia A and vWD not treatment of choice where virally inactivated concentrates are available. May still have a role in acquired vWD when purified VIII products are ineffective.
- Hypo/dysfibrinogenaemia eg in DIC and liver disease/liver transplantation is used to treat and prevent bleeding.
- Of no proven value as empirical treatment in post-op or uraemic bleeding.

Instructions for use

- Keep frozen until required.
- Thaw at room temperature/37°C (takes 5–10 min); *use immediately.*
- ABO compatibility not required.
- Give through filter needle.
- Dose depends on the indications for use and desired increment
  – hypofibrinogenaemia: severe 2–4 bags/10kg body wt

  less severe 1–2 bags.
- Aim to keep fibrinogen >1g/l.
- Factor VIII minimum adult dose 5 bags.

Complications

Viral transmission – rare but reported. Reactions, fever, chills, allergic reactions.

Blood transfusion

Intravenous immunoglobulin

Used as antibody replacement in 1° and 2° antibody deficiency states, and as immune modulator.

Preparations of intravenous IgG (IVIg)
- Contain predominantly IgG (with small amounts of IgA and IgM).
- Prepared from large pool of normal donors eg >1000 (>20,000 in BPL IVIg).
- Contain all subclasses of IgG encountered in normal population.

Uses
1. Antibody replacement

1° immune deficiency	*2° immune deficiency*
Transient hypogammaglobulinaemia of infancy	CLL
	Non-Hodgkin's lymphoma
Common variable immune deficiency	Multiple myeloma
Sex-linked hypogammaglobulinaemia	Post-BMT
Late-onset hypogammaglobulinaemia	
Hypogammaglobulinaemia with thymoma	

2. Immune modulation

Autoimmune diseases	*Antiviral activity*
ITP	Prophylaxis/treatment of CMV in BMT patients
Autoimmune haemolytic anaemia	Red cell aplasia induced by parvovirus B19
Autoimmune neutropenia	Haemophagocytic syndromes (viral)
Red cell aplasia	
Coagulation factor inhibitors	
Post-transfusion purpura (PTP)	
Neonatal platelet alloimmunisation	
Thrombocytopenia in pregnancy	

Mechanisms of action
Not fully understood: natural anti-idiotypic antibodies suppress antibody production in patient; Fc receptor blockade on macrophages (thereby blocking RE function) and T/B lymphocytes (inhibits autoantibody production); suppression of production of inflammatory mediators (eg TNF, IL-1) produced by macrophages.

Administration
Usual dose 0.4g/kg/d × 5d (eg ITP, etc) or 0.2–0.4g/d × 1 day monthly (CLL, myeloma, etc). Check TPR and BP pre-infusion. With first infusion check TPR and BP ½ hourly for the first hour only. *Side-effects are more likely at the start of an infusion and in the first hour.* (*See pack insert and BNF for details.*)

Complications
- Fevers, chills.
- Backache.
- Myalgic symptoms.
- Flushing.
- Nausea ± vomiting.
- Severe allergic reactions in IgA deficient patients (due to small amount of IgA in IVIg preparation).

Autologous blood transfusion

System allows patient to be transfused with his/her own red cells, avoiding (some) problems associated with transfusion of allogeneic (ie donor) blood, eg immunological incompatibility, risks of transmission of infection, and transfusion reactions. Useful for patients who wish not to receive allogeneic blood or who have irregular antibodies that make crossmatching difficult. Can be *pre-deposit* or *intraoperative red cell salvage*.

Pre-deposit system

Involves collection of 2–4 units of blood: the first unit is collected ~2 weeks before the operation and the second is taken 7–10d prior to surgery. Iron replacement usually given. Some pre-deposit programmes use rHuEPO (enables a larger number of units to be collected but *expensive*).

Advantages

- Can store RBCs up to 5 weeks at 4°C.
- May donate 2–4 units pre-op.
- Avoids many problems associated with allogeneic blood transfusion.

Disadvantages

- Generally requires Hb ≥11.0g/dl.
- Patients must be 'fit' for pre-donation programme (eg to donate 450ml 2–4×pre-op) and live near transfusion centre.
- Requires close coordination between surgeon, patient and transfusion lab and fixed date for surgery.
- Little/no reduction in workload – blood must be treated in same way as regular donor units (including microbiological screening, grouping, compatibility testing, etc).
- Cost is high.
- Transfusion should be to donor *only.*
- Bacterial contamination of blood units may still occur.
- Patient may still require additional allogeneic units.
- Blood may be wasted if operation cancelled.
- Patients with epilepsy excluded (risk of seizures).

Intraoperative blood salvage

Allows blood lost during surgery to be reinfused into patients using suction catheters and filtration systems. Expensive and not widely used in the UK at present. Intraoperative blood salvage useful in cardiovascular surgery but may be used for almost any surgical procedure (provided no faecal contamination or risk of tumour dissemination).

1. Single use disposable canisters (eg Solcotrans™) where the patient is heparinised and anticoagulated blood is collected into ACD anticoagulant in the canister. Red cells reinfused after filtration through a microaggregate filter.
2. Automated or semi-automated salvage (eg Hemonetics Cell Saver™). Blood is collected, washed centrifugally, filtered and red cells held for reinfusion.

Other physical methods – pre-operative haemodilution

Involves reducing the Hb concentration prior to surgery. Reduces blood viscosity and red cell loss (through reduced haematocrit). Provides a bank of freshly collected autologous whole blood for return later.

- 2–3 units of blood are collected with replacement using crystalloids or colloid solutions.

Blood transfusion

- Hb is reduced to ~10 g/dl and haematocrit to 30% (0.3).
- O_2 transport improves (increased cardiac output).
- Used mainly in younger patients and in those with no pre-existing cardiopulmonary disease.

Pharmacological methods of blood saving

- Various drugs used to modify the coagulation and fibrinolytic systems, eg DDAVP.
- Platelet inhibitory drugs eg prostacyclin.
- Aprotinin widely used in cardiovascular surgery, liver transplantation and other surgical procedures.

Jehovah's witnesses

- Religious sect numbering 120,000 in the UK.
- Pose ethical and management difficulties due to their refusal of blood transfusion, derived from a literal interpretation of a number of biblical passages (*Acts* 15:28-29).
- JW still die during both elective and emergency surgery due to their beliefs.

Elective surgery – discuss
1. Risks of surgery and the specific risk of refusing blood.
2. Extent of religious belief (preferably alone to prevent any external pressure).
3. What blood derived products they personally are willing to accept eg albumin, FFP, platelets, etc?

If the surgeon agrees to an operation, communication then becomes paramount and the JW should be referred to both an anaesthetist and haematologist – preferably when the patient is placed on the waiting list to allow time for any optimisation and for further counselling with their family.

Pre-operative considerations
- Timing (eg liver transplantation before clotting function deteriorates).
- Autologous blood transfusion – not permitted but may be acceptable to some.
- Morning list – to allow post-op observations during 'office hours'.
- Admission to ITU for invasive monitoring if required.
- Stop anticoagulants and NSAIDs.
- Optimise Hb – nutrition, B_{12}, folate, Fe, erythropoietin.

Operative considerations
- **Surgeon**
  - Consultant
  - Positioning of patient – to prevent venous congestion
  - Tourniquets if possible
  - Speed
  - Meticulous haemostasis
- **Anaesthetist**
  - Consultant
  - Regional blocks
  - Hypotensive anaesthesia
  - Hypothermia
  - Isovolaemic haemodilution – permitted as long as blood remains linked to circulation
  - Hypervolaemic haemodilution
  - Intraoperative blood scavenging eg cellsavers
  - Blood substitutes (fluorocarbons)
  - Pharmacological methods to improve clotting eg DDAVP, tranexamic acid, aprotinin
- **Post-operative considerations**
  - Observation for re-bleed – HDU, senior surgeon review
  - Optimise Hb – nutrition enteral or parental feeding, B_{12}, folate, Fe, erythropoietin
  - Severe anaemia – IPPV to reduce oxygen demand
  - Reduce phlebotomy & use paediatric vials
  - Acid suppression to reduce GIT bleeding.

Emergency surgery
- Advanced directives.
- Early investigations CT, USS abdo, pelvis.
- Low threshold to theatre.

Children

- Communication with parent.
- Judicial intervention if required.

Phone numbers and addresses 17

CancerBACUP

A major British Cancer Information and Support Charity; aims to provide clear, accurate, up-to-date information as well as sensitive and confidential support for patients and their families. Also provides assistance to health care professionals with specific enquiries relating to patients in their care.

CancerBACUP services for patient's and their families
- A national freephone cancer information service (tel 0800-181199), staffed by specialist oncology nurses.
- Cancer counselling service offering people the chance to talk through their concerns face to face
  - 0171-696-9003 (London)
  - 0141-553-1553 (Glasgow)
- CancerBACUP produces excellent written information eg booklets on specific cancers, treatments and aspects of living with cancer and factsheets on specific chemotherapy drugs, hormonal therapies, brain tumours and rare tumours. Available from CancerBACUP's administration, tel 0171-696-9003.

CancerBACUP services for health professionals
Medical Advisory Committee Statements produced by an expert panel on controversial or complex oncology issues including
- Clinical trials.
- Cancer screening – cervical, breast, prostate, colorectal and ovarian cancer.
- Breast cancer, the pill and hormone replacement therapy.
- Information on
  - Support groups
  - Sources of help
- Lists of booklets and factsheets.

Internet
CancerBACUP web site: *http://www.cancerbacup.org.uk*

Phone numbers and addresses

Leukaemia Research Fund (LRF)

The LRF is one of the major UK based research charities in the field of leukaemia and related conditions. It supports leukaemia research in major academic institutions, work supported ranges from basic science relating to the molecular genetics of leukaemogenesis to extensive case controlled studies into epidemiology of leukaemia and related disorders.

In addition to funding major research it provides information booklets on a range of (mainly) malignant blood disorders which are suitable for patients, their relatives and carers and also appropriate for non-specialist professional staff who become involved in specific aspects of the clinical care of the patient with leukaemia or related disorder.

The stated aim of the fund is to improve treatments, find cures and prevent all forms of leukaemia and related cancers through a programme of nationally funded, high calibre research activities.

Booklets are available on the acute and chronic leukaemias, lymphomas including Hodgkin's disease, myeloma and related disorders, myelodysplasia myeloproliferative disorders & aplastic anaemia. A revised series of booklets was produced in 1997. Availability of such information on the wards or in the clinic is vary helpful to patients and their carers.

Address for the Leukaemia Research Fund
43 Great Ormond Street, London, WC1N 3JJ
Telephone   0171 405 0101
Fax   0171 242 1488
e-mail   info@leukaemia.research.org.uk
WWW   *http://www.leukaemia.research.org.uk*

Phone numbers and addresses

Clinical Trials Service Unit (CTSU)

For randomisation/entry into MRC trials.

CTSU
Freepost
Oxford OX2 6BR

tel 01865-240972
fax 01865-726003

Phone numbers and addresses

Medical Research Council

20 Park Crescent
London W1N 4AL

tel 0171-636-5422

Phone numbers and addresses

Haematology on-line

There are many Internet resources available for haematology, including organisations, journals, atlases, conference proceedings, and newsgroups. The main difficulty with Internet resources is that they change so frequently and they are constantly being updated and outdated.

Major prerequisites for browsing the Internet include: computer with modem or network link. If a modem is used you will need an Internet Service Provider (ISP) – basically this is a commercial organisation that will allow you access to the Internet at variable cost (£10+/month) with local access telephone numbers. If you intend to download or upload large (eg graphics) files regularly it is worth considering an Integrated Services Digital Network line (ISDN, useful also for videoconferencing). Full details of how to set up your computer is covered in McKenzie's book (*below*).

Searching routines

The key is to search frequently and learn how to search effectively. The best search engine currently is Metacrawler. This engine involves 6 'sub-engines' (eg Yahoo, AltaVista, and 4 others) which will maximise your 'hits'. Address is http://www.metacrawler.com/.

The most useful specialist index is OMNI (http://omni.ac.uk/), which is operated by a consortium including BMA Library, MRC, Wellcome Centre for Medical Science, and others.

Useful books

Medicine and the Internet, 2nd edition, Bruce C McKenzie, Oxford, 1997.
Internet Starter Kit for Macintosh, 4th edition, Adam C Engst, Hayden Books, 1996 (includes CD ROM containing all software you need to get on-line).

Magazines

Wired, *.net*, and several others. Not aimed at medical community but contain details of new web sites, software updates, etc.

Haematology on-line

Organisation

	WWW address
American Society of Hematology	http://www.hematology.org/
BACUP	http://www.cancerbacup.org.uk/
Bloodline	http://www.cjp.com/blood/cjp.morph?ForceTrackID=tid4602
Blood journal	http://www.bloodjournal.org/
British Journal of Haematology	http://www.blacksci.co.uk/products/journals/toc/bjh.htm
British Medical Journal	http://www.bmj.com/bmj/
British Society for Haematology	http://www.blacksci.co.uk/uk/society/bsh/
Cancer journal	http://www.ca-journal.org/
Cancer Research Campaign	http://www.freepages.co.uk/canres/
European Bone Marrow Transplant Association	http://bmdw.leidenuniv.nl/ebmt/ebmt.html/
Haematologica journal	http://www.haematologica.it
Imperial Cancer Research Fund	http://www.icnet.uk/
Lancet	http://www.thelancet.com/
Leukemia Research Fund	http://dspace.dial.pipex.com/lrf-//
Medical Matrix	http://www.medmatrix.org/Index.asp
Medical Research Council	http://www.nimr.mrc.ac.uk/MRC/
MRC Molecular Haematology Unit	http://immwww.jr2.ox.ac.uk:80/groups/mrc_molhaem
Meducation	http://www.meducation.com/
Medweb	http://www.gen.emory.edu/MEDWEB/keyword/hematology.html
National Blood Service	http://uk-commerce.com/bloodservice/
National Library of Medicine	http://www.nlm.nih.gov
Nature	http://www.nature.com/
New England Journal of Medicine	http://www.nejm.org/JHome.htm
Oncolink	http://cancer.med.upenn.edu
Oxford Haemophilia Centre	http://www.medicine.ox.ac.uk/ohc/
Oxford Regional Blood Club	http://btinternet.com/~phm/BloodClub.html
Royal College of Pathologists	http://rcpath.org
Royal College of Physicians	http://rcplondon.ac.uk
Royal Society of Medicine	http://www.roysocmed.ac.uk
Science	http://www.sciencemag.org/index-alt.html
Sickle Hut	http://homepages.ihug.co.nz/~jfung.medical.htm
The Hematology Site	http://geocities.com/HotSprings/5340/
Wellcome Trust	http://www.wellcome.ac.uk/
World Federation of Hemophilia	http:www.wfh.org/

Atlases/morphology

	WWW address
Atlas of Hematology	http://medic.bgu.ac.il/mirrors/pathy/Pictures/atoras.html
Atlas of Hematology (Nagoya)	http://www.med.nagoya-u.ac.jp/pathy/Pictures/atlas.html
Hematology Image Atlas	http://hms.medweb.harvard.edu/HS_Heme/AtlasTOC.htm
Introduction to Blood Morphology	http://hslib.washington.edu/courses/blood/intro.html

Charts and nomograms 19

Karnofsky performance status

Normal, no complaints; no evidence of disease	100%
Able to carry on normal activity; minor signs or symptoms of disease	90%
Normal activity with effort; some signs or symptoms of disease	80%
Cares for self; unable to carry on normal activity or to do active work	70%
Requires occasional assistance but is able to care for most of his needs	60%
Requires considerable assistance and frequent medical care	50%
Disabled; requires special care and assistance	40%
Severely disabled; hospitalisation is indicated although death is not imminent	30%
Very sick; hospitalisation necessary	20%
Moribund; fatal processes progressing rapidly	10%
Dead	0%

WHO/ECOG performance status

0 Fully active; able to carry on all pre-disease performance without restriction.

1 Restricted in physically strenuous activity, but ambulatory and able to carry out work of a light or sedentary nature, eg light housework, office work.

2 Ambulatory and capable of all self-care but unable to carry out any work activities; up and about more than 50% of waking hours.

3 Capable of only limited self care, confined to bed or chair more than 50% of waking hours.

4 Completely disabled; cannot carry on any self care; totally confined to bed or chair.

Oken MM *et al* Am J Clin Oncol 1982 5 649

Charts and nomograms

WHO haematological toxicity scale

Parameter	Grade 0	Grade 1	Grade 2	Grade 3	Grade 4
Haemoglobin (g/dl)	≥11.0	9.5–10.9	8.0–9.4	6.5–7.9	<6.5
Leucocytes ($\times10^9$/l)	≥4.0	3.0–3.9	2.0–2.9	1.0–1.9	<1.0
Granulocytes ($\times10^9$/l)	≥2.0	1.5–1.9	1.0–1.4	0.5–0.9	<0.5
Platelets ($\times10^9$/l)	≥100	75–99	50–74	25–49	<25
Haemorrhage	none	petechiae	mild blood loss	gross blood loss	debilitating blood loss

Body surface area nomogram

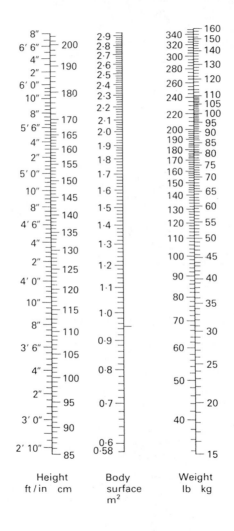

Height ft / in cm	Body surface m²	Weight lb kg

From *Oxford Handbook of Acute Medicine*, P Ramrakha & K Moore, OUP, 1997 (*with permission*)

Gentamicin dosage nomogram

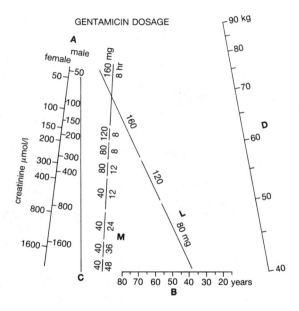

GENTAMICIN DOSAGE

from *Oxford Handbook of Clinical Medicine 3E*, RA Hope *et al.*, OUP, 1993 (*with permission*)

Charts and nomograms

Normal ranges (adults)

Haematology

Hb	13.0–18.0 g/dl (♂)
	11.5–16.5 g/dl (♀)
Haematocrit	0.40–0.52 (♂)
	0.36–0.47 (♀)
RCC	$4.5–6.5 \times 10^{12}/l$ (♂)
	$3.8–5.8 \times 10^{12}/l$ (♀)
MCV	77–95 fl
MCH	27.0–32.0 pg
MCHC	32.0–36.0 g/dl
WBC	$4.0–11.0 \times 10^9/l$
Neutrophils	$2.0–7.5 \times 10^9/l$
Lymphocytes	$1.5–4.5 \times 10^9/l$
Eosinophils	$0.04–0.4 \times 10^9/l$
Basophils	$0.0–0.1 \times 10^9/l$
Monocytes	$0.2–0.8 \times 10^9/l$
Platelets	$150–400 \times 10^9/l$
Reticulocytes	0.5–2.5% (or $50–100 \times 10^9/l$)
ESR	2–12 mm/1st hour (Westergren)
Serum B_{12}	150–700 ng/l
Serum folate	2.0–11.0 µg/l
Red cell folate	150–700 µg/l
Serum ferritin	15–300 µg/l (varies with sex and age)
	14–200 µg/l premenopausal female
INR	0.8–1.2
PT	12.0–14.0 s
APTT ratio	0.8–1.2
APTT	26.0–33.5 s
Fibrinogen	2.0–4.0 g/l
Thrombin time	± 3 s of control
XDPs	<250 µg/l
Factors II, V, VII, VIII, IX, X, XI, XII	50–150 i.u./dl
RiCoF	45–150 i.u./dl
vWF: Ag	50–150 i.u./dl
Protein C	80–135 u/dl
Protein S	80–135 u/dl
Antithrombin III	80–120 u/dl
APCR	2.12–4.0
Bleeding time	3–9 min

Biochemistry

Serum urea	3.0–6.5 mmol/l
Serum creatinine	60–125 µmol/l
Serum sodium	135–145 mmol/l
Serum potassium	3.5–5.0 mmol/l
Serum albumin	32–50 g/l
Serum bilirubin	<17 µmol/l
Serum alk phos	100–300 i.u./l
Serum calcium	2.15–2.55 mmol/l
Serum LDH	200–450 i.u./l
Serum phosphate	0.7–1.5 mmol/l
Serum total protein	63–80 g/l
Serum γ-GT	10–46 i.u./l
Serum iron	♂ 14–33 µmol/l
	♀ 11–28 µmol/l
Serum TIBC	45–75 µmol/l
Serum ALT	5–42 i.u./l
Serum AST	5–42 i.u./l
Serum free T_4	9–24 pmol/l
Serum TSH	0.35–5.5 mU/l

Immunology

IgG	5.3–16.5 g/l
IgA	0.8–4.0 g/l
IgM	0.5–2.0 g/l

Complement
C3	0.89–2.09 g/l
C4	0.12–0.53 g/l
C1 esterase	0.11–0.36 g/l
CH_{50}	80–120%

C-reactive protein   <6 mg/l

Serum β_2-microglobulin 1.2–2.4 mg/l

CSF proteins
IgG	0.013–0.035 g/l
Albumin	0.170–0.238 g/l

Urine proteins
Total protein	<150 mg/24h
Albumin (24h)	<20 mg/24h

Paediatric normal ranges

Haemostasis

Parameter	Neonate	Adult level
Platelet count	$150–400 \times 10^9/l$	as adult
Prothrombin time	few sec longer than adult	up to 1 week
APTT	up to 25% increase	by 2–9 months
Thrombin time		as adult
Bleeding time	2–10 min	as adult
Fibrinogen	2.0–4.0g/l	as adult
Vit K factors		
Factor II	30–50% adult level	up to 6 months
Factor VII	30–50% adult level	by 1 month
Factor IX	20–50% adult level	up to 6 months
Factor X	30–50% adult level	up to 6 months
Factor V		as adult
Factor VIII	Variable: 50–200% adult level	
VW Factor	usually raised (up to $3 \times$ adult level)	
Factor XI	20–50% adult level	6–12 months
Factor XII	20–50% adult level	3–6 months
Factor XIII	50–100% adult level	1 month
FDP/XDP	up to twice adult level	by 7 days
AT	50–80% adult level	6–12 months
Protein C	30–50% adult level	up to 24 months
Protein S	30–50% adult level	3–6 months
Plasminogen	30–80% adult level	2 weeks

Normal FBC values at various ages from birth to 12 years

Age	Hb (g/dl)	Hct (l/l)	MCV (fl)	WBC (× 10⁹/l)	Neutrophils (× 10⁹/l)	Lymphocytes (× 10⁹/l)
Birth cord blood	13.5–19.5	0.42–0.60	98–118	9–30	6–26	2–11
1–3 days	16.0–21.0	0.45–0.67	95–121	9.4–34	5–21	2–11.5
1 week	15.2–19.8	0.42–0.66	88–126	5–21	1.50–10	2–17
2 weeks	14.0–19.0	0.39–0.63	86–124	5–20	1–9.5	2–17
1 month	11.9–16.1	0.31–0.55	85–123	5–19.5	1–9	2.5–16.5
2–6 months	10.5–12.5	0.28–0.42	86–102	6–17.5	1–8.5	4–13.5
0.5–2 years	10.5–13.5	0.33–0.39	70–86	6–17.5	1.5–8.5	4–10.5
2–6 years	11.5–13.5	0.34–0.40	75–87	5.5–15.5	1.5–8.5	2–8
6–12 years	11.5–15.5	0.35–0.45	77–95	4.5–13.5	1.5–8.0	1.5–6.8

*Guidelines only: wide range in first weeks of life. Platelet count as adult.
Reference: *Practical Paediatric Haematology*, Hinchliffe & Lilleyman (eds) John Wiley & Sons, 1987.

Index